H.-J. Gertz and Th. Arendt (eds.)

Alzheimer's Disease –
From Basic Research to
Clinical Applications

SpringerWienNewYork

Prof. Dr. H.-J. Gertz
Klinik und Poliklinik für Psychiatrie, Universität Leipzig,
Bundesrepublik Deutschland
Prof. Dr. Th. Arendt
Paul-Flechsig-Institut für Hirnforschung, Universität Leipzig,
Bundesrepublik Deutschland

© 1998 Springer-Verlag/Wien
Softcover reprint of the hardcover 1st edition 1998

Printing: A. Holzhausens Nfg., A-1070 Wien
Graphic design: Ecke Bonk
Printed on acid-free and chlorine-free bleached paper
SPIN: 10673041

With 52 (partly coloured) Figures

ISBN-13:978-3-211-83112-0   e-ISBN-13:978-3-7091-7508-8
DOI: 10.1007/978-3-7091-7508-8

Preface

As human longevity continues to be extended, so will the impact of age-associated dementia on individual lives and society. Alzheimer's disease as the most common cause of dementia in the elderly remains a seminal problem and its underlying pathology is still poorly understood. Available therapeutic strategies require considerable refinement and the development of new therapeutic strategies need input from basic research. Thus continued efforts are necessary both to understand basic mechanisms of the condition and to achieve more powerful therapies.

From June 5 to 7, 1997 the international conference "Alzheimer's Disease – From Basic Research to Clinical Applications" was held in Leipzig. This conference brought together experts from clinical and basic science fields. Their contributions are collected in this volume. The issue bridges the gap between laboratory work in basic science and the development of urgently needed therapeutic strategies. Areas presented are the molecular and cellular biology of the disease, pathogenetic mechanisms and potential therapeutic targets, genetics, risk factors, strategies of prevention and treatment as well as practical aspects of medical and social care for patients with Alzheimer's disease.

Leipzig, August 1998   **H.-J. Gertz**
                                                        Th. Arendt

Contents

VIII   Contents

Listed in Current Contents / Life Sciences

Alzheimer's disease: the size of the problem, clinical manifestation and heterogeneity

H. Förstl

Department of Psychiatry, TU Munich, Federal Republic of Germany

Summary. Age is the major demographic risk factor for the development of Alzheimer's disease (AD) and the ageing of our society has contributed to the growing importance of AD. The problem of AD has been tackled from numerous clinical and scientific angles. The traditional clinico-pathological disease concept, which relies on the manifestation of a dementia syndrome and the elimination of other relevant systemic and brain diseases for a diagnosis of AD, accommodates a number of genetically and clinically heterogenous conditions, but cannot promote our understanding of the preclinical pathogenetic processes and their interaction. If new molecular biological discoveries cannot be integrated with this traditional clinico-pathological model, it may have outlived its usefulness.

The size of the problem

Alzheimer's disease (AD) on paper

Thirty years ago, when the term AD was still reserved for the presenile cases of a primary degenerative dementia, the problem seemed almost forgotten. Since then we have seen a steady increase of publications on all aspects of AD, particularly in the basic sciences. Table 1 compares the publications on AD, its diagnosis, therapy, genetics and metabolism with papers on other dementing diseases which have been listed in Current Contents since 1966. The number of publications on vascular dementia, the AIDS dementia complex, and Creutzfeldt-Jakob's disease is also increasing, but at a more modest level, whereas the research output on various aspects of neurosyphilis appears to be in a steady state since 1966.

At the last turn of the century, progressive paralysis represented a conundrum of great clinical and literary importance, which may perhaps be compared with today's most prevalent dementia, AD. After a rising flood of publications, the discovery of treponema pallidum, its significance, and of ways to avoid and defeat it, a swelling stream of research turned into a mere trickle. It is possible, that the present flood of Alzheimer research, reflects a genuine increase of relevant information, but it is unlikely that we will dis-

Table 1. Publications on Alzheimer's disease, other forms of dementia and neurosyphilis as listed in Current Contents since 1966

Keywords	1966–70	1971–75	1976–80	1981–85	1986–90	1991–95
AD-total	2	61	332	1,565	4,602	6,937
AD-diagnosis	1	12	42	318	704	1206
AD-drug ther.	—	1	25	146	387	613
AD-genetics	—	2	26	96	400	943
AD-metabolism	—	6	48	232	1,045	1,711
Dementia, vasc.	—	—	—	—	127	407
ADRC (AIDS)	—	—	—	—	232	819
CJD	22	196	247	295	387	569
Neurosyphilis	137	122	144	196	210	200

AD Alzheimer's disease, *ADRC* AIDS dementia related complex, *CJD* Creutzfeldt-Jakob disease, Creutzfeldt Jakob syndrome

cover another ignominious saprophyte responsible for this condition and that a scientific breakthrough will lead to a cure as effective as in progressive paralysis. However, we will probably learn how to influence the course of this process more effectively, perhaps even before its clinical manifestation.

Ageing and AD

AD is a process which does affect more of us the older we get and which may start much earlier than we tend to assume. Bickel (1997) summarised the major demographic changes of the twentieth century. Around 1900, fertility and mortality were high. Today low fertility and mortality rates are characteristic of developed countries. Decreased mortality has led to a larger number of elderly people and decreased fertility has pushed the proportion of old people in our society even higher (Table 2). Ten percent of men and nineteen percent of women are older than 65. In comparison to the early years of the 20th century, there are twice as many over 65-, four times as many over 80-, ten times as many over 90-year olds, and we have every reason to assume that this development will continue. This will lead to increased morbidity and an increased need for hospital and nursing care. Age is the single most important demographic risk factor for AD and other forms of dementia and AD is the single most important mental health problem in an ageing society.

Most studies estimate the prevalence of moderate to severe dementia over 65 as 4%–8%. The prevalence, incidence and morbidity risk for moderate to severe dementia appears to grow with every year of age (meta-analysis by Bickel, 1997; Table 3). It is presently unclear whether the risk of developing dementia may level off after age ninety (Ritchie and Kildea, 1995), but this consideration may appear theoretical in view of the extreme elite character of today's over 90-year olds. There are other risk factors apart from age (van Duijn, 1996): other causes of dementia; Parkinson's disease and Down's syndrome in the patient's family; a previous history of depression; perhaps

Table 2. Demographic changes in Germany between 1900 and 1990 (according to Bickel et al., 1997)

	1900	1990
>65 yrs.	3.2 Mio (5%)	12.2 Mio (15%)
Life expectancy (male:female)	45/48 yrs	73/79 yrs
Proportion reaching age 65 (m:f)	36/44%	77/88%
age 80 (m:f)	9/12%	37/59%
age 90 (m:f)	1/1%	7/19%

Table 3. A meta-analysis of field studies on the prevalence, incidence and morbidity risk for moderate to severe dementia in different age groups (according to Bickel et al., 1997)

	Prevalence	Incidence	Morbidity risk
65–69 yrs.	2%	0.1–0.8%	1–5% ≤ 70 yrs.
75–79 yrs.	5–7%	1–3.8%	10–18% ≤ 80 yrs.
85–89 yrs.	16–23%	2–7%	40–56% ≤ 90 yrs.
>90 yrs.	25–42%	(7.4–8.2%)	90% ≤ 100 yrs.

head trauma and hypothyroidism. Molecular biologists have successfully pinned down several genetic correlates of "familiality": the ApoE4 allele, which increases the risk for AD in heterozygous and more so in homozygous carriers; the mutations of the preseniline genes on chromosomes 1 and 14, and of the amyloid precursor protein (APP) gene on chromosome 21. The term "risk factor" would be a light-hearted euphemism for the preseniline- and APP-mutations which are autosomal dominant and show near complete penetrance.

AD leads to an greater than 2-fold increase of mortality and allegedly causes one third of the deaths in people over 75. The duration of illness is 5 to 8 years. It lasts longer in younger patients (10 years under 65) and shorter in older patients (4 years over 80). These estimates rely on retrospection and refer to the earliest surmised clinical manifestation before a first diagnosis of dementia or, more specifically, of probable AD has been made.

The manifestation of AD according to current diagnostic criteria

Diagnosis, syndromal and differential

One of the interesting and irritating issues about AD is, that a positive clinical diagnosis based on positive, on characteristic clinical findings cannot be made, — at least not according to the current criteria. An abbreviated version of the Diagnostic Criteria for Research (DCR) from the ICD-10 is given in Table 5

Table 4. Predictors of cognitive decline from selected studies

	Demographic	Disease	Symptoms
Burns et al. (1991)	↓ familiality ↔ age, gender	↓ short duration ↔ onset	↓ moderate stage ↔ aphasia
Förstl et al. (1996)	↔ age, ApoE	↓ atrophy, EEG-changes	↓ cognitive deficits
Haupt et al. (1992)	↔ sporadic/familial	↔ onset	
Lopez et al. (1991)		↓ EEG-changes	↓ delusions, hallucinations, aggression, aphasia
Mielke et al. (1994)	↔ familiality, gender	↔ onset, duration	
Miller et al. (1991)			↓ extrapyramidal s.
Morris et al. (1993)			↓ cognition
Mortimer et al. (1992)			↓ cognition, insomnia, aggression
Teri et al. (1990)			↓ agitation, wandering

↓ predicts cognitive decline, ↔ no significant influence

Table 5. The (obligatory) manifestation of Alzheimer's disease according to DCR (Diagnostic Criteria Research according to the International Classification of Diseases, 10th revision)

Obligatory	required [excluding] features
1. Decline of memory:	most evident in the learning of new information
2. Decline of ≥ 1:	judgement and thinking; general processing of information
3. Presence of ≥ 2:	emotional lability; irritability; apathy; coarsening of social behaviour
4. Awareness of environment	[absence of clouded consciousness]
5. Six months duration	[otherwise tentative diagnosis only]
6. No other causes	[brain or systemic disease, alcohol or drug abuse]

as one example of such diagnostic instruments. I could have chosen another set of criteria, but the essence would have a similar taste. The authors of such traditional clinical criteria have pronounced their tentative nature and the need for further revisions. The daily use of these instruments nevertheless misleads us to believe that they represent a well-established fact, in this case a disease entity with obvious and natural boundaries. However, traditional diagnostic criteria and our diagnostic process are an intricate mixture of modest clinical evidence and unwarranted assumptions about the underlying neuropathology. The high rates of cross-validation between a clinical and a neuropathological diagnosis of AD is largely due to the low specificity of both clinical and neuropathological criteria and to the high prevalence of plaques and tangles in elderly people, many of whom are demented. Genetic markers will need to be integrated into future criteria and this new angle may lead to a fundamental revision of the diagnostic approach, which may no longer be based on clinical symptoms, but on the biological factors at least in an important subgroup of dementing individuals. Meanwhile we will have to wrestle with a number of problems inherent in the traditional clinico-pathological model and its application to patients with cognitive impairment: (a) the focus is on the "dementia syndrome" instead of the underlying process; (b) the obligatory elimination of any other relevant systemic or brain disease in the diagnostic process as a modest common denominator for the "primary degenerative forms" of dementia.

(a) The dementia syndrome. Once a diagnosis of AD can be made, there is already a highly significant difference between the brain atrophy in a group of patients with mild dementia, according to Clinical Dementia Rating (Berg, 1982), and the brain volume in a matched elderly control sample (Förstl et al., 1995a). A diagnosis relying on the late manifestations of a disease process will necessarily come too late in order to enter the battle before the patient's brain has taken decades of pounding and suffered irreversibly; this is clearly different from other diseases, e.g. diabetes mellitus, where we do not have to wait until the kidneys, the eyes, the brain etc. have been severely damaged before we make a diagnosis and take the appropriate countermeasures. Beyreuther (1997) estimated an onset of amyloid plaque formation — considered a prime suspect responsible for the destruction of synapses and neurons — 30 years or more before the first clinical signs of the disease. As the plaque formation and other mechanisms contributing to neurodegeneration appear to be slow processes, there should be ample time to interfere with the pathogenesis of AD long before the clinical manifestation of dementia. Dementia appears to be a late phenomenon, only occurring after our brains' capacity for compensation is eventually worn out. We have tried to predict the development of cognitive impairment in non-demented elderly individuals and found that molecular biological risk markers (e.g. ApoE4), quantitative measures of global brain and hippocampal atrophy — the "early after-effects" of the underlying disease process — were better predictors of future cognitive impairment, than the patients' subjective complaints and mild cognitive impairment at first examination (Förstl et al., 1995b).

(b) Homogeneity and heterogeneity. The diagnostic process relies on inclusion (dementia syndrome) and exclusion criteria which require the elimination of other relevant systemic and brain disease. The purity of the diagnosis does not reflect reality in everyday practice where the majority of elderly patients are multimorbid and are treated for a number of medical conditions, all of whom may interact with cognitive performance and potentially with the neurodegenerative process. We have demonstrated in an earlier study, that demented patients satisfying neuropathological criteria for AD can show evidence of numerous other medical diseases (Förstl et al., 1991). According

6

H. Förstl

to clinical diagnostic criteria, AD has to be the pure version of dementia, the pristine syndrome without evidence of another underlying specific and relevant cause. A diagnosis of AD represents the virtual immunization of a patient against any other relevant illness. On the other hand, the common diagnostic denominator of AD according to these criteria is so small, that clinically very heterogenous conditions can be accomodated under the heading of AD, some of this variability is listed in Table 6. There are patients with presenile and patients with a senile onset of AD. The distribution of the age of onset is not bi-modal but multi-modal and this is partly explained by some of the underlying molecular biological risk factors which have been identified in recent years. Accordingly the over-simlifying concept of familiality versus non-familiality is currently undergoing similar revisions brought about by new revelations about the background of familial clustering.

Amnesia is an early and — according to traditional diagnostic criteria — obligatory element of the dementia syndrome. In some of the patients other cognitive disturbances, e.g. aphasia, may precede other disturbances and remain predominantly severe in the course of illness. The pattern of neuropsychological deficits can be heterogenous on cross-sectional examination and deterioration may show a great deal of variability before an endstage is reached. Most of the patients show other psychopathological, behavioural and neurological disturbances during some stage of their illness. None of these individual "non-cognitive" features listed in table 6 is obligatory for the diagnosis and as individual features can be predominant or completely absent they contribute a large part to the clinical heterogeneity of AD.

Table 6. The variability and heterogeneity of AD accomodated under DCR criteria

Dimensions	Examples
Demographic	
Age	presenile/senile
Familiality	familial/sporadic
Clinical	
Neuropsychology	predominant amnesia, aphasia, . . .
Psychopathology	depression, delusions, hallucinations, . . .
Behaviour	apathy, agitation, aggrssion, wandering, . . .
Neurology	rigidity, myoclonus, cerebral seizures, . . .
Localization	
Neuroimaging	temporoparietal/other atrophy, perfusion & metabolic changes
Macropathology	temporoparietal/other atrophy
Histology	
Standard stains	plaque and tangle numbers, neuronal shrinkage, Lewy bodies, . . .
Specific stains	synaptic changes, . . .
Molecular biology	
Risk markers	ApoE4
Diagnostic markers	preseniline 1, 2; APP-mutations

The severity of clinical impairment is associated with the severity of functional and also of morphological brain changes as examined radiologically or neuropathologically. The clinical symptom-pattern can be related to the distribution of functional and morphological alterations. Controversy surrounds the influence of clinical features on the course of AD.

Different variants of AD have been described characterised by "typical" symptoms, for example a benign course, rigidity or myoclonus (Chui et al., 1985; Mayeux et al., 1985), by pronounced parietal or frontal lobe symptoms (Girling and Berrios, 1991; McDonald, 1969) and by diverse neuropathological features e.g. the number of neurofibrillary tangles or the areas of severe neuronal change (Alzheimer, 1911; Bondareff et al., 1987). However, none of these clusters of features is so distinctive and stable over time to warrant the definition of a "subtype".

A wider angle of research

The research on dementing conditions is currently handicapped by its entrenched categorical focus on the dementia syndrome. The advantage of such studies is their easy feasibility with small convenience samples of patients examined during short periods of time. Their disadvantage is that such samples and results will always be subject to biases, that little proactive interventions are possible in the late stages of illness. It would be of great scientific and practical merit to take a more developmental and comprehensive view of the long run and not only a snapshot of the loosers at the finishing line. The difficulties of such an approach are obvious: long study periods and large sample sizes are required. Such approaches are costly and they lack immediate professional reward.

Results from molecular biological research will revolutionize our understanding of dementing conditions and the integration of these findings with our traditional clinico-pathological concepts may prove a difficult exercise.

References

Alzheimer A (1911) Über eigenartige Krankheitsfälle des späteren Alters. Z Ges Neurol Psychiat 4: 356–385

Baumgart P, Helgenberger F, Weyerer S, Pfeifer-Kurda M, Förstl H (1995) The course of cognition and depression in the elderly patients with affective disturbances and mild cognitive impairment. Int J Geriat Psychiat 10: 419–421

Berg L (1984) Clinical dementia rating. Br J Psychiatry 145: 339

Beyreuther K (1997) Molekularbiologie der Alzheimer Demenz. Lehrbuch der Gerontopsychiatrie. Enke, Stuttgart

Bickel H (1997) Epidemiologie psychischer Erkrankungen im Alter. Lehrbuch der Gerontopsychiatrie. Enke, Stuttgart

Bondareff W, Mountjoy CQ, Roth M, Rossor MN, Iversen L, Reynolds GP (1987) Age and histopathological heterogeneity in Alzheimer's disease: evidence for subtypes. Arch Gen Psychiatry 44: 412–417

Burns A, Jacoby R, Levy R (1991) Progression of cognitive impairment in Alzheimer's disease. J Am Geriatr Soc 39: 39–45

Chui HC, Teng EL, Henderson VW, Moy AC (1985) Clinical subtypes of dementia of the Alzheimer type. Neurology 35: 1544–1550

van Duijn CM (1996) Epidemiology of the dementia: recent developments and new approaches. J Neurol Neurosurg Psychiatry 60: 478–488

Förstl H, Hentschel F, Sattel H, Geiger-Kabisch C, Besthorn C, Czech C, Mönning U, Beyreuther K (1995) Age-associated memory impairment and early Alzheimer's disease — only time will tel the difference. Drug Res 45: 394–397

Förstl H, Zerfass R, Geiger-Kabisch C, Sattel H, Besthorn C, Hentschel F (1995) Brain atrophy in normal ageing and Alzheimer's disease — volumetric discrimination and clinical correlations. Br J Psychiatry 167: 739–746

Förstl H, Sattel H, Besthorn C, Daniel S, Geiger-Kabisch C, Hentschel F, Sarochan M, Zerfass R (1996) Longitudinal cognitive, electroencephalographic and morphological brain changes in ageing and Alzheimer's disease. Br J Psychiatry 168: 280–286

Girling DM, Berrios GE (1991) Extrapyramidal signs, primitive reflexes and frontal lobe functional in senile dementia of the Alzheimer type. Br J Psychiatry 157: 888–893

Haupt M, Kurz A, Romero B, et al (1992) Symptomprogression bei Alzheimerscher Krankheit: gibt es einen Zusammenhang mit dem Manifestationsalter oder der familiären Belastung. Z Gerontopsychol -psychiat 4: 91–98

Lopez OL, Becker JT, Brenner RP, et al (1991) Alzheimer's disease with delusions and hallucinations: neuropsychological and electroencephalographic correlates. Neurology 41: 906–912

Mayeux R, Stern Y, Spanton S (1985) Heterogeneity in dementia of the Alzheimer type: evidence of subgroups. Neurology 35: 53–61

McDonald C (1969) Clinical heterogeneity in senile dementia. Br J Psychiatry 115: 267–271

McKhann G, Drachman D, Folstein M, Katzman R, Price D, Stadlan EM (1984) Clinical diagnosis of Alzheier's disease: report of the NINCDS-ADRDA work group under the auspices of the Department of Health and Human Services Task Force on Alzheimer's disease. Neurology 34: 939–944

Mielke R, Herholz K, Grond M, et al (1994) Clinical deterioration in probable Alzheimer's disease correlates with progressive metabolic impairment of association areas. Dementia 5: 36–41

Miller TP, Tinklenberg JR, Brooks JO, Fenn HH, Yesavage JA (1991) Selected psychiatric symptoms associated with rate of cognitive decline in patients with Alzheimer's disease. J Geriat Psychiat Neurol 6: 235–238

Morris JC, Rubin EG (1993) Clinical diagnosis and course of Alzheimer's disease. Psychiatr Clin North Am 14: 223–236

Mortimer JA, Ebbit B, Jun S, et al (1992) Predictors of cognitive and functional progression in patients with probable Alzheimer's disease. Neurology 42: 1689–1696

Ritchie K, Kildea D (1995) Is senile dementia "age-related" or "ageing-related"? — Evidence from meta-analyis of dementia prevalence in the oldest old. Lancet 346: 931–934

Teri L, Hughes JP, Larson EB (1990) Cognitive deterioration in Alzheimer's disease: behavioural and health factors. J Gerontol 45: 58–63

WHO (1993) The ICD-10 classification of mental and behavioural disorders: diagnostic criteria for research. WHO, Geneva

Author's address: Prof. Dr. H. Förstl, Department of Psychiatry, Technical University, Ismaninger Strasse 22, D-81675 München, Federal Republic of Germany

Progression of Alzheimer's disease: variability and consistency: ontogenic models, their applicability and relevance

B. Reisberg, E. H. Franssen, L. E. M. Souren, S. Auer, and **S. Kenowsky**

Zachary and Elizabeth M. Fisher Alzheimer's Disease Education and Resources Program, New York University Medical Center, New York, NY, U.S.A.

Summary. Much has been learned about the clinical symptomatology of Alzheimer's disease (AD) and ontogenic reciprocal relationships in the past few decades. It is now possible to describe and verify inexorable symptomatic sequences and corresponding temporal relationships. It is also possible to identify more variable symptoms in AD. Ontogenic models can be useful in providing a clearer understanding of the nature of AD symptomatology in terms of both consistency and variability. These models can also be informative in explicating the management needs of AD patients and the treatment possibilities of AD symptoms as well as the etiology of variability in AD symptoms.

Nature and import of AD symptomatology: developmental reciprocals

Functionally, 16 successive stages in AD progression can be described using the Functional Assessment Staging (FAST) procedure (Reisberg et al., 1984; Reisberg, 1988) (Table 1). Studies have verified that in AD uncomplicated by concomitant morbidity, the sequence of these 16 FAST stages in AD fulfill the Guttman statistical criteria for ordinality (Guttman, 1950; Sclan and Reisberg, 1992). These 16 FAST stages in AD progression occur in an inverse sequence from the order of the acquisition of the same functions in normal human development (Reisberg et al., 1986; Reisberg, 1986) (Table 2). Just as these functional markers are robust indicators of normal development, generally more useful in describing the developmental human course than, for example, IQ testing, similarly, the FAST sequence is a robust indicator of the degenerative course of AD, more useful than for example, mental status assessment. For instance, just as infants generally might be expected to achieve only bottom scores (zero) on the Mini-Mental State Examination (MMSE) (Folstein et al., 1975), stage 7 AD patients generally achieve only bottom scores (zero) on the MMSE (Sclan and Reisberg, 1992; Auer et al., 1994). Similarly, just as one would apply special psychological tests for the assessment of cognition in infancy and childhood, the same tests, with some modifications, have proven useful for the assessment of residual cognition in

Table 1. Functional assessment staging (FAST)[1] (Check highest consecutive level of disability)

1.	☐		No difficulty, either subjectively or objectively.
2.	☐		Complains of forgetting location of objects. *Subjective work difficulties.*
3.	☐		Decreased job functioning evident to co-workers. Difficulty in traveling to new locations. *Decreased organizational capacity.**
4.	☐		*Decreased ability to perform complex tasks,* (e.g. planning dinner for guests), handling personal finances (e.g. forgetting to pay bills), difficulty marketing, etc.*
5.	☐		*Requires assistance in choosing proper clothing* to wear for the day, season, or occasion, e.g. patient may wear the same clothing repeatedly, unless supervised.*
6.	☐	(a)	*Improperly putting on clothes without assistance or cuing* (e.g. may put street clothes on over night clothes, or put shoes on wrong feet, or have difficulty buttoning clothing) occasionally or more frequently over the past weeks.*
	☐	(b)	Unable to bathe properly without assistance (e.g., *difficulty adjusting bath-water temperature*) occasionally or more frequently over the past weeks.*
	☐	(c)	*Inability to handle mechanics of toileting* (e.g., forgets to flush the toilet, does not wipe properly or properly dispose of toilet tissue) occasionally or more frequently over the past weeks.*
	☐	(d)	*Urinary incontinence* (occasionally or more frequently over the past weeks; or must be guided in toileting to prevent occurrence of urinary incontinence).
	☐	(e)	*Fecal incontinence* (occasionally or more frequently over the past weeks; or must be guided in toileting to prevent occurrence of fecal incontinence).
7.	☐	(a)	Ability to speak limited to approximately a half *a dozen different intelligible words or fewer*, in the course of an average day or *in the course of an intensive interview.*
	☐	(b)	Speech ability limited to the use of *a single intelligible word* in an average day or in the course of an intensive interview (the person may repeat the word over and over).
	☐	(c)	Ambulatory ability lost (cannot *walk without personal assistance*).
	☐	(d)	Ability to sit up without assistance lost (e.g., the individual *will fall over if there are no lateral rests* [arms] *on the chair*).
	☐	(e)	Loss of the ability to smile.
	☐	(f)	Loss of the ability to hold up head independently.

AD patients (Sclan et al., 1990; Auer et al., 1994). In accordance with these observations, prospective longitudinal study has indicated that the FAST staging sequence can account for approximately two times the temporal variance in AD course explained by the MMSE (Reisberg et al., 1996a).

Each functional stage in AD can be described in terms of a corresponding developmental age (DA) (Reisberg et al., 1986, 1996b). In the course of AD, cognitive, praxic and feeding changes can be described which appear to

Table 2. Functional stages in normal human development and Alzheimer's disease[1,2]

Developmental age	Acquired abilities	Lost abilities	Alzheimer stage
12+ years	Hold a job	Hold a job	3 — Incipient
8–12 years	Handle simple finances	Handle simple finances	4 — Mild
5–7 years	Select proper clothing	Select proper clothing	5 — Moderate
5 years	Put on clothes unaided	Put on clothes unaided	6 — Moderately severe
4 years	Shower unaided	Shower unaided	
4 years	Toilet unaided	Toilet unaided	
3–4½ years	Control urine	Control urine	
2–3 years	Control Bowels	Control Bowels	
15 months	Speak 5–6 words	Speak 5–6 words	7 — Severe
1 year	Speak 1 word	Speak 1 word	
1 year	Walk	Walk	
6–10 months	Sit up	Sit up	
2–4 months	Smile	Smile	
1–3 months	Hold up head	Hold up head	

[1] Reisberg B (1986) Dementia: a systematic approach to identifying reversible causes. Geriatrics 41(4): 30–46. [2] Reisberg B (1988) Functional Assessment Staging (FAST). Psychopharmacol Bull 24: 653–659.

approximate the capacities in the corresponding DA_s (Auer et al., 1994; Reisberg et al., 1988, 1990, 1992).

So called "primitive" or "developmental" neurologic reflexes have been known to occur in what was believed to be normal aging (Paulson and Gottlieb, 1968; Jacobs and Gossman, 1980) and in AD (Huff et al., 1987). Research in recent years has indicated that these developmental neurologic reflexes emerge in AD at a point which might be anticipated from the corresponding DA (Franssen et al., 1991, 1993). Furthermore, recent studies have found that just as these developmental neurologic reflexes serve as robust indicators of normal nervous system development in normal infancy and early childhood, they can also serve as powerful markers of the degenerative course of AD (Franssen et al., 1997; Franssen and Reisberg, 1997).

For example, a recent study found that the emergence of the tactile sucking reflex, palmar and plantar grasp reflex and the plantar extensor reflex (Babinski reflex), distinguished activity of daily living (ADL) deficient AD patients who are not yet incontinent (i.e., FAST stage 6a to 6c patients). From ADL deficient permanently doubly incontinent AD patients who are still ambulatory (i.e., FAST stage 7a and 7b patients), with a specificity, sensitivity and overall accuracy each greater than 85% (Franssen et al., 1997). Consequently, the emergence of these developmental reflexes marks a specific epoch in the degenerative course of AD. Developmental reflexes are also useful in delineating the degenerative course of AD, particularly in stages 6 and 7, in other ways, just as they would be in the corresponding DA_s (i.e., birth to 5 years of age) (Franssen et al., 1991, 1993; Franssen and Reisberg, 1997).

Electrophysiologic changes in AD have also been found to reverse the normal developmental patterns. For example, in terms of electroencephalogic (EEG) changes, there is a gradual increase in fast alpha and beta activity in normal development. Just the opposite seems to occur in AD. In AD there is initially a progressive increase in theta activity, and then in both theta and delta, with corresponding decrements in beta and fast alpha wave activity as the degenerative process of AD advances (Cioni et al., 1992; Prichep et al., 1994). These processes, i.e., developmental increases in fast wave EEG frequencies and progressive decrements in slow wave EEG frequencies in AD, appear to be approximately symmetrical based upon the corresponding DA_s. Recently, Braak and Braak have noted that the sequential topography of neurodegenerative change in AD in terms of the Braak and Braak stages of neurofibrillary pathology, mirrors inversely the sequential topography of myelin deposition in normal brain development (Braak and Braak, 1996, 1991; Flechsig, 1920).

Myelin is the fatty substance that forms the sheath about certain nerve fibers. Previously, McGeer et al. (1990) had noted that the areas most retarded in myelinization in normal development are those most prone to neuronal loss in AD based upon Brun and Englund's observations of neuronal loss in AD (Brun and England, 1981). McGeer et al. (1990) also noted that the areas most retarded in myelinization in normal development are the areas showing the greatest decrement in glucose metabolism in AD.

Consequently, it is now clear that in terms of functional progression, cognitive loss, and praxic disturbance, the progression of AD mirrors corresponding developmental landmarks. Similarly, developmental landmarks can be described corresponding to neurologic and physiologic aspects of AD degeneration. Finally, anatomic explanations for the observed homologies have been noted. These developmental reciprocals can also assist in elucidating other symptoms in AD such as so-called behavioral disturbance symptoms (Table 3) (Reisberg et al., 1998).

Management import of ontogenic symptomatic models

The DA of the AD patient can provide a rapid and accurate appreciation of the AD patients care requirements (Reisberg et al., 1996b) (Table 4). Each FAST stage corresponds very closely to the Global Deterioration Scale (GDS) stage from which the FAST was originally derived (Reisberg et al., 1982). Specifically, a 0.9 correlation has been noted between these closely related measures (Reisberg et al., 1985a, 1993). The management needs and care requirements of the AD patients at each stage can be determined with great accuracy by the corresponding DA as shown in Table 4.

Table 3. Behavioral pathologic symptoms in Alzheimer's disease (AD) and developmental age (DA) analogies

BEHAVE-AD symptomatic category*	AD stage when most manifest	Corresponding DA	Corresponding behavioral symptom at DA*
Delusions- Not firmly held and transient false beliefs in AD.	5 & 6	2–7 years	Fantasy- Not firmly held and transient false beliefs in children.
If they cannot locate objects, may accuse "people" of stealing them.	5	5–7 years	When unable to locate objects or when asked for an object, may accuse people of taking them.
Imagine dead parents or other relatives are alive and/or physically present.	6	2–5 years	Imaginary friends.
May derive comfort from and talk to dolls.	6	2–5 years	May derive comfort from and talk to dolls.
May develop the anxiety and/or belief that their family will no longer care for them.	5 & 6	2–7 years	May develop the anxiety and/or belief that their family will no longer care for them.
Hallucinations- Uncommon in AD.	Variable (4 to 6)	2–12 years	Uncommon in children.
May experience shadows as people, may "hear" an imaginary ring.			May perceive shadows as people, may "hear" imaginary noises.
Activity disturbances- May wander away if not supervised.	6	2–5 years	May wander away if not supervised.
Insistent repetition of demands or questions.			Insistent repetition of demands or questions.
Storing or hiding objects in inappropriate places.			Storing or hiding objects in inappropriate places.

(continued)

Table 3. *Continued*

BEHAVE-AD symptomatic category*	AD stage when most manifest	Corresponding DA	Corresponding behavioral symptom at DA*
Aggressivity- Verbal outbursts which may be accompanied by anger. Physical threats and occasional violence such as grabbing or scratching. Occasional negativity such as refusal to bathe, dress, etc.	6	2–5 years	Verbal outbursts which may be accompanied by anger. Physical threats and occasional violence such as grabbing or scratching. Occasional negativity such as refusal to bathe, dress, etc.
Affective disturbances- Episodes of tearfulness Occasional pessimistic or negative statements, such as, "I wish I were dead" or "I'm going to kill myself", or "I feel like nothing", without clear affective component or true suicidal intent.	5 & 6 4 & 5	2–7 years 5–12 years	Episodes of tearfulness. Occasional pessimistic or negative statements, such as, "I'm going to hurt myself" without pathologic component or true destructive intent.
Anxieties and phobias- Anxiety regarding upcoming events with repetitive statements, such as, "When are we going?" Vocalized anxiety or fear regarding being left alone. Fear of darkness, bathing, etc.	5 5 & 6 6	5–7 years 2–7 years 2–5 years	Anxiety regarding upcoming events with repetitive statements, such as, "When are we going?" Vocalized anxiety or fear regarding being left alone. Fear of darkness, bathing, etc.

*Symptoms, although common and characteristic, are not universal and do not occur in all AD patients or children. ©1997 by Barry Reisberg, M.D. All rights reserved

Table 4. Management needs in normal development and of the Alzheimer's patient at the corresponding developmental age (DA)

Global deterioration and FAST stage of aging and AD	Developmental age (DA)	Management needs of aged and AD patients
1	Adult	None
2	Adult	None
3	12+ years	None
4	8–12 years	Independent survival still attainable.
5	5–7 years	Patient can no longer survive in the community without part-time assistance.
6	2–5 years	Patient requires full time supervision.
7	0–2 years	Patient requires continuous care.

For example, the stage 7 AD patient, has a corresponding DA of 2 years or less. The stage 7 AD patient requires full time, around-the-clock assistance just as an infant would. The stage 6 AD patient has a corresponding DA of 2 to 5 years, and requires approximately the same amount of care and supervision as a 2 to 5 year old.

Knowledge of the DA of the AD patient can assist clinicians in rapidly recognizing care needs of the AD patient and in rapidly resolving problems posed by the AD patient's care requirements.

For example, in response to the practical care question, "can one leave the stage 6 AD patient alone?", knowledge of the DA results in the immediate answer, "one can no sooner leave the stage 6 AD patient alone than one can leave a 2 to 5 year old child alone".

Similarly, one can pose the question, "can the stage 5 AD patient survive in the community independently?". Knowledge of the DA of the stage 5 patient results in the answer "a stage 5 AD patient can manage in the community with approximately the same success as a 5 to 7 year old child, i.e., they had better be watched over or they will get into very serious difficulty". This is precisely what happens to stage 5 patients who live alone in the community. They are preyed upon by less scrupulous societal elements, they can't pay their own rent, they can't independently market or prepare adequate meals, etc. Basically, a stage 5 AD patient requires approximately the same amount of community support as a 5 to 7 year old.

Can the stage 4 patient survive independently in the community? Stage 4 corresponds to a DA of approximately 8 to 12 years. Like the 8 to 12 year old, the stage 4 patient can manage on their own to a large extent, however, they require someone to pay the rent on time and to watch over personal finances and similarly complex aspects of modern life survival.

Finally, just as a teenager can mange on their own if necessary in the community, the same is true of the stage 3 patient with mild memory impairment and decreased ability in executive functional tasks.

Implications of ontogenic models for symptomatic consistency and variability

Capacities which proceed in a consistent and seemingly inexorable manner in normal human development are lost in a similarly consistent and seemingly inexorable manner with the progression of AD.

For example, the consistency and variability of acquisition of the 16 functional capacities described in the FAST is entirely mirrored by the consistency and variability of the loss of these same functions in the degenerative dementia of AD. In general, these functions are acquired consistently and universally in normal development and the loss of these functions in AD is similarly consistent and has been found to fulfill the Guttman criteria for an ordinal scaling procedure of progressive loss (Guttman, 1950; Sclan and Reisberg, 1992). However, just as there is some variability in the order of acquisition of these functions in normal development, there is similar variability in the order of loss of these same functions in the degenerative dementia of AD (Reisberg et al., 1985b; Sclan and Reisberg, 1992). For example, just as the ability to dress and to bathe are acquired at virtually the same time in normal development and either ability may be acquired first, the loss of these same abilities in AD occurs at virtually the same time and either loss may occur initially (Sclan and Reisberg, 1992).

The same patterns of consistency and variability of capacity acquisition and symptomatic loss can be described for various cognitive skills in development and AD. However, importantly, symptoms which are variable in normal development are also variable in AD. For example, the behavioral symptoms described in Table 3 are variable in normal development. To cite a few examples, although fantasies are very common in young children, not all children will derive comfort from and talk to dolls. Similarly, although so-called delusions are very common in stage 5 and 6 AD patients, not all AD patients will derive comfort from and talk to dolls (Reisberg et al., 1989a). Similarly, not all young children will wander away unless supervised, although this is very common, and conversely, not all AD patients will wander away unless supervised, although this is common (Reisberg et al., 1989a). Aggressive behaviors are common in children aged 2 to 5, marked by verbal outbursts, physical threats or violence, (grabbing, scratching, etc.) and/or negativity with refusal to do things. Aggressivity marked by the same symptoms, i.e., verbal outbursts, physical threats or violence, and/or negativity with refusal to do things, is similarly common in stage 6 AD. Just as not all children aged 2 to 5 are violent, not all stage 6 AD patients are violent.

Apart from the utility of ontogenic models in pointing to the variability of symptomatology in AD, these models also point to the conditions which can produce this variability. For example, a 2 to 5 year old child who is frustrated or mistreated will frequently respond with a "temper tantrum". A stage 6 AD patient who is frustrated or mistreated will frequently respond with what has been termed a "catastrophic reaction". A 2 to 7 year old child who is insecure, whose pride has been wounded, or who experiences their current life as intolerable, will frequently retreat into fantasy. A stage 5 or 6 AD patient who is insecure, whose pride has been wounded, or who experiences their current life as intolerable, will frequently develop delusions (e.g. that people have taken things from them, that they are still working, or that their parents are still alive). Just as we might consider treating a child's temper tantrums by removing the source of frustration or mistreatment, we might consider treating the AD patient's catastrophic reactions by removing the sources of frustration or mistreatment. Just as we use fantasy therapy to explore and treat the source of a child's insecurity, etc., we might use "delusion therapy" in AD to explore and treat the source of the AD patients insecurity, wounded pride, etc.

Ontogenic models can also be useful in identifying symptoms which should not occur in AD. For example, just as a 2 to 3 year old child who is speaking in sentences should be able to walk without assistance, a stage 6e AD patient who is generally capable of speaking in sentences, should be able to ambulate independently. If the 2 year old child cannot walk, then some other pathologic process has interfered with normal development producing excess disability. If the stage 6e AD patient cannot walk, then some other pathologic process has interfered with the AD degenerative process producing excess morbidity.

Just as infants and, to a lesser extent, small children, are very vulnerable, stage 7 AD patients, and, to a lesser extent, stage 6 AD patients, are very vulnerable. If we do not provide an infant with any love and attention, they develop a failure to thrive syndrome or a so-called anaclitic depression. If we do not provide a stage 7 AD patient with any love and attention, they withdraw and develop a condition very similar to the failure to thrive syndrome or an anaclitic depression like condition. If we do not take the time to feed an infant, they become emaciated. If we do not take the time to feed a stage 7 AD patient, they become emaciated. If an infant does not move regularly and properly, they may develop deformities. If a stage 7 AD patient does not move regularly and properly, they develop contractures (Souren et al., 1995). If we do not clean an infant properly, they develop rashes and sores. If a stage 7 AD patient is not cleaned properly, they develop stage 1 to stage 4 ulcerations, i.e., rashes and sores.

Etiopathogenic import of ontogenic observations for AD

Selective vulnerability of the brain myelin can explain the observed striking developmental relationships in AD. As noted by McGeer et al. (1990) and Braak and Braak (1996), the last brain areas to be myelinated in normal human development are the first to be involved with AD pathology. Interestingly, myelinization of the brain is an ongoing process which continues to increment from the fetal period well into adult life. Brain areas which are myelinated first have the thickest myelin deposition; those brain areas which are developmentally most recent have the least myelin deposition. Consequently, developmentally recent, thinly myelinated brain regions, may be the most vulnerable to the AD pathologic process. Supporting this pathogenic model is the observation that apolipoprotein genotype conveys risks and vulnerability in AD. Apolipoproteins are molecules responsible for lipid transportation in various organs and may thus play some role in myelin preservation.

One interesting aspect of the developmental model of AD which is not readily explained by the myelin vulnerability model alone, is the temporal reciprocal relationships which have been noted. Specifically, it has been noted that until stage 7 of AD, the time course of symptomatic loss in AD is mirrored by the temporal course of symptomatic acquisition in AD (Reisberg et al., 1989b, 1990, 1996a). Stage 7 of AD is very much longer than the corresponding DA, i.e., infancy. However, until stage 7, the duration of AD is approximately the same as the duration of the corresponding DA interval. To cite one example, AD patients go from loss of ability to select clothing properly to double incontinence over approximately the same five year interval as a child goes from achieving fecal continence (approximately age 2), to achieving the ability to properly select clothing, for example for school, at approximately 7 years of age. What is producing these temporal reciprocals? One possibility is that fundamental mechanisms which govern development are also operant in AD. Specifically, myelin may protect the neurons or, alternatively, the last brain regions to be myelinated may simply point to the most vulnerable neurons. Growth factors, mitogens, or related factors, may be producing the developmental reciprocals observed.

Conclusion

Striking developmental reciprocals for AD symptoms have been well described. These reciprocal relationships can promote clinical knowledge of AD management and treatment, and advance scientific knowledge of etiopathogenesis. Better understanding of AD can possibly also improve knowledge of potentials in normal human development, and can help to uncover the pathophysiology of normal and pathologic human maturation.

Acknowledgments

This work was supported in part by United States Department of Health and Human Services grants AG03051, AG08051, AG09127, and AG11505 from the National Institute on Aging of the US National Institutes of Health and by the Zachary and Elizabeth M. Fisher Alzheimer's Disease Education and Resources Program at the New York University Medical Center.

References

Auer SR, Sclan SG, Yaffee RA, Reisberg B (1994) The neglected half of Alzheimer disease: cognitive and functional concomitants of severe dementia. JAGS 42: 1266–1272

Braak H, Braak E (1991) Neuropathological stageing of Alzheimer-related changes. Acta Neuropathol 82: 239–259

Braak H, Braak E (1996) Development of Alzheimer-related neurofibrillary changes in the neocortex inversely recapitulates cortical myelogenesis. Acta Neuropathol 92: 197–201

Brun A, Englund E (1981) Regional pattern of degeneration in Alzheimer's disease: neuronal loss and histopathological grading. Histopathology 5: 549–564

Cioni G, Biagioni E, Cipolloni C (1992) Brain before cognition: EEG maturation in pre-term infants. In: Kostovic I, Knezevic S, Wisniewski HM, Spillich GJ (eds) Neurodevelopment, aging and cognition. Birkhäuser, Boston, pp 75–98

Flechsig P (1920) Anatomie des menschlichen Gehirns und Rückenmarks auf myelogenetischer Grundlage. Thieme, Leipzig

Folstein MF, Folstein SE, McHugh PR (1975) Mini-mental state: a practical method for grading the cognitive state of patients for the clinician. J Psychiat Res 12: 189–198

Franssen EH, Reisberg B (1997) Neurologic markers of the progression of Alzheimer disease. Int Psychogeriat 9 [Suppl 1]: 297–306

Franssen EH, Reisberg B, Kluger A, Sinaiko E, Boja C (1991) Cognition-independent neurologic symptoms in normal aging and probable Alzheimer's disease. Arch Neurol 48: 148–154

Franssen EH, Kluger A, Torossian CL, Reisberg B (1993) The neurologic syndrome of severe Alzheimer's disease: relationship to functional decline. Arch Neurol 50: 1029–1039

Franssen EH, Souren LEM, Torossian CL, Reisberg B (1997) Utility of developmental reflexes in the differential diagnosis and prognosis of incontinence in Alzheimer disease. J Geriat Psychiat Neurol 10: 22–28

Guttman L (1950) The basis for scalogram analysis. In: Stouffer SA, Guttman L, Suchman EA, Lazersfeld PF, Starr SA, Clausen JA (eds) Measurement and prediction. Princeton University Press, Princeton

Huff FJ, Boller F, Luchelli F, Querriera R, Beyer J, Belle S (1987) The neurologic examination in patient's with probable Alzheimer's disease. Arch Neurol 44: 929–932

Jacobs L, Gossman MD (1980) Three primitive reflexes in normal adults. Neurology 30: 184–188

McGeer PL, McGeer EG, Akiyama H, Itagaki S, Harrop R, Peppard R (1990) Neuronal degeneration and memory loss in Alzheimer's disease and aging. Exp Brain Res [Suppl] 21: 411–426

Paulson G, Gottlieb G (1968) Developmental reflexes: the reappearance of foetal and neonatal reflexes in aged patients. Brain 91: 37–52

Prichep LS, John ER, Ferris SH, Reisberg B, Alper K, Almas M, Cancro R (1994) Quantitative EEG correlates of cognitive deterioration in the elderly. Neurobiol Aging 15: 85–90

Reisberg B (1986) Dementia: a systematic approach to identifying reversible causes. Geriatrics 41: 30–46

Reisberg B (1988) Functional assessment staging (FAST). Psychopharmacol Bull 24: 653–659

Reisberg B, Ferris SH, de Leon MJ, Crook T (1982) The Global Deterioration Scale for assessment of primary degenerative dementia. Am J Psychiat 139: 1136–1139

Reisberg B, Ferris SH, Anand R, de Leon MJ, Schneck MK, Buttinger C, Borenstein J (1984) Functional staging of dementia of the Alzheimer's type. Ann NY Acad Sci 435: 481–483

Reisberg B, Ferris SH, Anand R, de Leon MJ, Schnek MK, Crook T (1985a) Clinical assessment of cognitive decline in normal aging and primary degenerative dementia: concordant ordinal measures. In: Pichot P, Berner P, Wolf R, Thau K (eds) Psychiatry, vol 5. Plenum Press, New York, pp 333–338

Reisberg B, Ferris SH, de Leon MJ (1985b) Senile dementia of the Alzheimer type: diagnostic and differential diagnostic features with special reference to functional assessment staging. In: Traber J, Gispen WH (eds) Senile dementia of the Alzheimer type, vol 2. Springer, Berlin Heidelberg New York Tokyo, pp 18–37

Reisberg B, Ferris SH, Franssen EH (1986) Functional degenerative stages in dementia of the Alzheimer's type appear to reverse normal human development. In: Shagass C, et al (eds) Biological psychiatry 1985, vol 7. Elsevier Science, New York, pp 1319–1321

Reisberg B, Ferris SH, de Leon MJ, Sinaiko E, Franssen EH, Kluger A, Mir P, Borenstein J, George AE, Shulman E, Steinberg G, Cohen J (1988) Stage-specific behavioral, cognitive, and in vivo changes in community residing subjects with age-associated memory impairment (AAMI) and primary degenerative dementia of the Alzheimer type. Drug Dev Res 15: 101–114

Reisberg B, Franssen EH, Sclan SG, Kluger A, Ferris SH (1989a) Stage specific incidence of potentially remediable behavioral symptoms in aging and Alzheimer's disease: a study of 120 patients using the BEHAVE-AD. Bull Clin Neurosci 54: 95–112

Reisberg B, Ferris SH, de Leon MJ, Kluger A, Franssen EH, Borenstein J, Alba R (1989b) The stage specific temporal course of Alzheimer's disease: Functional and behavioral concomitants based upon cross-sectional and longitudinal observation. In: Iqbal K, Wisniewski HM, Winblad B (eds) Alzheimer's disease and related disorders: progress in clinical and biological research, vol 317. Alan R Liss, New York, pp 23–41

Reisberg B, Pattschull-Furlan A, Franssen EH, Sclan S, Kluger A, Dingcong L, Ferris SH (1990) Cognition-related functional, praxis and feeding changes in CNS aging and Alzheimer's disease and their developmental analogies. In: Beyreuther K, Schettler G (eds) Molecular mechanisms of aging. Springer, Berlin Heidelberg New York Tokyo, pp 18–40

Reisberg B, Ferris SH, Torossian CL, Kluger A, Monteiro I (1992) Pharmacologic treatment of Alzheimer's disease: a methodologic critique based upon current knowledge of symptomatology and relevance for drug trials. Int Psychogeriat 4 [Suppl 1]: 9–42

Reisberg B, Sclan SG, Franssen EH, de Leon MJ, Kluger A, Torossian CL, Shulman E, Steinberg G, Monteiro I, McRae T, Boksay I, Mackell JA, Ferris SH (1993) Clinical stages of normal aging and Alzheimer's disease: the GDS staging system. Neurosci Res Commun 13 [Suppl 1]: 551–554

Reisberg B, Ferris SH, Franssen EH, Shulman E, Monteiro I, Sclan SG, Steinberg G, Kluger A, Torossian CL, de Leon MJ, Laska E (1996a) Mortality and temporal course of probable Alzheimer's disease: a five-year prospective study. Int Psychogeriat 8: 291–311

Reisberg B, Kenowsky S, Franssen EH, Souren L, Shulman E, Steinberg G, Aronstein Z, Auer SR (1996b) Slowing the progression of Alzheimer's disease: towards a science of Alzheimer's disease care. The Fifth National Alzheimer's Disease Education Conference Proceedings. Alzheimer's Association, Chicago

Reisberg B, Auer SR, Monteiro I, Franssen E, Kenowsky S (1998) A rational psychological approach to the treatment of behavioral disturbances and symptomatology in Alzheimer's disease based upon recognition of the developmental age. Int Acad Biomed Drug Res 13: 102–109

Sclan SG, Reisberg B (1992) Functional assessment staging (FAST) in Alzheimer's disease: reliability, validity and ordinality. Int Psychogeriat 4 [Suppl 1]: 55–69

Sclan SG, Foster JR, Reisberg B, Franssen EH, Welkowitz J (1990) Application of Piagetian measures of cognition in severe Alzheimer's disease. Psychiatr J Univ Ottawa 15: 221–226

Souren LEM, Franssen EM, Reisberg B (1995) Contractures and loss of function in patients with Alzheimer's disease. JAGS 43: 650–655

Authors' address: Dr. B. Reisberg, Alzheimer's Disease Education and Resources Program, New York University Medical Center, New York, NY 10016, U.S.A.

Mild cognitive impairment — an early stage of Alzheimer's disease?

O. Almkvist[1,2], **H. Basun**[1,2], **L. Bäckman**[2,3], **A. Herlitz**[2,4], **L. Lannfelt**[1], **B. Small**[2], **M. Viitanen**[1,2], **L. O. Wahlund**[1], and **B. Winblad**[1,2]

[1] Division of Geriatric Medicine, Department of Clinical Neuroscience and Family Medicine, Karolinska Institute, University Hospital, Huddinge, [2] Stockholm Gerontology Research Center, Stockholm, [3] Department of Psychology, University of Göteborg, and [4] Department of Psychology, University of Stockholm, Sweden

Summary. The hypothesis that mild cognitive impairment (MCI) represents an early stage of Alzheimer's disease (AD) was investigated by reviewing recent research from three sources: asymptomatic and symptomatic individuals carrying mutations that cause AD, hospital-samples of non-demented patients with MCI at the initial examination that are followed longitudinally, and community-based incident cases of AD.

Studies with asymptomatic mutation carriers of the amyloid precursor protein and presenilin 1 gene have shown a linear and disease-related decline in most cognitive functions that begins approximately 10 years before the expected clinical onset of AD. However, there is considerable overlap between the level of impairment for mutation carriers and non-carriers of the same age during the early preclinical stage of AD. Hospital-based longitudinal studies have shown that non-demented individuals with isolated mild episodic memory impairment may develop clinically diagnosed AD with widespread cognitive deficits in a few years time. Community-based epidemiological studies on the incidence of AD demonstrate that indices of episodic memory, in addition to measures of general cognitive functioning, are useful in predicting early AD. In contrast, subjective memory impairment or age-associated memory impairment are less powerful predictors of future dementia development.

In summary, there is converging evidence to demonstrate that preclinical AD is characterized by a common behavioral phenotype, with cognitive decline in several domains, predominantly in episodic memory. The decline appears to start many years before the clinical onset of AD. Moreover, the progression of the impairment appears to be continuous. Finally, this pattern of performance generalizes across etiology of AD (familial or sporadic), clinical onset (early or late), sample composition (hospital or community), and method of assessment.

Introduction

Alzheimer's disease (AD) is characterized by neuropathological findings such as senile plaques and neurofibrillary tangles that have specific distributions in terms of brain regions affected. In addition, these distributions change in a specific manner during the course of the disease. The earliest changes in the preclinical phase of the disease are found only in the transentorhinal region only, an area located between the entorhinal region and the adjoining temporal cortex. In mild clinical AD, these changes become more severe and radiate into neighboring regions as well as to the posterior cortical association areas of the brain. By contrast, the primary sensory and motor projection areas are relatively spared from neuropathological changes during this stage. Finally, during the end stage of the disease, the advanced stage, the neuropathological abnormalities become even more severe in the previously affected regions and the extrapyramidal system becomes affected as well. This three stage model of neuropathological changes in AD has been described by several researchers (Braak and Braak, 1992; Brun and Gustafsson, 1976; Fewster et al., 1991; Price, 1991; Tomlinson, 1970). In the present paper, we will focus on the preclinical and the early clinical stage of the disease and describe the cognitive impairments that are observed in these two stages.

In reviewing recent research addressing these issues, we describe information from three sources: a) asymptomatic and symptomatic individuals carrying mutations that cause AD, b) hospital-based longitudinal studies of healthy elderly adults or non-demented patients with mild cognitive impairment (MCI) who eventually develop AD, and c) community-based studies targeting on the incidence of AD. Cross-sectional studies are not included because they typically include patients with more severe impairment. We will argue that information obtained from these three classes of studies converges into a common pattern of cognitive impairment that are stage-distinct and stage-differentiated.

In brief, the preclinical stage of AD involves an impairment of episodic memory that may be relatively mild and comparable to what is found in many normal elderly individuals. In addition, the deficits that are apparent on this stage may last for several years. In the early clinical stage, episodic memory becomes more severely disturbed and, simultaneously, impairments will appear in multiple cognitive domains such as verbal and visuospatial processes as well as attention and executive functioning. By contrast, primary memory and procedural memory, as well as sensory and motor abilities may be relatively well preserved. However, there may be considerable interindividual variability in the pattern of cognitive deficits, with not all domains being affected in all persons. In many cases, there is a marked asymmetry in cognitive impairment, showing verbal versus spatial predominance or sparing as one example. This stage, may also last for several years.

Studies on carriers of AD-causing mutations

In the preclinical stage of AD, studies of asymptomatic carriers of the amyloid precursor protein (APP) and presenilin-1 (PS1) mutations demonstrate that episodic memory (i.e., encoding, storage, and conscious retrieval of information with a temporal-spatial personal referent) is clearly impaired (Almkvist, 1996; Almkvist et al., 1995; Farlow et al., 1994; Karlinsky et al., 1992; Kennedy et al., 1995; Newman et al., 1994; Smalley et al., 1992). The impairment may be observed several years before the expected clinical onset (Almkvist et al., 1997a,b). In addition to the changes in episodic memory, some deficits among gene-carriers have been observed in other domains including visuospatial abilities, attention, and executive functions (Almkvist et al., 1995, 1997a; Farlow et al., 1994; Karlinsky et al., 1992; Newman et al., 1994). In the preclinical stage, no changes have been reported in sensory and motor function, primary memory, procedural memory, or verbal skills.

The trajectory of decline appears to be linear in the preclinical and early clinical stages of persons carrying APP and PS1 mutations (Almkvist et al., 1997a,b). Our data indicate that the decline starts more than 10 years before the clinical onset stage of the disease, when the clinical diagnosis is possible. Further evidence regarding this pattern is provided by the fact that there is a linear relationship between cognitive functioning and the duration of the disease, as well as levels of proteins in cerebrospinal fluid (e.g., APP metabolites and tau) that are associated with the disease process (Almkvist et al., 1997a,b).

Clinical studies of incident AD

In clinical studies on incident AD cases, healthy elderly adults or non-demented memory impaired subjects are followed until some of them develop dementia. Afterwards, the baseline performance of the incident cases is compared to the non-incident cases to identify possible cognitive markers of dementia development. Using comprehensive neuropsychological batteries, a number of factors have been found to be related to the future development of dementia. Among these significant predictors are verbal ability such as naming and category fluency (Devanand et al., 1997; Flicker et al., 1991). In addition, indices of psychomotor speed such as the Digit Symbol test (Devanand et al., 1997; Flicker et al., 1991, 1993b; Tierney et al., 1996) and visuospatial functioning as exemplified by the Block Design test (Devanand et al., 1997) have been found to be sensitive markers for dementia development. However, the most salient predictor appears to be different measures of episodic memory functioning (Bondi et al., 1994; Devanand et al., 1997; Flicker et al., 1991, 1993b; Fuld et al., 1990; Masur et al., 1990; Tierney et al., 1996; Tuokko et al., 1991). In light of objective episodic memory deficits in those individuals who develop dementia, it is interesting to note that there is conflicting evidence concerning the predictive power of subjective memory complaints for later development of dementia in otherwise healthy elderly individuals. Some studies are negative (Flicker et al., 1993a; O'Brien et al., 1992), although also positive results have been presented (Schmand et al., 1996). Furthermore, it has been demonstrated that memory deficit denoted as age-associated memory impairment (AAMI) does not predict the future development of AD or dementia (Hänninen et al., 1995; Snowdon and Lane, 1994). Hypothetically, a more serious episodic memory deficit than subjective or AAMI appears to be required to predict development of AD.

Although episodic memory tasks appear to have the best predictive power to indicate early dementia development, it is unclear which aspect of episodic memory is most vulnerable to dementia. For example, it is not known whether the deficits in memory performance of AD patients result from impairments in encoding, storage, or retrieval processes. Although conclusive evidence regarding the nature of the episodic memory impairment in preclinical AD is lacking, some tentative suggestions can be offered. First, given that the size of the impairment in preclinical AD is equally large, or even larger, in recognition compared with free recall (Small et al., in press a), it seems unlikely that retrieval problems are a major source of the difficulty in this stage of the disease. Rather, such results suggest that encoding difficulty may predominate. In addition, data indicating that delayed recall may be particularly sensitive in identifying persons in the preclinical stage of the disease (e.g., Tierney et al., 1996), suggests that storage and consolidation processes may be implicated as well.

Neuropsychological tests may differ in terms of their sensitivity because of varying task difficulty rather than the specific process tapped by the memory task. Tests may differ in terms of material to be remembered, presentation format, retrieval format, instruction, support at encoding and retrieval, pacing, and time of testing (e.g., immediate or delayed). All of these factors influence performance. Therefore, the range of cognitive deterioration in the specific sample of subjects is important, and test difficulty and level of cognitive dysfunction has to be properly matched.

Epidemiological studies of incident AD

Results from epidemiological studies on incident AD have demonstrated that a variety of measures of episodic memory performance (Grober and Kawas, 1997; Herlitz et al., 1997; Jacobs et al., 1995; Johansson and Zarit, 1997; Linn et al., 1995; Masur et al., 1994; Small et al., 1997) are reliable predictors of individuals, who will develop AD within some years. In addition, other cognitive functions may be important. For example, verbal abilities such as naming (Jacobs et al., 1995), fluency (Aronson et al., 1990; Masur et al., 1994), and abstraction (Jacobs et al., 1995; Small et al., 1997a). In addition, psychomotor speed as indexed by the Trailmaking test (Herlitz et al., 1997; Masur et al., 1994), as well as general level of cognitive functioning (Herlitz et al., 1997; Johansson and Zarit, 1997; Small et al., 1997b; Yoshitake et al., 1995) have proven to be sensitive for early dementia development. Thus, longitudinal studies of clinical samples and epidemiological research converge in suggesting that several cognitive domains are affected in preclinical AD, with the greatest sensitivity seen for tasks assessing episodic memory.

Comment

There is converging evidence to indicate that preclinical AD is characterized by a common behavioral phenotype, with cognitive deficits appearing primarily in episodic memory. In the early clinical stage of the disease, evidence points to the fact that AD is characterized by numerous impairments affecting multiple cognitive domains including episodic memory, verbal abilities, visuospatial function, attention, and executive functions. However, some abilities may be spared by the disease including primary and procedural memory, sensory and motor performance. It is important to note that individuals with preclinical AD and AD in the early clinical stage are relatively well functioning in activities of daily living. The development from preclinical to very mild AD appears to be the natural course for a large proportion of persons with MCI. However, it is necessarily true that not all individuals with isolated memory impairment will develop AD (Smith et al., 1996).

The decline associated with the disease appears to start many years before a clinical diagnosis is possible, given current criteria of AD. There is evidence to indicate that the preclinical manifestations of the disease appear at least 5 to 10 years prior to the clinical onset of dementia (Almkvist and Bäckman, 1993; Almkvist et al., 1995; LaRue and Jarvik, 1987; Linn et al., 1995). It has been argued that preclinical cases of AD, when not identified, may contaminate conclusions from studies that focus on "normal aging". For example, Sliwinski and colleagues (1996) have demonstrated that the inclusion of persons in preclinical AD may result in an underestimation of the true mean and an overestimation of the true variance in cognitive functions for normal elderly individuals.

Although the cognitive phenotype, that is, type and degree of impairment, is known both in the preclinical and the early clinical stages of the disease, the shape of this decline is unclear. For example, is progression best described as a linear and continuous trajectory, or is the progression phasic in nature? There are data to suggest that the decline process is biphasic (Haxby et al., 1992), triphasic (Brooks et al., 1993; Gray and Della Sala, 1996), or varies across the disease course in a specific manner (Stern et al., 1996) among patients with mild to moderate sporadic AD. However, this type of change could be due to ceiling or floor effects in the assessment instruments as they may not be fully sensitive to very early and very late changes of the disease process (Stern et al., 1996). By contrast, data on carriers of APP and PS1 mutations from our laboratory indicate a linear decline in neuropsychological tests covering a preclinical period of 20 years and a clinical period of 10 years. Furthermore, there is no indication of a non-linear trend in our data. It is interesting to note that the linear relationship holds not only with regard to cognitive functioning and duration of the disease, but also with regard to biochemical markers of the disease such as cerebrospinal fluid levels of APP metabolites (Almkvist et al., 1997a) and tau (Almkvist et al., 1997b), the former related to senile plaques and the latter to neurofibrillary tangles. However, awaiting further evidence, the issue of the shape of the decline process remains unresolved. Possibly, there are subtypes of AD that differ in terms of etiology and the nature of decline.

The cognitive phenotype appears to be consistent across sporadic and familial AD (Almkvist et al., 1996), although there is strong evidence showing variability in onset age as well as duration. For some PS1 mutations, the onset age is in the thirties and the duration is approximately five. On the other hand, AD caused by APP mutations typically has a much later onset age and a longer duration. However, in familial AD due to different mutations, the pattern of cognitive impairment across the disease process appears to be qualitatively similar.

In summary, a large proportion of patients with MCI, most frequently manifested as isolated episodic memory dysfunction, will develop into early AD with multiple cognitive deficits.

Acknowledgement

This research was supported by a grant from the Swedish Medical Research Council (12 245) to the first author.

References

Almkvist O (1996) Neuropsychological features of early Alzheimer's disease: preclinical and clinical stages. Acta Neurol Scand [Suppl] 165: 63–71

Almkvist O, Bäckman L (1993) Progression in Alzheimer's disease: sequencing of neuropsychological decline. Int J Geriatr Psychiatr 8: 755–763

Almkvist O, Basun H, Wahlund LO, Lannfelt L (1995) Cognitive functions of familiy members with and without the APP670/671 mutation. In: Iqbal K, Mortimer JA, Winblad B, Wisniewski HH (eds) Research advances in Alzheimer's disease and related disorder. John Wiley, New York, pp 251–259

Almkvist O, Jelic V, Lannfelt L, Nordberg A, Shigeta M, Wahlund LO, Winblad B (1996) Alzheimer's disease with and without familial aggregation: a case for phenotypical similarity. In: Turner JD, Beyreuther K, Theuring F (eds) Alzheimer's disease: etiological mechanisms and therapeutic possibilities (Ernst Schering Research Foundation, Workshop 17). Springer, Berlin Heidelberg New York Tokyo, pp 1–15

Almkvist O, Basun H, Wagner S, Wahlund LO, Lannfelt L (1997a) Impaired cognitive functions are strongly related to low cerebrospinal fluid levels of α-cleaved amyloid precursor protein in the Swedish Alzheimer mutation family. Arch Neurol 54: 641–644

Almkvist O, Jensen M, Basun H, Wahlund LO, Amberla K, Viitanen M, Lannfelt L (1997b) Elevated cerebrospinal fluid tau correlates with Alzheimer disease symptoms in apolipoprotein E ε4(+) carriers. (submitted)

Aronson MK, Ooi WL, Morgenstern H, Hafner A, Masur D, Crystal H, Frishman WH, Fisher D, Katzman R (1990) Women, myocardial infarction, and dementia in the very old. Neurology 40: 1102–1106

Bondi MW, Monsch AU, Galasko D, Butters N, Salomon DP, Delis DC (1994) Preclinical markers of dementia of the Alzheimer type. Neuropsychol 8: 374–384

Braak H, Braak E (1992) Neuropathological stageing of Alzheimer-related changes. Acta Neuropathol 82: 239–259

Brooks J, Kraemer HC, Tanke ED, Yesavage JA (1993) The methodology of studying decline in Alzheimer's disease. J Am Geriatr Soc 41: 623–628

Brun A, Gustafson L (1976) Distribution of cerebral degeneration of Alzheimer's disease. Arch Psychiatr Nervenkrank 223: 15–23

Devanand DP, Folz M, Gorlyn M, Moeller JR, Stern Y (1997) Questionnable dementia: clinical course and predictors of outcome. J Am Geriatr Soc 45: 321–328

Farlow M, Murrell J, Ghetti B, Unverzagt F, Zeldenrust S, Benson M (1994) Clinical characteristics in a kindred with early-onset Alzheimer's disease and their linkage to a G⇒T change at position 2149 of the amyloid precursor protein gene. Neurology 44: 105–111

Fewster PH, Griffin-Brooks S, MacGregor J, Ojalvo-Rose E, Ball MJ (1991) A topographical pathway by which histopathological lesions disseminate through the brain of patients with Alzheimer's disease. Dementia 2: 121–132

Flicker C, Ferris SH, Reisberg B (1991) Mild cognitive impairment in the elderly: predictors of dementia. Neurology 41: 1006–1009

Flicker C, Ferris SH, Reisberg B (1993a) A longitudinal study of cognitive function in elderly persons with subjective memory complaints. J Am Geriatr Soc 41: 1029–1032

Flicker C, Ferris SH, Reisberg B (1993b) A two-year longitudinal study of cognitive function in normal aging and Alzheimer's disease. J Geriatr Psychiatr Neurol 6: 84–96

Fuld PA, Masur DM, Blau AD, Crystal H, Aronson MK (1990) Object-memory evaluation for prospective detection of dementia in normal functioning elderly: predictive and normative data. J Clin Exp Neuropsychol 12: 520–528

Gray C, Della Sala S (1996) Charting decline in dementia. In: Morris RG (ed) The cognitive neuropsychology of Alzheimer-type dementia. Oxford University Press, Oxford, pp 23–46

Grober E, Kawas C (1997) Learning and retention in preclinical and early Alzheimer's disease. Psychol Aging 12: 183–188

Haxby JV, Raffaele K, Gillette J, Schapiro MB, Rapoport SI (1992) Individual trajectories of cognitive decline in patients with dementia of the Alzheimer type. J Clin Exp Neuropsychol 14: 575–592

Hänninen T, Hallikainen M, Koivisto K, Helkala EL, Reinikainen KJ, Soininen H, Mykkänen L, Laakso M, Pyörälä K, Riekkinen PJ (1995) A follow-up study of age-associated memory impairment: neuropsychological predictors of dementia. J Am Geriatr Soc 43: 1007–1015

Herlitz A, Small BL, Fratiglioni L, Almkvist O, Bäckman L (1997) Detection of mild dementia in community surveys: is it possible to increase the accuracy of our diagnostic instruments? Arch Neurol 54: 319–324

Jacobs DM, Sano M, Doonief G, Marder K, Bell T, Stern Y (1995) Neuropsychological detection and characterization of preclinical Alzheimer's disease. Neurology 45: 957–962

Johansson B, Zarit SH (1997) Early cognitive markers of the incidence of dementia and mortality: a longitudinal population-based study of the oldest old. Int J Geriatr Psychiatr 12: 53–59

Karlinsky H, Vaula G, Haines JL, Ridgley J, Bergeron C, Mortilla M, Tupler RG (1992) Molecular and prospective phenotypic characterization of a pedigree with familial Alzheimer's disease and a missense mutation in codon 717 of the beta-amyloid protein gene. Neurology 42: 1445–1453

Kennedy AM, Newman SK, Frackowiak RSJ, Cunningham VJ, Roques P, Stevens J, Neary D, Bruton CJ, Warrington EK, Rossor MN (1995) Chromosome 14 linked familial Alzheimer's disease: a clinico-pathological study of a single pedigree. Brain 118: 185–205

LaRue A, Jarvik L (1987) Cognitive function and prediction of dementia in old age. Int J Aging Hum Dev 25: 79–88

Linn RT, Wolf PA, Bachman DL, Knoefel JE, Cogg JL, Belanger AJ, Kaplan EF, D'Agostino RB (1995) The preclinical phase of probable Alzheimer's disease. Arch Neurol 52: 485–490

Masur DM, Fuld PA, Blau AD, Crystal H, Aronson MK (1990) Predicting development of dementia in the elderly with selective reminding test. J Clin Exp Neuropsychol 12: 529–538

Masur DM, Sliwinski M, Lipton RB, Blau AD, Crystal HA (1994) Neuropsychological prediction of dementia and the absence of dementia in healthy elderly persons. Neurology 44: 1427–1432

Newman SK, Warrington EK, Kennedy AM, Rossor MN (1994) The earliest cognitive change in a person with familial Alzheimers disease: presymptomatic neuro-psychological features in a pedigree with familial Alzheimer's disease confirmed at necropsy. J Neurol Neurosurg Psychiatry 57: 967–972

O'Brien JT, Beats B, Hill K, Howard R, Sahakian B, Levy R (1992) Do subjective memory complaints precede dementia? A three-year follow-up of patients with supposed "benign senescent forgetfulnes". Int J Geriatr Psychiatr 7: 481–486

Price JL, Davis PB, Morris JC, White DL (1991) The distribution of tangles, plaques and related immunohistochemical markers in healthy aging and Alzheimer's disease. Neurobiol Aging 12: 295–312

Schmand B, Jonker C, Hoijer C, Lindeboom J (1996) Subjective memory complaints may announce dementia. Neurology 46: 121–125

Sliwinski M, Lipton RB, Buschke H, Stewart W (1996) The effects of preclinical dementia on estimates of normal cognitive functioning in aging. J Gerontol Psychol Sci 51B: P217–P225

Small BJ, Herlitz L, Bäckman L (1997) Cognitive development in Alzheimer's disease: charting the decline process. In: Edelstein B (ed) Comprehensive clinical psychology: clinical geropsychology, vol 1. Elsevier Science Ltd, Oxford

Small BJ, Herlitz L, Fratiglioni L, Almkvist O, Bäckman L (1997a) Cognitive predictors of incident Alzheimer's disease: a prospective longitudinal study Neuropsychol 11: 1–8

Small BJ, Viitanen M, Bäckman L (1997b) Mini-mental state examination item scores as predictors of Alzheimer's disease: incidence data from the Kungsholmen Project, Stockholm. J Gerontol Med Sci 52: 299–304

Smalley SL, Wolkenstein BH, LaRue A, Woodward JA, Jarvik LF, Matsuyama SS (1992) Commingling analysis of memory performance in offspring of Alzheimer patients. Genet Epidemiol 9: 333–345

Smith GE, Petersen RC, Parisi JE, Ivnik RJ, Kokmen E, Tangalos EG, Waring S (1996) Definition, course and outcome of mild cognitive impairment. Aging Neuropsychol Cogn 3: 141–147

Snowdon J, Lane F (1994) A longitudinal study of age-associated memory impairment. Int J Geriatr Psychiatr 9: 779–787

Stern Y, Liu X, Albert M, Brandt J, Jacobs DM, Del Castillo-Castaneda C, Marder K, Bell K, Sano M, Bylsma F, Lafleche G, Tsai W-Y (1996) Application of a growth curve approach to modeling the progression of Alzheimer's disease. J Gerontol Med Sci 51A: M179–M184

Tierney MC, Szalai JP, Snow WG, Fisher RH, Nores A, Nadon G, Dunn E, St. George-Hyslop PH (1996) Prediction of probable Alzheimer's disease in memory-impaired patients: a prospective longitudinal study. Neurology 46: 661–665

Tomlinson BE, Blessed G, Roth M (1970) Observations on the brains of demented people. J Neurol Sci 11: 205–242

Tuokko H, Vernon-Wilkinson R, Weir J, Beattie BL (1991) Cued recall and early identification of dementia. J Clin Exp Neuropsychol 13: 871–879

Yoshitake T, Kiyohara Y, Kato I, Ohmura T, Iwamoto H, Nakayama K, Ohmori S, Nomiyama K, Kawano H, Ueda K, Sueishi K, Tsuneyosh M, Fujishima M (1995) Incidence and risk factors of vascular dementia and Alzheimer's disease in a defined elderly Japanese population: the Hisayama study. Neurology 45: 1161–1168

Authors' address: Dr. O. Almkvist, Division of Geriatric Medicine B84, Huddinge Hospital, S-14186 Huddinge, Sweden

The prognosis of mild cognitive impairment in the elderly

H. Wolf[1]**, M. Grunwald**[1]**, G. M. Ecke**[1]**, D. Zedlick**[1]**, S. Bettin**[2]**,
C. Dannenberg**[2]**, J. Dietrich**[3]**, K. Eschrich**[4]**, T. Arendt**[5]**, and H.-J. Gertz**[1]

Departments of [1]Psychiatry, [2]Nuclear Medicine, [3]Radiology, [4]Biochemistry, and
[5]Paul Flechsig Institute for Brain Research, University of Leipzig,
Federal Republic of Germany

Summary. *Purpose:* To determine whether or not subtypes of intellectual functioning are suitable to predict further cognitive decline in individuals with mild cognitive impairment. *Design:* naturalistic longitudinal study (mean interval 2.7 years). *Patients:* 41 subjects with mild cognitive impairment who attended a memory clinic. *Methods:* SIDAM, CT, SPECT, and ApoE genotype. *Results:* At follow-up, 8 out of 41 patients (19.5%) with MCI had progressed to dementia, 8 patients (19.5%) had improved to normal levels of cognitive functioning, 25 patients (61%) had remained stable within the MCI group. At baseline the two prognostic groups differed significantly with regard to age, memory functions, orientation, and the degree of atrophy of the left medial temporal lobe on CT scan. *Conclusion:* The majority of MCI patients in this study remained cognitively stable within the observation period. Patients with older age, poorer test performance on memory tasks and orientation deficits are at higher risk of progressive decline to dementia. CT measures of medial temporal lobe atrophy may be a sensitive parameter of group discrimination.

Introduction

International criteria for the diagnosis of dementia require the presence of multiple cognitive deficits, among which memory impairment is essential. There must be evidence of decline from a previously higher level, and the deficits must be severe enough to interfere with social or occupational functioning. The ICD 10 (WHO, 1990) stipulates a duration of at least 6 months. To exclude delirium, the cognitive deficits must be present in clear consciousness. Alzheimer's disease (AD) represents the most common cause of dementia, followed by vascular dementia (VaD).

The term "Mild Cognitive Impairment" (MCI) can be used to describe the intermediate state of cognitive functioning in which a decline from a previously higher level has occured which is not severe enough to fulfil the criteria of dementia. A variety of terms and concepts has been introduced in the psychiatric literature to describe this grey area of cognitive functioning in the elderly (Table 1).

The existing concepts can be divided into three groups. MCI is regarded as 1.) a preliminary stage of dementia (Roth et al., 1986; O'Connor et al., 1991; Gurland, 1982), 2.) a benign age-related cognitive decline with no other aetiological background than ageing (Crook et al., 1988; Kral, 1962, 1978; Reisberg et al., 1982), and 3.) an intermediate category to describe the transitional zone between dementia and normal ageing without aetiological presumptions (Henderson and Huppert, 1984; Hughes et al., 1982; Zaudig et al., 1991, 1992).

Table 1. Mild cognitive impairment — an overview of terms and concepts

Term/authors	Concept
"Benign senescent forgetfulness" Kral (1962)	memory dysfunction in the elderly which progresses slowly and is characterised by the inability to recall on certain occasions relatively unimportant experiences of the past, equally frequent in both sexes, expression of *a senium naturale* as opposed to *senium ex morbo* in "malignant senescent forgetfulness"
"age assosiated memory impairment" Crook et al. (1986)	form of benign senescent forgetfulness. Diagnostic criteria: aged over 50, complaints of memory loss reflected in everyday problems (misplacing objects, difficulty remembering telephone numbers, names of individuals following introduction, difficulty remembering multiple items to be purchased etc), gradual onset of memory problems, memory test performance that is at least 1 SD below the mean established for young adults,exclusion of any other psychiatric or physical disease associated with cognitive decline
"limited dementia" Gurland et al. (1982)	memory dysfunction which is not severe enough to interfere with the patient's capability to live independently. Criteria: 1. subjective report of memory decline, 2. increased reliance on notes and reminders, 3. occasionally forgets names of aquaintances, forgets appointments or misplaces objects, 4. occasionally has destructive or dangerous memory lapses such as burning cooking or leaving on gas taps, and 5. has one or two errors on cognitive testing: forgets current or past President, exact date, phone number, post code, dates of marriage or moving to present location, or cannot remember interviewer's name, even on third challenge
"questionable dementia" Hughes et al. (1982)	based on Clinical Dementia Rating Scale (CDR), consistent slight forgetfulness, partial recollection of events, but fully orientated except for slight difficulty with time relationships, slight impairment in solving problems, slightly impaired functioning in job, shopping and social groups, life at home, hobbies and interests slightly impaired

Table 1. *Continued*

"minimal dementia" Roth et al. (1986)	= CAMDEX category, refers to individuals with a mild impairment of recall, minor and variable errors in orientation, a blunted capacity to follow arguments and solve problems, and occasional errors in everyday tasks
"mild cognitive decline" Reisberg et al. (1982)	= GDS 3, cognitive test performance at least 1SD below mean of their age group (equivalent of AAMI) plus memory complaint, 85% do not convert to dementia within 3 years of observation
"mild dementia" Henderson and Huppert (1984)	not a diagnosis itself but a rubric for the early stages of several neuropatholological disorders, the single common feature is "the presence of cognitive deficits, presumed to be a decline from a formerly higher level of functioning", it is not known whether or not these individuals will eventually become demented
"mild cognitive decline" (ICD 10)	accomodates a range of conditions in which subjective and objective loss of intellectual abilities has occured which is not severe enough to fulfil the criteria of dementia, may precede, accompany, or follow a wide variety of infectious and physical disorders. Diagnostic criteria: 1. presence of a physical disorder, 2. the report of cognitive disorder by the patient or a reliable informant, 3. an abnormality or decline in performance in quantified cognitive assessment, nor specifically intended for use in the elderly, 4. exclusion of dementia, organic amnesic syndrome, delirium and other brain organic syndromes associated with cognitive decline
"mild cognitive impairment" Zaudig (1991, 1992)	impaired cognitive functioning, based on the performance in the neuropsychological test battery of the SIDAM, exclusion of dementia, no other specific aetiological concept, SIDAM-Score (SISCO) 34–49

However, no general concept of MCI has been determined so far. Certainly, cognitive impairment in the elderly is an aetiologically heterogeneous condition. Additionally, a variety of factors which may contribute to the diagnosis of MCI have to be borne in mind: 1. In the elderly, physical illness is frequent. Multimorbidity can be associated with -often temporary-cognitive decline (Clarfield, 1988). 2. Psychiatric conditions, in particular depressive syndromes, are commonly accompanied by considerable cognitive dysfunction and may mistakenly be diagnosed as dementia ("Pseudodementia", Reifler et al., 1982). 3. Poor education, low intelligence, and very old age influence test performance and may lead to a falsely positive diagnosis of MCI (Bleecker et al., 1988).

Diagnostic approaches

In clinical psychiatry, a diagnosis is usually made on the basis of defined criteria (categorial approach). Henderson (1986) emphasised the priority of categorial approaches to the diagnosis of a disease, since the severity of a condition can only be measured after it has been defined. However, with regard to MCI no feasible categorial definition is available to date. Furthermore, most of the aforementioned concepts are insufficiently operationalised to be suitable for scientific use. Thus, at this stage of our knowledge it seems more useful to follow Gurland et al. (1983) who pointed out that it is methodically imprecise to solely base the diagnosis of MCI on a definition. These authors suggested that quantitative scales should be preferred (dimensional approach), since cognitive impairment is characterised by a continuous decline from normal cognitive functioning to dementia. Based on these considerations, we have used the Structured Interview for the Diagnosis of Dementia of Alzheimer Type, Multi-Infarct Dementia and Dementias of other aetiologies according to ICD-10 and DSM-III-R (SIDAM, Zaudig et al., 1991, 1992), and applied cut-off points on the SIDAM-Score (SISCO) for a dimensional approach to the diagnosis of MCI.

Prognosis

From a clinical point of view, the prognosis of MCI is the most puzzling question: the condition can either remain stable or progress to dementia. In particular, the progression to dementia has most important implications for the patient and his or her relatives. Few longitudinal studies have been carried out to assess the outcome of MCI. Cooper et al. (1996) could demonstrate from a general-praxis based sample that about one fifth of the patients with mild cognitive deficits at initial observation had developed dementia after a mean interval of 27 months. All incident cases of clinical dementia in this study had arisen from the group with initial mild cognitive impairment. Table 2 gives an overview of progression rates of MCI reported in previous studies.

Predicting the prognosis

In recent years, much emphasis has been placed on the search for reliable predictors of progressive cognitive decline in patients with MCI. The identification of neuropsychological signs, structural changes and biological markers which may reliably predict the prognosis of cognitive impairment is crucial for an early diagnosis of Alzheimer's disease and other dementing conditions. Different approaches have been undertaken to predict the outcome of MCI, such as neuropsychological assessment (Tierney, 1996a; Petersen et al., 1994, 1995; Masur, 1994; Linn et al., 1995; Flicker et al., 1991; Tröster et al., 1994), neuroimaging modalities, in particular CT, MRI (De Leon et al., 1993; Smith and Jobst, 1996) and functional neuroimaging (Small et al., 1995; Haxby et al.,

Table 2. Progression rates to dementia in non-demented memory-impaired patients reported in a number of previous studies

Authors	Inclusion criteria	Number of patients	Follow up at	% of patients who progressed to dementia
Kral et al. (1978)	benign senescent forgetfulness	n = 20	4 years	5
Rubin et al. (1989)	"questionable dementia" CDR 0.5	n = 16	up to 7 years	69
Devanand (1997)	"questionable dementia" CDR 0.5	n = 75	mean 2.5 years	41
Bowen et al. (1997)	individuals with isolated memory loss vs. group of memory complainers	n = 21	2.3 years	48 vs. 18
Cooper et al. (1996)	minimal dementia and mild dementia	n = 106	27 months	20
O'Connor et al. (1991)	"minimal dementia" according to CAMDEX	n = 29	1 year 2 years	21 50
Tierney et al. (1996a,c)	memory-impaired, non-demented	n = 123	2 years	24
Petersen et al. (1995)	MCI, more than 1.5 SD below age-appropriate norms on memory tests, CDR 0.5	n = 66	1.5 years 3 years 4.5 years	24 44 55
Tröster et al. (1996)	non-demented cognitively normal subjects with memory complaint	n = 35	4 to 6 years	13
Linn et al. (1995)	free of dementia	n = 1045	7 to 13 years	3.8
Masur et al. (1995)	non-demented	n = 317	at least 4 years	20

1987), and ApoE genotyping (Tierney et al., 1996b; Petersen et al., 1996; Small et al., 1996; Nalbantoglu et al., 1994). For all of these methods, some value could be demonstrated in the prediction of further decline to dementia in MCI patients.

In our present study, we have examined a sample of patients with MCI attending a memory clinic. In order to determine whether subtypes of intellectual functioning are suitable to predict the clinical outcome of cognitive impairment, we applied the test battery of the SIDAM (Zaudig et al., 1991). We hypothesized that patients who later develop dementia are already compromised in memory function at initial observation. In addition, cranial computed tomography (CT), cranial single photon emission computed tomography (SPECT), and apolipoprotein E (ApoE) genotyping were used to address the issue of possible predictors.

Method

Subjects

Initially (baseline = t_0), 117 subjects who consecutively attended the memory clinic of the Department of Psychiatry of the University of Leipzig were examined. After an average of 2,7 years, 80 cases could be re-examined (mean age at baseline 66,5 years, range 51–84). The SIDAM interview was used for the quantitative assessment of cognitive functioning. Regardless of aetiological considerations, subjects were defined as demented (De) when their SIDAM scores were 32 and below, and as mildly cognitively impaired (MCI) when their SIDAM scores ranged between 33 and 51. At baseline (T_0), 41 out the 80 patients who could be re-examined fulfilled our criteria for MCI, 8 were demented, and 32 patients showed no cognitive impairment. All patients underwent CT and SPECT. The apolipoprotein E (ApoE) status was analysed in a large subset of patients.

Instruments

The Structured Interview for the Diagnosis of Dementia of Alzheimer Type, Multi-Infarct Dementia and Dementias of other aetiologies according to ICD-10 and DSM-III-R (SIDAM). The SIDAM (Zaudig et al., 1991; Zaudig, 1992) is a short diagnostic screening instrument which has been deliberately constructed to service each element of the DSM-III-R and ICD-10 criteria for dementia. The SIDAM contains a short test battery which includes all MMSE items (Folstein et al., 1975), as well as the items of the Expanded Mini-Mental State (Farmer and Helzer, 1986). The 55 questions can be summed up, resulting in the SIDAM score (SISCO), which ranges from 0 (the worst cognitive impairment) to 55 (no cognitive impairment). The SISCO covers a broader range of cognitive functions than the MMSE does and detects mild degrees of cognitive decline as well. It can be divided into 10 subscores which describe subtypes of intellectual functioning. In addition to the test performance, a SIDAM-ADL scale, the Hachinski Score (Hachinski et al., 1975) and the Modified Ischaemic Score (Rosen et al., 1980) are imbedded into the diagnostic algorithm. The SIDAM has been primarily designed to differentiate between the presence and absence of dementia. However, with respect to the group with mild cognitive impairment, standard criteria and case finding methods could be devised according to DSM-III-R (American Psychiatric Association, 1987) and ICD-10 (World Health Organisation, 1991). The use of cut-off points on the SISCO for the diagnosis of mild cognitive impairment, no cognitive impairment and dementia could be successfully validated by means of GDS and CDR (Zaudig, 1992).

SPECT. Photons were registered using a dual detector scintillation camera (ADAC Laboratories, Vertex) equipped with a high resolution low-energy parallel hole collimator. A symmetric 20% energy window at 140 KeV was used. In addition to numerical quantitation of activity distribution, tomograms were visually classified using the following scoring system: 0 = homogeneous distribution, 1 = inhomogeneities, not definitely abnormal, 2 = definitely abnormal (activity deficits), 3 = severe defects.

CT. The whole intracranial space was assessed by basis-parallel 5 mm slices, 500 mAs with Somatom-Plus or Somatom-Plus-S. The following indices were assessed using linear measurements: cisterna insularis (left/right), cella media index, Evan's ratio, frontal horn index (max skull diameter at frontal horn level: max frontal horn distance), Huckman index, medial temporal lobe (interuncle/left/right), posterior horn index.

ApoE Genotypes. In a subsample of 66% of our patients, the ApoE genotype was assessed. From whole blood, 227 bp region of DNA that spans ApoE polymorphic signs was amplified using the polymerase chain reaction (PCR). The PCR product was digested with Cfol, and the products of the restriction digestion were separated on a polyacryla-mide gel as described by Wenham et al. (1991).

Results

At follow-up, 8 out of 41 patients (19,5%) with MCI had progressed to dementia (referred to as MCI-De), 8 patients (19,5%) had improved to normal levels of cognitive functioning (MCI-NCI, NCI = No Cognitive Impairment), 25 patients (61%) had remained stable within the MCI group (MCI-MCI). Using the diagnostic algorithm which is part of the SIDAM, all patients who had progressed to dementia at follow-up received the clinical diagnosis of Alzheimer's disease according to ICD-10 criteria. Three of them were male and five female.

Due to the small number of patients, parametric rank tests could not be used for statistical analysis. Therefore, we applied the non-parametric rank test by Mann and Whitney (U-test) for the descriptive analysis of our data.

Table 3 shows the characteristics of the stable group (MCI-MCI) and the decliners (MCI-De). Patients in the MCI-De group were significantly older than those who remained cognitively stable (74.5 vs. 65.0 years, $p = 0.003$). Furthermore, the two prognostic groups differed significantly in their baseline MMSE and SIDAM scores ($p = 0.017$, $p = 0.009$).

Neuropsychological parameters (SIDAM-Subscores)

At baseline (T_0), significant group differences were present on the SIDAM subscales "memory" ($p = 0.0078$) and "orientation" ($p = 0.0002$). Of the SIDAM subscales which assess memory function, significant group differences could be found on the scale "long term memory" ($p = 0.003$) and "short term memory" ($p = 0.027$) (Table 4).

CT and SPECT findings

Tables 5 and 6 show the results of the descriptive analyses comparing the two prognostic groups retrospectively. At T_0, significant group differences could be observed in one CT parameter: The group of patients who eventually progressed to dementia showed significantly lower scores on the index "left medial temporal lobe" (i.e., higher degrees of temporal lobe atrophy) than the

38   H. Wolf et al.

Table 3. Baseline characteristics of the two prognostic groups of MCI, *sd* standard deviation

Prognostic group	MCI-MCI n = 25			MCI-De n = 8			Mann-Whitney 2-tailed p-value
	mean	range	sd	mean	range	sd	
Age (to)	65.0	51–81	7.50	74.5	67–84	5.60	0.0032
SISCO (to)	46.2	35–51	4.86	40.2	33–47	5.01	0.0093
MMSE-Score (to)	26.4	20–30	2.83	23.6	19–27	2.67	0.0174
Years of school education	9.5	8–12	1.66	10.5	8–12	1.77	0.1642

Table 4. Baseline differences in SIDAM-subscores in the two prognostic groups, m% = mean percentage of maximum score

SISCO Subscore (to)	max. Score = 100%	MCI-MCI m%	MCI-De m%	Δ Diff. %	p-value (2-tailed) Mann-Whitney
Higher cortical functions	20	82.20	81.87	0.33	0.7823
Aphasia/Apraxia	10	94.00	92.50	1.50	0.6754
Verbal abilities/calculation	7	70.85	71.42	−0.57	0.6201
Constructional abilities	3	69.33	70.83	−1.50	0.7512
Intellectual abilities	5	87.20	80.00	7.20	0.3982
Memory	20	79.20	60.62	18.58	0.0078
Long-term memory	7	89.14	64.28	24.86	0.0031
Immediate recall	5	84.00	95.00	−11.00	0.0530
Short-term memory	8	67.50	35.93	31.57	0.0278
Orientation	10	95.20	77.50	17.70	0.0002

cognitively stable group (p = 0.011). The same trend was observed for the right medial temporal lobe (p = 0.077). No significant group differences on the assessed SPECT parameters were present at T_0.

ApoE genotype

One ApoE 4 allele was carried by 2 out of 6 patients (33%) of the MCI-De group and 5 out of 17 patients (29%) of the stable group. There were no patients homozygotic for ApoE 4 in our population. We do not know the ApoE genotype in about one third of patients in either group (Table 7).

At T_0, the two groups of patients overlap too much to permit a reliable prediction of the prognosis by use of cut-off points on SIDAM subscores or CT measures at baseline. In Figure 1, the baseline overlap of the two prognostic groups and interindividual differences in the course of MCI are demon-

Table 5. SPECT — mean rating scores in the two prognostic groups at baseline examination, *sd* standard deviation

SPECT (to)	MCI-MCI mean rating score	sd	MCI-De mean rating score	sd	p-value (2-tailed) Mann-Whitney
Frontal left	0.39	0.58	0.71	0.56	0.1434
Frontal right	0.37	0.49	0.21	0.39	0.4635
Temporo-parietal left	1.02	0.85	1.57	0.97	0.1471
Temporo-parietal right	0.60	0.67	1.14	0.85	0.1131

Table 6. Baseline differences between the two prognostic groups in CT parameters, *sd* standard deviation

CT scan (to)	MCI-MCI mean (mm)	sd	MCI-De mean (mm)	sd	p-value (2-tailed) Mann-Whitney
Cisterna insularis (left)	4.95	2.18	6.49	2.67	0.1262
Cisterna insularis (right)	4.80	2.06	5.57	2.86	0.4738
Cella media index	3.45	0.044	3.29	0.32	0.2730
Evan's ratio	0.25	0.03	0.26	0.03	0.6463
Frontal index	3.19	0.49	3.01	0.40	0.3455
Huckman	56.74	8.79	61.66	8.64	0.1775
Medial temporal lobe (interuncle)	27.08	3.35	28.84	3.80	0.3148
Medial temporal lobe (left)	10.74	3.38	6.81	3.01	0.0116
Medial temporal lobe (right)	10.53	3.00	7.80	3.70	0.0775
Posterior horn index	1.91	0.16	1.83	0.17	0.1323

Table 7. Apolipoprotein E genotype in the two prognostic groups

ApoE	MCI-MCI number of cases	MCI-De number of cases
e3e3	9	3
e3e4	4	2
e2e3	2	1
e2e4	1	—
Mutation	1	—

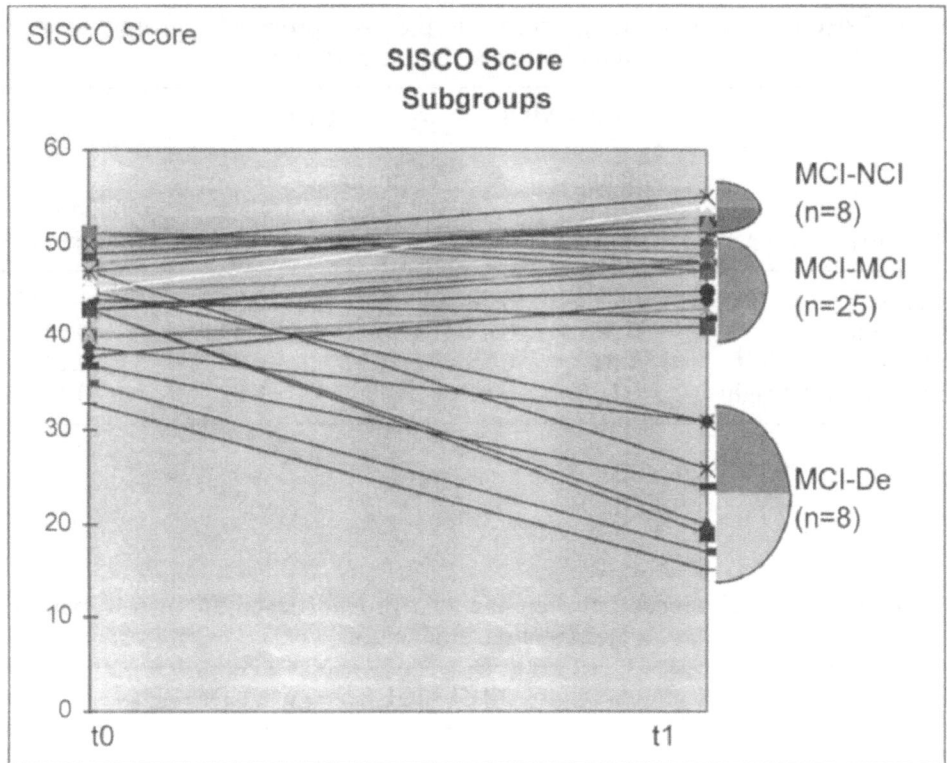

Fig. 1. SIDAM Scores (SISCO) of all individuals. Changes between baseline (t0) and follow-up examination (t1) and formation of subgroups

strated by means of the SISCO scores obtained by each individual at baseline and follow-up examination.

Rate of progression

The crossover group (MCI-De) declined on the SISCO within the observation period by a mean score of 17.4 SISCO points, whereas the stable group showed a slight overall improvement on the SISCO by 1.4 points over a mean interval of 2.7 years. Figures 2 and 3 show the change in test performance on the SIDAM subscales between T_0 and T_1 for both groups.

Fig. 2 and **3.** Cognitive change in individuals with constant mild cognitive impairment (MCI-MCI) and the individuals who progressed to dementia (MCI-De). Development of subtypes of intellectual functioning (SIDAM subscores, percentage of maximum score on each subscale) between baseline (t_0) and follow up examination (t_1). Lines characterise mean change over time for each SIDAM subscale, each symbol represents one individual patient

SISCO Subscore

MCI-MCI

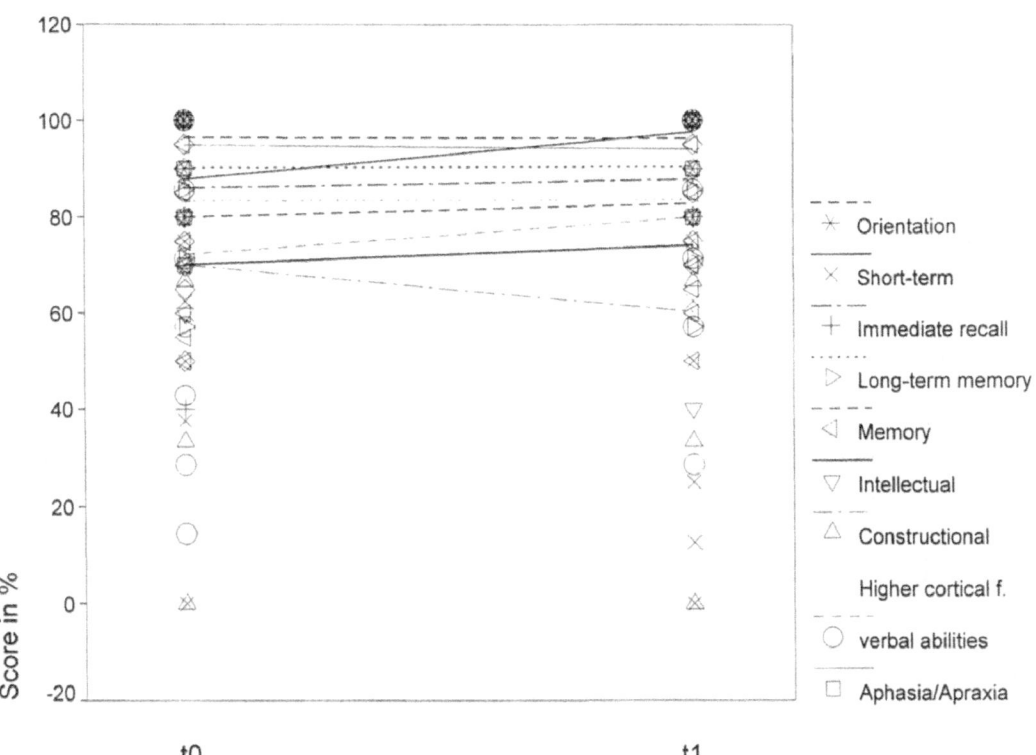

Legend:
- ✳ Orientation
- ✕ Short-term
- ✛ Immediate recall
- ▷ Long-term memory
- ◁ Memory
- ▽ Intellectual
- △ Constructional
- Higher cortical f.
- ○ verbal abilities
- ☐ Aphasia/Apraxia

SISCO Subscore

MCI-De

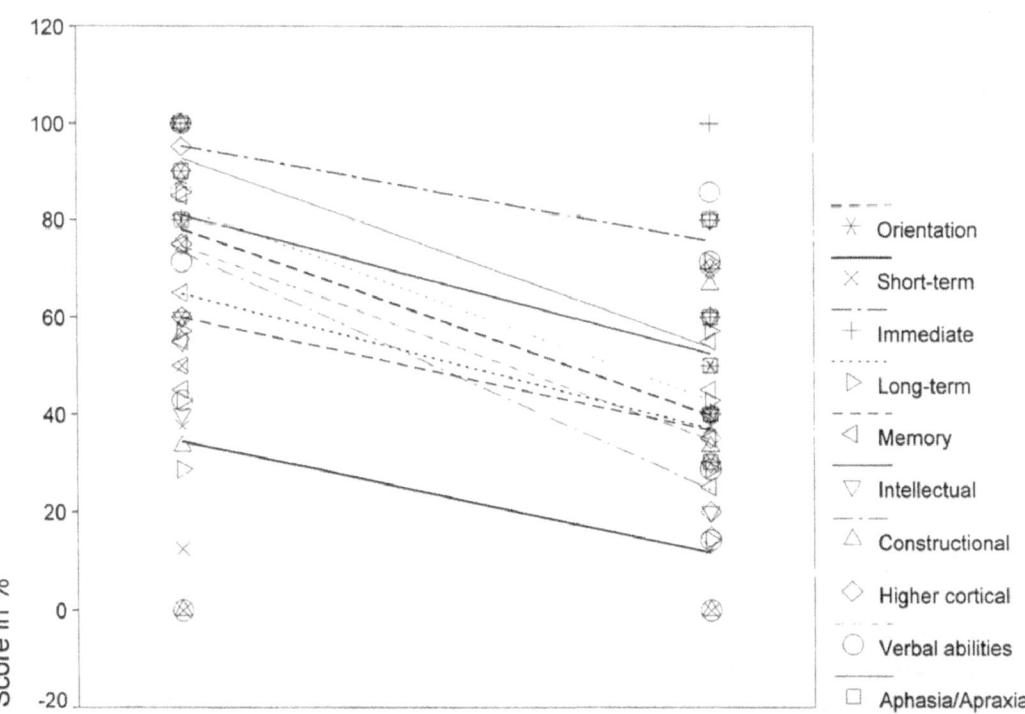

Legend:
- ✳ Orientation
- ✕ Short-term
- ✛ Immediate
- ▷ Long-term
- ◁ Memory
- ▽ Intellectual
- △ Constructional
- ◇ Higher cortical
- ○ Verbal abilities
- ☐ Aphasia/Apraxia

Discussion

Prognosis

In our study, the majority of patients with MCI remained stable within a mean interval of 2.7 years. Of the rest of our patients, one fifth progressed to dementia, and one fifth improved to normal cognitive function. The progression rate to dementia in our study compares to the findings described by Cooper et al. (1996) who used similar criteria. Furthermore, our results suggest that improvement to normal levels of cognitive functioning in the group of cognitively impaired patients may occur as frequently as further decline to dementia. Dawe et al. (1992) estimated that the annual incidence rate of dementia in the MCI population ranges from 1 to 25%. The considerable variation in prognostic outcome of MCI in previous studies may be due to different concepts used for the definition of MCI. A recent study by Devanand et al. (1997), which evaluated the clinical course and outcome of patients with questionable dementia (QD, CDR 0.5) revealed great heterogeneity in prognostic outcome with most patients in the "dementia" and "no dementia" categories at follow up (mean interval 2.5 years). The authors suggest that this heterogeneity may even enhance the feasibility of further development of potential predictors of outcome in cognitively impaired patients.

In our unselected population of memory clinic attenders, all patients who eventually became demented happened to have Alzheimer's disease according to the clinical criteria of ICD 10. Generally, it may be presumed that it is more difficult to predict further decline to dementia in pathogenetically heterogeneous populations. However, some possible predictors of AD have been shown to be associated with other causes of dementia as well (Horn et al., 1996; Gustafson et al., 1997; St. Clair et al., 1994; Helsiami et al., 1996; Almkvist et al., 1993, 1994).

Age

As in other studies (Devanand et al., 1997; Cooper et al., 1996; Linn et al., 1995; Petersen et al., 1995) patients who progressed to dementia (MCI-De) were significantly older than subjects with constant mild impairment (MCI-MCI). Although one is tempted to correct age differences by statistical means, this finding is of practical relevance. Clearly, age is a major risk factor for AD (Rubin et al., 1993). Since some of the parameters characteristic for the early stages of AD (such as temporal lobe atrophy and decline in memory function) also occur with normal ageing, it is more difficult to make an early diagnosis of AD in persons of more advanced age. Furthermore, the progression rates to dementia in different populations can be expected to be a function of age, a fact which might also explain the variance in prognostic outcome observed in previous studies.

Cognitive functions — memory and orientation

Our results support the contention that memory measures are the cognitive measures most sensitive to progressive cognitive decline (Terry and Katzmann, 1983; Christensen et al., 1991; Welsh et al., 1992; Petersen et al., 1994, 1995; Devanand et al., 1997; Bowen et al., 1997).

The observed overlap of decliners and nondecliners at baseline in all areas of cognitive functioning implies that a reliable prediction of the prognosis of MCI on an individual basis is not possible. Repeated testing in relatively short intervals might be useful, in particular since the MCI-MCI group showed a slight overall improvement, whereas the MCI-De group declined significantly on all subscores of the SIDAM. Similar effects (an actual improvement of test performance in "nondecliners" at repeated testing) have been observed by other investigators (Small et al., 1995; Mitrushina and Satz, 1991). It has been suggested that intervals of three or more years may be needed to avoid practice effects in elderly subjects with age associated memory impairment (Youngjohn and Crook, 1993). However, the presence of learning effects (or even the absence of improvement) at repeated tests might be used to predict a benign outcome. Since differing premorbid levels of intelligence may significantly contribute to the observed overlap, information about individual's premorbid functioning or informant's perception of change could essentially improve the predictive accuracy of psychometric tests (Tierney et al., 1996c).

It should be borne in mind that changes in other areas than memory and even noncognitive symptoms may precede memory problems in early AD and other dementing disorders. Richards et al. (1993) demonstrated that mild extrapyramidal abnormalities, such as changes in posture, hypomimia, monotonous speech, tremor, muscular hypertension and bradykinesia may predict the development of dementia in elderly inidviduals. Oppenheim (1994) found that noncognitive changes of the psychiatric, neurological and noncoping type make up the earliest signs of the disease in 53% of AD patients. His findings, which suggest that the earliest clinical manifestations of Alzheimer's disease may, in many cases, significantly predate objective signs of memory impairment, should be borne in mind but require replication in longitudinal settings.

The observed memory deficits can be linked with higher degrees of temporal lobe atrophy. Neuropsychological experiments in human diseases (Zola-Morgan et al., 1986) suggest that the integrity of ventromedial temporal lobe structures is essential for normal memory. Braak and Braak (1991) could demonstrate that the pattern of Alzheimer-related changes disrupts projections among the entorhinal cortex, hippocampal formation, and amygdala at multiple sites, and also disrupts projections between these structures and cortical and subcortical targets. The progressive accumulation of structural alterations in the ventromedial temporal lobe, and in neocortical areas closely related to it, likely contributes to the worsening of memory impairment. The degree of temporal lobe atrophy has been considered to have potential as a screening tool in the population. It has been proposed that measurement of the rate of atrophy in asymptomatic or MCI cases may be a predictor of AD

and could be used to monitor the effectiveness of therapies designed to retard
the rate of degeneration (Smith and Jobst, 1996). Small et al. (1995) who
prospectively assessed a population with age associated memory impairment
found no significant group differences between decliners and nondecliners

Table 8. Recent studies assessing possible predictors of future cognitive decline in non-demented subjects
and association of increased age and final diagnosis of dementia/progressive decline

	Number of patients	Mean age	Prediction of	Predictors	Decline associated with increased age
Devanand et al. (1997) CDR 0.5	75	aged over 40	dementia (DSM-III-R)	MMSE: delayed recall plus neuropsychological tests	yes
Flicker et al. (1991) GDS 3	32	71.3	increase in GDS rating	verbal recall, visuospatial recall, language	no
Tierney et al. (1996a,c) cognitively impaired, not demented	123	73.9/ 71.5	AD NINCDS-ADRDA	delayed recall, attention, informant's perception	no
Petersen et al. (1995) CDR 0.5	66	79.8	dementia (DSM-III-R) AD (NINCDS-ADRDA)	ApoE status	yes
Small et al. (1995) patients with memory complaints	42	60	1. decline in visual-spatial memory 2. decline in verbal memory	1. parietal asymmetry on PET, baseline visual-spatial memory, female gender 2. education, basal verbal memory	no
Linn et al. (1995) free of dementia	1045	65–88	probable AD	verbal memory, immediate auditory attention span	yes
Masur et al. (1995)	317	75 to 85	dementia (DSM-III)	delayed recall, verbal fluency	no
Förstl et al. (1995) modified AAMI	32	67.0	progressive cognitive decline	degree of brain atrophy (enlarged lateral ventricles)	not reported

with regard to measures of brain atrophy. Interestingly, parietal asymmetry on PET -one of the earliest metabolic changes observed in patients with AD-turned out to be predictive of future decline in visual-spatial memory in this relatively mildly impaired population. In our present study, SPECT findings did not seem to be useful in predicting further cognitive decline in MCI. This is in acccordance with previous studies which demonstrated the absence of characteristic flow deficits in the early stages of degenerative diseases (Reed et al., 1989). It has been argued that the lack of early signs in the parieto-temporal regions might reflect the presence of compensatory mechanisms for ongoing neuronal or microvascular disintegration (Knapp et al., 1996).

Of course, the observed higher degrees of medial temporal lobe atrophy in the MCI-De group might be enhanced by the fact that individuals in this group were significantly older. However, there is evidence from a recent study that medial temporal lobe atrophy in normal elderly individuals occurs indepently of age (Launer et al., 1995). In other studies, the frequency of atrophy of hippocampal structures was found to be strongly related to age in normal elderly subjects but not in subjects with MCI or AD (Meyer et al., 1997; de Leon et al., 1997).

Furthermore, one might question the diagnostic value of relatively simple linear measures. Previous studies using MRI demonstrated the value of linear measures of atrophy in the temporal lobe structures in the diagnosis of AD (Erkinjuntti et al., 1993; Frisoni et al., 1996). Linear measures differed significantly between patients with early AD and normal controls but with considerable overlap.

It has to be borne in mind that the aforementioned findings are not specific and even though their predictive value can be demonstrated in statistical group comparisons, they can not reliably predict subsequent development of dementia in any individual patient. Neuropathological findings as well as other neuroimaging studies suggest that differences between normal ageing and early dementia are more quantitative than qualitative in nature. Radiological measures of temporal lobe and hippocampal atrophy which have been found sensitive in identifying early AD (de Leon et al., 1993), could also be shown to occur in nondemented elderly individuals (Launer et al., 1995; Meyer et al., 1997). Neuropathologically, the same hierarchical deposition of neurofibrillary tangles which has been described in Alzheimer's disease seems to occur in normal ageing but in a less pronounced fashion (Braak and Braak, 1991; Gertz et al., 1996, 1997).

ApoE

In our study, the two prognostic groups appear to have a similar frequency of carrier status of the ApoE4 allele. The observed frequencies of the ApoE4 allele in both prognostic groups are above the reported rates for normal controls in several studies (Strittmatter et al., 1993; Poirier et al., 1993; Kurz et al., 1995; Petersen et al., 1995; Blesa et al., 1996; Tsai et al., 1993). Reported ApoE4 frequencies in MCI populations vary between 27% and 58%

(Petersen et al., 1995; Förstl et al., 1995). Few longitudinal studies on memory-impaired patients have included the ApoE carrier status in their predictor analysis (Petersen et al., 1996; Tierney et al., 1996a). Our finding that the ApoE4 allele frequency is not different in the two prognostic groups is in contrast with results obtained by other investigators (Petersen et al., 1995). Furthermore, our results do not support the thesis that ApoE is a very strong predictor of cognitive change within a 2 to 3 observation period. Possible reasons for these contradictory findings might be sought in selection bias effects (Kurz et al., 1995; Poirier et al., 1993), and regional and ethnic variability of ApoE4 frequency (Hallmann et al., 1991). To draw a definite conclusion, more cases and post mortem confirmation of AD diagnosis are required. In any case, our findings support the position that although ApoE genotyping may be useful in evaluating the differential diagnosis of AD, it should not be used to predict the development of AD (Tierney et al., 1996b).

References

Almkvist O (1994) Neuropsychological deficits in vascular dementia in relation to Alzheimer's disease: reviewing evidence for functional similarity or divergence. Dementia 5(3–4): 203–209

Almkvist O, Backman L, Basun H, Wahlund LO (1993) Patterns of neuropsychological performance in Alzheimer's disease and vascular dementia. Cortex 29(4): 661–673

American Psychiatric Association (1987) Diagnostic and statistical manual of mental disorders, 3rd ed rev. American Psychiatric Association, Washington DC

Bleecker ML, Bolla-Wilson K, Kawas C, Agnew J (1988) Age-specific norms for the Mini-Mental State Exam. Neurology 38(10): 1565–1568

Blesa R, Adroer R, Santacruz P, Ascaso C, Tolosa E, Oliva R (1996) High apolipoprotein E epsilon 4 allele frequency in age-related memory decline. Ann Neurol 39(4): 548–551

Bowen J, Teri L, Kukull W, McCormick W, McCurry SM, Larson EB (1997) Progression to dementia in patients with isolated memory loss. Lancet 15;349(9054): 763–765

Braak H, Braak E (1991) Neuropathological stageing of Alzheimer-related changes. Acta Neuropathol (Berl) 82(4): 239–259

Christensen H, Birrell P (1991) Explicit and implicit memory in dementia and normal ageing. Psychol Res 53(2): 149–161

Clarfield AM (1988) The reversible dementias: do they reverse? Ann Intern Med 15;109(6): 476–486

Cooper B, Bickel H, Schäufele M (1996) Early development and progression of dementing illnesss in the elderly: a general praxis based study. Psychol Med 26: 411–419

Crook T, Larrabee GJ (1988) Age-associated memory impairment: diagnostic criteria and treatment strategies. Psychopharmacol Bull 24(4): 509–514

Dawe B, Procter A, Philpot M (1992) Concepts of mild memory impairment in the elderly and their relationship to dementia: a review. Int J Geriatr Psychiatry 443–449

de Leon MJ, Golomb J, George AE, Convit A, Tarshish CY, McRae T, De Santi S, Smith G, Ferris SH, Noz M, et al (1993) The radiologic prediction of Alzheimer disease: the atrophic hippocampal formation. AJNR Am J Neuroradiol 14(4): 897–906

de Leon MJ, George AE, Golomb J, Tarshish C, Convit A, Kluger A, de Santi S, McRae T, Ferris SH, Reisberg B, Ince C, Rusinek H, Bobinski M, Quinn B, Miller DC,

Wisniewski HM (1997) Frequency of hippocampal formation atrophy in normal aging and Alzheimer's disease. Neurobiol Aging 18: 1–11

Devanand DP, Folz M, Gorlyn M, Moeller JR, Stern Y (1997) Questionable dementia: clinical course and predictors of outcome. J Am Geriatr Soc 45(3): 321–328

Erkinjuntti T, Lee DH, Gao F, Steenhuis R, Eliasziw M, Fry R, Merskey H, Hachinski VC (1993) Temporal lobe atrophy on magnetic resonance imaging in the diagnosis of early Alzheimer's disease. Arch Neurol 50(3): 305–310

Flicker C, Ferris SH, Reisberg B (1991) Mild cognitive impairment in the elderly: predictors of dementia. Neurology 41: 1006–1009

Folstein MF, Folstein SE, McHugh PR (1975) "Mini-mental state". A practical method for grading the cognitive state of patients for the clinician. J Psychiatr Res 12/3: 189–198

Forstl H, Hentschel F, Sattel H, Geiger-Kabisch C, Besthorn C, Czech C, Monning U, Beyreuther K (1995) Age-associated memory impairment and early Alzheimer's disease. Only time will tell the difference. Arzneimittelforschung 45(3A): 394–397

Frisoni GB, Beltramello A, Weiss C, Geroldi C, Bianchetti A, Trabucchi M (1996) Linear measures of atrophy in mild Alzheimer disease. AJNR Am J Neuroradiol 17(5): 913–923

Gertz HJ, Xuereb JH, Huppert FA, Brayne C, Kruger H, McGee MA, Paykel ES, Harrington CR, Mukaetova-Ladinska EB, O'Connor DW, Wischik CM (1996) The relationship between clinical dementia and neuropathological staging (Braak) in a very elderly community sample. Eur Arch Psychiatry Clin Neurosci 246(3): 132–136

Gertz HJ, Xuereb J, Huppert F, Brayne C, McGee MA, Paykel E, Harrington C, Mukaetova-Ladinska E, Arendt T, Wischik CM (1998) Examination of the validity of the hierarchical model of neuropathological staging in normal aging and Alzheimer's disease. Acta Neuropathol 95: 154–156

Gurland BJ, Dean L, Copeland J, Gurland B, Golden R (1982) Criteria for diagnosis of dementia in the communitiy elderly. Gerontologist 22: 180–186

Gurland BJ, Copeland JRM, Kuriansky J, Kelleher M, Sharpe L, Dean LL (1983) The mind and mood of ageing: mental health problems in the communitiy elderely in New York and London. Haworth Press, New York

Gustafson L, Abrahamson M, Grubb A, Nilsson K, Fex G (1997) The impact of apolipoprotein E4 on cause of death in Alzheimer's disease. Neurology 49(1): 76–81

Hachinski VC, Iliff LD, Zilkha E, Boulay GA du, McAllister VL, Marshall J, Roth M, Russell RW Symon L (1975) Cerebral blood flow in dementia. Arch Neurol 32: 632–637

Hallman DM, Boerwinckle E, Saha N, et al (1991) Apolipoprotein E polymorphism: a comparison of allele frequencies and effects in nine populations. Am J Hum Genet 49: 338–349

Haxby JV, Grady CL, Friedland RP, Rapoport SI (1987) Neocortical metabolic abnormalities precede nonmemory cognitive impairments in early dementia of the Alzheimer type: longitudinal confirmation. J Neural Transm [Suppl] 24: 49–53

Helisalmi S, Linnaranta K, Lehtovirta M, Mannermaa A, Heinonen O, Ryynanen M, Riekkinen P Sr, Soininen H (1996) Apolipoprotein E polymorphism in patients with different neurodegenerative disorders. Neurosci Lett 16;205(1): 61–64

Henderson AS (1986) Epidemiology in mental illness. In: Häfner H, Moschell G, Sartorius N (eds) Mental health in the elderly. Springer, Berlin Heidelberg New York Tokyo, pp 29–34

Henderson AS, Huppert FA (1984) The problem of mild dementia. Psychol Med 14: 5–11

Horn R, Ostertun B, Fric M, Solymosi L, Steudel A, Moller HJ (1996) Atrophy of hippocampus in patients with Alzheimer's disease and other diseases with memory impairment. Dementia 7(4): 182–186

Hughes CP, Berg L, Danziger WL, Coben LA, Martin RL (1982) A new clinical scale for the staging of dementia. Br J Psychiatry 140: 566–572

Knapp WH, Dannenberg C, Marschall B, Zedlick D, Löschmann K, Bettin S, Barthel H, Seese A (1996) Changes in local cerebral blood flow by neuroactivation and vasoactivation in patients with impaired cognitive function. Eur J Nucl Med 23: 878–888

Kral VA (1962) Senescent forgetfulness: benign and malignant. Can Med Assoc J 86: 257–260

Kral VA (1978) Benign senile forgetfulness. In: Katzman R, Terry RD, Bick KL (eds) Alzheimer's disease: senile dementia and related disorders, vol 7. Ageing. Raven, New York, pp 47–51

Kurz A, Egensperger R, Lautenschlager N, Haupt M, Altland K, Graeber MB, Muller U (1995) The apolipoprotein E gene and Alzheimer disease phenotype. Z Gerontol Geriatr 28(3): 195–199

Launer LJ, Scheltens P, Lindeboom J, Barkhof F, Weinstein HC, Jonker C (1995) Medial temporal lobe atrophy in an open population of very old persons: cognitive, brain atrophy, and sociomedical correlates. Neurology 45(4): 747–752

Linn RT, Wolf PA, Bachman DL, Knoefel JE, Cobb JL, Belanger AJ, Kaplan EF, D'Agostino RB (1995) The "preclinical phase" of probable Alzheimer's disease. A 13-year prospective study of the Framingham cohort. Arch Neurol 52(5): 485–490

Masur DM, Sliwinski M, Lipton RB, Blau AD, Crystal HA (1994) Neuropsychological prediction of dementia and the absence of dementia in healthy elderly persons. Neurology 44: 1427–1432

Mattis S (1988) Dementia rating scale. Anonymous Psychological Assessment Resources, Odessa, FL

Meyer JS, Shirai T, Akiyama H (1997) Frequency of hippocampal formation atrophy in normal aging and Alzheimer's disease. Neurobiol Aging 18: 1–11

Mitrushina M, Satz P (1991) Effect of repeated administration of a neuropsychological battery in the elderly. J Clin Psychol 47(6): 790–801

Nalbantoglu J, Gilfix BM, Bertrand P, Robitaille Y, Gauthier S, Rosenblatt DS, Poirier J (1994) Predictive value of apolipoprotein E genotyping in Alzheimer's disease: results of an autopsy series and an analysis of several combined studies. Ann Neurol 36(6): 889–895

O'Connor DW, Pollitt PA, Hyde JB, Fellows JL, Miller ND, Roth M (1990) A follow-up study of dementia diagnosed in the community using the Cambridge Mental Disorders of the Elderly Examination. Acta Psychiatr Scand 81(1): 78–82

O'Connor DW, Pollitt PA, Jones BJ, Hyde JB, Fellowes JL, Miller ND (1991) Continued clinical validation of dementia diagnosed in the community using the Cambridge Mental Disorders of the Elderly Examination. Acta Psychiatr Scand 83(1): 41–45

Oppenheim G (1994) The earliest signs of Alzheimer's disease. J Geriatr Psychiatry Neurol 7: 116–120

Petersen RC (1995a) Normal aging, mild cognitive impairment, and early Alzheimer's disease. The Neurologist 1: 326–344

Petersen RC, Smith GE, Ivnik RJ, Kokmen E, Tangalos EG (1994) Memory function in very early Alzheimer's disease. Neurology 44: 867–872

Petersen RC, Smith GE, Ivnik RJ, Tangalos EG, Schaid DJ, Thibodeau SN, Kokmen E, Waring SC, Kurland LT (1995b) Apolipoprotein E status as a predictor of the development of Alzheimer's disease in memory-impaired individuals. JAMA 273: 1274–1278

Petersen RC, Waring SC, Smith GE, Tangalos EG, Thibodeau SN (1996) Predictive value of ApoE genotyping in incipient Alzheimer's disease. Ann NY Acad Sci 802: 58–69

Poirier J, Davignon J, Bouthillier D, Kogan S, Bertrand P, Gauthier S (1993a) Apolipoprotein E polymorphism and Alzheimer's disease. Lancet 342: 697–699

Reed BR, Jagust WJ, Scab JP, Ober BA (1989) Memory and regional blood cerebral blood flow in mildly symptomatic Alzheimer's disease. Neurology 39: 1537–1539

Reifler BV (1982) Arguments for abandoning the term pseudodementia. J Am Geriatr Soc 30(10):665–668

Reisberg B, Ferris SH, de Leon MJ, Crook T (1982) The Global Deterioration Scale for assessment of primary degenerative dementia. Am J Psychiatry 139(9): 1136–1139

Richards M, Stern Y, Mayeux R (1993) Subtle extrapyramidal signs can predict the development of dementia in elderly individuals. Neurology 43: 2184–2188

Rosen WG, Terry RD, Fuld PA, Katzman R, Peck A (1980) Pathological verification of ischemic score in differentiation of dementias. Ann Neurol 7: 5, 486–488

Roth M, Tym E, Mountjoy CQ, Huppert FA, Hendrie H, Verma S, Goddard R (1986) CAMDEX. A standardised instrument for the diagnosis of mental disorder in the elderly with special reference to the early detection of dementia. Br J Psychiatry 149: 698–709

Rubin EH, Storandt M, Miller JP, Grant EA, Kinscherf DA, Morris JC, Berg L (1993) Influence of age on clinical and psychometric assessment of subjects with very mild or mild dementia of the Alzheimer type. Arch Neurol 50(4): 380–383

Small GW, La Rue A, Komo S, Kaplan A, Mandelkern MA (1995) Predictors of cognitive change in middle-aged and older adults with memory loss. Am J Psychiatry 152: 1757–1764

Small GW, Komo S, La Rue A, Saxena S, Phelps ME, Mazziotta JC, Saunders AM, Haines JL, Pericak-Vance MA, Roses AD (1996) Early detection of Alzheimer's disease by combining apolipoprotein e and neuroimaging. Ann NY Acad Sci 802: 70–78

Smith AD, Jobst KA (1996) Use of structural imaging to study the progression of Alzheimer's disease. Br Med Bull 52(3): 575–586

St Clair D, Norrman J, Perry R, Yates C, Wilcock G, Brookes A (1994) Apolipoprotein E epsilon 4 allele frequency in patients with Lewy body dementia, Alzheimer's disease and age-matched controls. Neurosci Lett 18; 176(1): 45–46

Strittmatter WJ, Saunders AM, Smechel D, et al (1993) Apolipoprotein E: high-avidity binding to the B-amyloid and increased frequency of type 4 allele in late onset familial Alzheimer's disease. Proc Natl Acad Sci USA 90: 1977–1981

Terry R, Katzmann R (1983) Senile dementia of the Alzheimer type: defining a disease. In: Katzmann R, Terry R (eds) The neurology of aging. F.A. Davis, Philadelphia

Tierney MC, Szalai JP, Snow WG, Fisher RH, Nores A, Nadon G, Dunn E, St. George-Hyslop PH (1996a) Prediction of probable alzheimer's disease in memory-impaired patients: a prospective longitudinal study. Neurology 46: 661–665

Tierney MC, Szalai JP, Snow WG, Fisher RH, Tsuda T, Chi H, McLachlan DR, St George-Hyslop PH (1996b) A prospective study of the clinical utility of ApoE genotype in theprediction of outcome in patients with memory impairment. Neurology 46(1): 149–154

Tierney MC, Szalai P, Snow GW, Fisher RH (1996c) The prediction of Alzheimer disease: the role of patient and informant perceptions of cognitive deficits. Arch Neurol 53: 423–427

Troster AI, Moe KE, Vitiello MV, Prinz PN (1994) Predicting long-term outcome in individuals at risk for Alzheimer's disease with the dementia rating scale. J Neuropsychiatry Clin Neurosci 6: 54–57

Tsai MS, Tangalos EG, Petersen RC, Smith GE, Schaid DJ, Kokmen E, Ivnik RJ, Thibodeau SN (1994) Apolipoprotein E: risk factor for Alzheimer disease. Am J Hum Genet 54(4): 643–649

Welsh KA, Butters N, Hughes JP, Mohs RC, Heyman A (1992) Detection and staging of dementia in Alzheimer's disease. use of the neuropsychological measures developed for the Consortium to Establish a Registry for Alzheimer's Disease. Arch Neurol 49: 448–452

Wenham PR, Price WH, Blundell G (1991) Apolipoprotein E genotyping by one-stage PCR. Lancet 337: 1158–1159

World Health Organisation (1990) International classification of diseases, 10th edition. WHO, Geneva

Youngjohn JR, Crook- TH 3d (1993) Learning, forgetting, and retrieval of everyday material across the adult life span. J Clin Exp Neuropsychol 15(4): 447–460

Zaudig M (1992) A new systematic method of measurement and diagnosis of "mild cognitive impairment" and dementia according to ICD-10 and DSM-III-R criteria. Int Psychogeriatr 4 [Suppl 2]: 203–219

Zaudig M, Mittelhammer J, Hiller W, Pauls A, Thora C, Morinigo A, Mombour W (1991) SIDAM — A structured interview for the diagnosis of dementia of the Alzheimer's type, multiinfarct dementia and dementias of other aetiology according to ICD-10 and DSM-III-R. Psychol Med 21: 225–236

Zola-Morgan S, Squire LR, Amaral DG (1986) Human amnesia and the medial temporal region: enduring memory impairment following a bilateral lesion limited to field CA1 of the hippocampus. J Neurosci 6(10): 2950–2967

Zola-Morgan S, Squire LR, Amaral DG (1986) Human amnesia and the medial temporal region: enduring memory impairment following a bilateral lesion limited to field CA1 of the hippocampus. J Neurosci 6(10): 2950–2967

Authors' address: Dr. H. Wolf, Department of Psychiatry, University of Leipzig, Emilienstrasse 14, D-04107 Leipzig, Federal Republic of Germany

Prevalence of mild cognitive impairment in an elderly community sample

J. Schröder[1], **B. Kratz**[1], **J. Pantel**[1], **E. Minnemann**[2], **U. Lehr**[2], and **H. Sauer**[3]

[1]Section of Geriatric Psychiatry, Department of Psychiatry, University of Heidelberg,
[2]German Center for Research on Aging, Heidelberg, and [3]Department of Psychiatry,
University of Jena, Jena, Federal Republic of Germany

Summary. The term "mild cognitive impairment" refers to cognitive deficits which exceed normal physiological aging processes, but do not fulfill the criteria for dementia. While recent studies indicate that the respective deficits can be reliably assessed, different diagnostic criteria have prevented a wide application of this diagnosis in clinical practice. The aims of the present study were (1) to assess the prevalence rates of four current diagnostic concepts and (2) to investigate mild cognitive impairment with respect to psychological and sociodemographic variables. Data from 202 probands recruited from the interdisciplinary longitudinal study on adult development were analyzed. On the time of examination, probands were between 60 to 64 years old and in a good health. The following prevalence rates were determined: 13.5% for age-associated memory impairment (AAMI), 6.5% for age-consistent memory impairment (ACMI), 1.5% for late-life forgetfulness (LLF), and 23.5% for aging-associated cognitive decline (AACD). Complaints of cognitive deficits were significantly correlated with higher scores on depression and neuroticism scales but with none of the neuropsychological measures. Reduced performance in neuropsychological tests was associated with a lower educational level and socioeconomic status. We conclude that the prevalence rates of mild cognitive impairment are highly dependant on the diagnostic criteria applied. In this respect the self-report of cognitive decline might be a less useful criteria. Longitudinal studies are warranted to further eludicate the predictive value of these diagnostic criteria.

Introduction

The concept of mild cognitive impairment refers to cognitive deficits which exceed normal physiological aging processes, but do not fulfill the criteria for dementia. Recent studies indicate that such minor cognitive deficits, in particular those involving mnestic functions characterize the initial stage of most dementing processes and may be decisive for early diagnosis (for review, see: Cooper et al., 1996).

Four major classifications were convened by different authors to operationalize the concept of "mild cognitive impairment": age-associated memory impairment (AAMI/Crook et al., 1986), age-consistent memory impairment (ACMI/Blackford and La Rue, 1989), late-life forgetfulness (LLF/Blackford and La Rue, 1989), and aging-associated cognitive decline (AACD/Levy, 1994).

The concept and the criteria for AAMI were developed by a workgroup of the National Institute of Mental Health in 1986. It denotes a condition in otherwise healthy middle age or elderly individuals (50 years and older) who complain about memory loss and who score at least 1 standard deviation below the mean established for young adults on neuropsychological tests of secondary (longterm) memory.

Blackford and La Rue (1989) criticized that AAMI criteria do not define the number of tests applied and that test performance was not compared to appropriate agenorms. To overcome these difficulties they proposed two further concepts: ACMI applies for a reduced performance within 1 standard deviation of the mean established for the respective agegroup on 75% or more of the tests administered, and LLF to denote test performance between 1 and 2 standard deviations below the age adjusted mean on 50% or more of the neuropsychological measures applied.

While these concepts solely refer to mnestic deficits, AACD as defined by a workgroup of the International Psychogeriatric Association (Levy, 1994) also refers to any subjective cognitive decline and objective evidence of reduced performance in any principle domain of cognition, such as attention, language, visuospatial functioning or deficits in abstract thinking. In addition, neuropsychological functioning should be assessed using well standardized tests on basis of norms adjusted for age and educational level.

Recent studies on mild cognitive impairment have yielded a wide variation of prevalence rates with estimates for AAMI ranging from 8.5% to 98% (Barker et al., 1995; Larrabee and Crook, 1994). Following Larrabee and Crook (1995) this variability may be attributed to the usage of different diagnostic criteria and failure to consider age as a variable in estimating prevalence. Inclusion of complaints of cognitive decline into the diagnostic criteria is another matter of discussion. While some authors found reports of memory loss to predict a reduced test performance (McGlone et al., 1990), others found cognitive complaints to be rather related to symptoms of depression or neurotic personality traits (Jorm et al., 1997).

We therefore investigated the prevalence rate of mild cognitive impairment in a cohort of otherwise healthy elderly subjects using the four diagnostic criteria mentioned above. The aims of our study were: (1) to assess the prevalence rates of four current concepts of mild cognitive impairment; and (2), to examine the importance of subjective memory complaints for diagnosing mild cognitive impairment.

Probands and methods

202 otherwise healthy subjects (97 females, 105 males) aged 60–64 were included. The sociodemographic characteristics of our sample are given in Table 1. The investigation

Table 1. Sociodemographic characteristics of the sample (age: 60–64)

	Male n = 105 (52%)	Female n = 97 (48%)
Educational level		
— no school-leaving certificate	10.5%	10.3%
— primary school	51.4%	53.6%
— secondary modern school	19.05%	19.6%
— grammar or professional school	19.05%	16.5%
Vocational training		
— no vocational training	7.6%	47.9%
— apprenticeship	58.1%	32.3%
— technical or master craftsman's school	17.1%	8.3%
— technical college or university degree	17.1%	11.5%
Employed at time of testing	29.8%	13%
Monthly net-income per household		
— 1,000–2,999 DM	10%	19.3%
— 3,000–4,999 DM	50%	56.8%
— 5,000–7,000 DM	40%	23.9%

was part of the interdisciplinary longitudinal study on adult development (ILSE) which was conducted in Bonn, Erlangen-Nürnberg, Heidelberg, Leipzig, and Rostock/F. R. Germany. Probands were selected from the community resident register which is a compulsory register of all residents. To increase the homogeneity of the sample and to facilitate follow-up investigations, only data from the Heidelberg subsample were used. Subjects were screened for health, by history, physical examination, electrocardiogramm, and laboratory testing. To exclude any psychiatric disorder, the standardized interview for the DSM-III-R (Wittchen et al., 1991) was applied. To address potential subclinical depressive mood changes, the self-rating depression scale (Zung, 1986) was used. In addition, the NEO five factor test (Borkenau and Ostendorf, 1993), the Nürnberger Alters-Inventar (Oswald and Fleischmann, 1991), and the Philadelphia Geriatric Center Morale Scale (Lawton, 1975) were used to investigate some important personality traits and attitudes towards aging.

Neuropsychological assessment: The neuropsychological test battery addressed primary and secondary memory, speed of processing, visuo-spatial orientation, and word fluency using the respective subtests of the Nürnberger-Alters-Inventar and the Leistungsprüfsystem (Horn, 1983), respectively. General intelligence was assessed by four subtests of the HAWIE-R (Tewes, 1991). Since cognitive performance may also vary with attentional performance, the latter was evaluated using the Aufmerksamkeits-Belastungs-Test (d2-Test; Brickenkamp, 1978).

At this point one methodological problem has to be stressed: Following the AAMI criteria test performance should be assessed using norm values for young adults. However, such values do hardly exist for neuropsychological measures constructed for use in old age. To overcome this difficulty, the respective results of the 697 probands aged 40 to 44 were drawn upon. Moreover, AACD criteria necessitate the application of norm values adjusted for educational level. Since the respective values were only available for some but not all neuropsychological measures applied, the results of the entire ageclass 1930–1932 (n = 697) were differentiated for high and low educational levels and used for comparison.

Data analysis: In a first step, the prevalence rates of AAMI, ACMI, LLF, and AACD were calculated. To address the potential impact of memory complaints, four subgroups of probands were identified: probands with cognitive complaints and deficits in test performance (at least 1 standard deviation below the mean value established for age), probands who complained cognitive decline without any indication of cognitive deficits in the neuropsychological tests applied ("memory complainers"), probands who did not complain any cognitive decline but showed a reduced cognitive performance ("non complainers"), and a control group who neither reported any impairment nor showed any neuropsychological deficits. Subsequently, these subgroups were compared for some important sociodemographic characteristics and personality traits.

Results

The prevalence rates determined are given in Table 2: 27 (13.5%) of the 202 probands examined fulfilled AAMI-criteria, 13 (6.5%) ACMI, 3 (1.5) LLF, and 47 (23.5%) AACD criteria. Moreover, a considerable overlap between the diagnostic criteria became apparent.

Cognitive decline was reported by 93 (46.5%) probands. 99 (49%) showed a reduced performance of at least one standard deviation below the age adjusted means in one or more of the neuropsychological tests applied. 44 probands reported a cognitive decline and showed a reduced performance in at least one of the neuropsychological tests administered. 49 (24.5%) probands complained cognitive decline but showed no deficits in any of the neuropsychological tests ("cognitive complainers"); 55 (27.5%) showed an impaired performance in one or more of the neuropsychological tests applied but did not report any subjective complaints ("non complainers"). 54 probands (27%) did not report any subjective memory complaints nor showed any neuropsychological deficits ("control group"). Among these subgroups, probands with a reduced neuropsychological test performance were characterized by significantly lower scores on intelligence measures, a lower educational level, and a lower income. In contrast, probands complaining cognitive decline, received higher scores on the Nürnberger Selfrating scale of the Nürnberger Altersinventar, the Self-Rating Depression Scale, the neuroticism scale of the NEO-FFI, and lower scores on the Philadelphia Geriatric Center Morale Scale, respectively (Table 3).

Table 2. Prevalence rates of the different diagnostic criteria

	AAMI	ACMI	LLF	AACD
AAMI	27 (13.5%)	6 (3%)	3 (1.5%)	17 (8.5%)
ACMI		13 (6.5%)	0 (0%)	0 (0%)
LLF			3 (1.5%)	3 (1.5%)
AACD				47 (23.5%)

AAMI age-associated memory impairment, *ACMI* age-consistent memory impairment, *LLF* late-life forgetfulness, *AACD* aging-associated cognitive decline

Table 3. Means and standard deviations of psychological and sociodemographic variables in probands with cognitive complaints and deficits in test performance, "cognitive complainers", "non complainers", and controls

	Complaints and deficits	"Non complainers"	"Complainers"	Controls		
	M (SD)	M (SD)	M (SD)	M (SD)	p <	Scheffe's test
NSL-NAI	44.7 (12.1)	33.1 (8.4)	39.1 (11.4)	31.9 (8.2)	0.0001	1 vs. 2, 4/ 3 vs. 2, 4
SDS	36.6 (7.3)	32.8 (5.9)	35.9 (7.5)	30.6 (5.6)	0.0001	1 vs. 2, 4/ 3 vs. 4
NEO-FFI: Neuroticism	1.58 (0.6)	1.38 (0.5)	1.61 (0.6)	1.32 (0.6)	0.04	
PGC: attitude towards aging	8.06 (1.7)	8.9 (1.3)	8.9 (1.3)	9.08 (1.3)	0.002	1 vs. 2, 3, 4
Mean of the four HAWIE-R subtests	9.79 (2.56)	9.38 (2.7)	11.79 (2.1)	12.16 (2.0)	0.0001	1 vs. 3, 4/ 2 vs. 3, 4
	n (%)	n (%)	n (%)	n (%)	p <	
Educational level:						not applicable
low	33 (75)	41 (74, 5)	27 (55)	26 (48)	0.007	
high	11 (25)	14 (25, 5)	22 (45)	28 (52)		
Monthly net-income per household						not applicable
1,000–2,999 DM	9 (22, 5)	6 (12)	9 (20)	3 (6)		
3,000–4,999 DM	21 (52, 5)	34 (68)	18 (39)	27 (52)	0.019	
5,000–7,000 DM	10 (25)	10 (20)	19 (41)	22 (42)		

NSL-NAI Nürnberger Selbsteinschätzungsliste, *SDS* Self-rating Depression Scale, *NEO-FFI* NEO Fünf Faktoren Inventar, *PGC* Philadelphia Geriatric Center Morale Scale, *HAWIE-R* Hamburg-Wechsler-Intelligenztest für Erwachsene

Discussion

The present study yielded three major findings: (1) evidence that the prevalence rates of "mild cognitive impairment" vary widely with the diagnostic concept applied; (2) an indication that cognitive complaints may be associated with depressive mood and neurotic personality traits in a subgroup of probands; and (3) support for an association of neuropsychological deficits with lower educational level and socioeconomic status.

Prevalence rates of mild cognitive impairment varied between 1.5% to 23.5% according to the diagnostic criteria applied. The lowest prevalence rate (1.5%) was found when LLF criteria were used; application of ACMI (6.5%) and AAMI (13.5%) criteria yielded considerable higher prevalence rates. On basis of AACD criteria the highest prevalence rate (23.5%) was found. The low prevalence rate of LLF corresponds with Smith et al. (1991) who did not found a single subject fulfilling the respective criteria among 99 probands with mild cognitive impairment. In contrast, the prevalence of AAMI reported in previous studies was estimated ranging from 35% to 98%, depending on the subjects' age (Larrabee and Crook, 1994). However, these numbers should be considered as an upperbound estimate of the prevalence of AAMI. Barker et al. (1995) found the prevalence rates of AAMI to range between 5.8% and 18.5% in a population of 50 to 95 years old probands. A comparable low prevalence rate was also communicated by Coria et al. (1993). Hence, the prevalence rates obtained for AAMI in the present study are well in this range. Up to now, rates for AACD were only evaluated in one epidemiological study (Hänninen et al., 1996) which involved 403 randomly selected probands (68–76 years of age). In all, 26.6% of the subjects fulfilled the AACD criteria, a value surprisingly close to the 23.5% found in the present study. The prevalence rates were only slightly related to age with somewhat lower rates in the oldest age group (20.5%). That the present study found the prevalence of AAMI to be lower than that of AACD corresponds to the different inclusion criteria of these classifications: While AAMI focuses on mnestic impairment, AACD also refers to any cognitive deficits. Moreover, to satisfy criteria for AAMI, subjects should present with verbal and performance Intelligence Quotient scores between 90 and 130. Therefore subjects with low intelligence measures are a priori excluded if AAMI criteria are used.

The selection of neuropsychological tests and the definition of reduced test performance have to be discussed as another potential confounding variables. Particular tests are only proposed in the AAMI criteria, while AACD criteria refer to domains of neuropsychological functioning without reference to certain tests. Both AAMI and AACD criteria do not define the number of neuropsychological tests applied. Following both AAMI and AACD criteria, a reduced test performance is defined by a reduced performance in a single or more test. One may argue that the likelihood of meeting this criterion by chance will increase when more tests are applied. In addition, none of the diagnostic criteria refers to the test-retest reliability of the neuropsychological tests used.

The present study indicates that complaints of cognitive and mnestic decline are rather related to depressive mood and neurotic personality traits than to a reduced test performance per se. Similar results were reported by Jorm et al. (1997) and McGlone et al. (1990). Jorm et al. (1997) found cognitive complaints to correspond to neurotic symptoms, in particular depression and anxiety rather than to future cognitive decline. McGlone et al. (1990) investigated memory complaints in 29 patients with dementia, 28 subjects with AAMI, and 35 healthy controls. Both self-assessment and relatives responses on a standardized questionnaire differentiated patients groups from healthy controls. While relatives' ratings corresponded with a reduced test performance, memory complaints correlated with depressive mood rather than objective mnestic deficits. However, the present study also demonstrated that cognitive complaints can not solely be explained by depressive mood changes: Probands with both complaints and a reduced test performance exhibited a tendency to score even higher on depression scales than those who complained cognitive decline, but did not show a reduced test performance. That mild cognitive impairment comprises a subgroup with pronounced depressive symptoms is supported by Ritchie et al. (1996). It is generally accepted that depressive symptoms may arise in a considerable percentage of patients with medical or neurological disorders (Creed, 1997). Therefore one may hypothesize that depressive symptoms may also result from mild cognitive impairment in a subgroup of probands.

Lastly, we found a clear association between neuropsychological deficits and lower measures of general intelligence, education, and socioeconomic status. In the AAMI, ACMI, and LLF criteria low Intelligence scores are considered as an exclusion criteria, while adjustment for levels of prior education are recommended by the AACD classification. Following Katzmann (1993) higher education might lead to an increased brain reserve capacity which would retard the onset of cognitive decline. However, this association might also refer to confounding factors such as different lifestyles. A significant increased risk of cognitive impairment associated with a lower educational level was recently reported by Kalmijn et al. (1997). However, this association only applied for subjects without an apolipoprotein e4 allele. That apolipoprotein E status has to be considered as a potential moderator variable is also supported by Petersen et al. (1995) who found apoliprotein e4 to be a strong predictor of clinical progression. These findings indicate that reduced levels of general intelligence, education, and socioeconomic status cannot be considered as confounding variables per se, but may refer to a particular subgroup of subjects with mild cognitive impairment.

In conclusion, the present study demonstrates that mild cognitive impairment is frequently found among otherwise healthy elderly. Further studies are necessary to standardize the different classifications and to investigate mild cognitive impairment as a potential predictor of dementing processes.

Acknowledgements

This study was supported by a grant from the Ministry of Science and Research of Baden-Württemberg and the Federal Ministry for Families, Seniors, Women, and Youth/F.R. Germany.

References

Barker A, Jones R, Jennison Ch (1995) A prevalence study of age-associated memory impairment. Br J Psychiatry 167: 642–648

Blackford RC, La Rue A (1989) Criteria for diagnosing age-associated memory impairment: proposed improvements from the field. Dev Neuropsych 5(4): 295–306

Borkenau O, Ostendorf F (1993) NEO-Fünf-Faktoren-Inventar nach Costar und McCrae. Hogrefe, Göttingen

Brickenkamp R (1978) Test d2. Aufmerksamkeits-Belastungs-Test. Hogrefe, Göttingen

Cooper B, Bickel H, Schäufele M (1996) Early development and progression of dementing illness in the elderly: a general-practice based study. Psychol Med 26: 411–419

Coria F, Gomez de Caso JA, Minguez L, Rodriguez Artalejo F, Claveria LE (1993) Prevalence of age-associated memory impairment and dementia in a rural community. J Neurol Neurosurg Psychiatry 56: 973–976

Creed F (1997) Assessing depression in the context of physical illness. In: Robertson MM, Katona CLE (eds) Depression and physical illness. John Wiley & Sons, Chichester New York Weinheim Brisbane Singapore Toronto

Crook T, Bartus RT, Ferris SH, Whitehouse P, Cohen GD, Gershon S (1986) Age-associated memory impairment: proposed diagnostic criteria and measures of clinical change (NIMH-Workgroup). Dev Neuropsych 2(4): 261–276

Crook TH (1989) Diagnosis and treatment of normal and pathologic memory impairment in later life. Semin Neurol 9: 20–30

Derousné C, Kalafat M, Guez D, Malbezin M, Poitrenaud J (1994) The age-associated memory impairment construct revisited. Int J Ger Psychiatry 9: 577–587

Ebly EM, Hogan DB, Parhad IM (1995) Cognitive impairment in the nondemented elderly: results from the Canadian study of health and aging. Arch Neurol 52: 612–619

Feher EP, Larrabee GJ, Sudilovsky A, Crook TH (1994) Memory self-report in Alzheimer's disease and in age-associated memory impairment. J Ger Psychiatry Neurol 7(1): 58–65

Hänninen T, Koivisto K, Reinikainen KJ, Helkala EL, Soininen H, Mykkänen L, Laakso M, Riekkinen PJ (1996) Prevalence of ageing-associated cognitive decline in an elderly population. Age Ageing 25: 201–205

Horn WC (1983) Leistungsprüfsystem. Hogrefe, Göttingen

Jolles J, Verhey FRJ, Riedel WJ, Houx PJ (1995) Cognitive impairment in elderly people. Predisposing factors and implications for experimental drug studies. Drugs Aging 7(6): 459–479

Jorm AF, Christensen H, Korten AE, Hendersson AS, Jacomb PA, Mackinnon A (1997) Do cognitive complaints either predict future cognitive decline or reflect past cognitive decline? A longitudinal study of an elderly community sample. Psychol Med 27: 91–98

Kalmijn S, Feskens EJM, Launer LJ, Kromhout D (1997) Longitudinal study of the effect of apolipoprotein e4 allele on the association between education and cognitive decline in elderly men. BMJ 314: 34–35

Katzmann R (1993) Education and the prevalence of dementia and Alzheimer's disease. Neurology 43: 13–20

Larrabee GJ, Crook III TH (1994) Estimated prevalence of age-associated memory impairment derived from standardized tests of memory function. Int Psychogeriatr 1: 95–104

Levy R (1994) Aging-associated cognitive decline. Int Psychogeriatr 6(1): 63–68

McGlone J, Gupta S, Humphrey D, Oppenheimer S, Mirsen T, Evans DR (1990) Screening for early dementia using memory complaints from patients and relatives. Arch Neurol 47: 1189–1193

Oswald WD, Fleischmann VM (1991) Nürnberger-Alters-Inventar. Universität Erlangen-Nürnberg, Erlangen-Nürnberg

Petersen RC, Smith GE, Ivnik RJ, Tangalos EG, Schaid DJ, Thibodeau SN, Kokmen E, Waring SC, Kurland LT (1995) Apolipoprotein E status as a predictor of the development of Alzheimer's disease in memory impaired individuals. JAMA 273: 1274–1278

Ritchie K, Leibovici D, Ledésert B, Touchon J (1996) A typology of sub-clinical senescent cognitive disorder. Br J Psychiatry 168: 470–476

Small GW, LaRue A, Komo S, Kaplan A (1997) Mnemonics usage and cognitive decline in age-associated memory impairment. Int Psychogeriatr 9: 47–56

Smith G, Ivnik RJ, Petersen RC, Malec JF, Kokmen E, Tangalos E (1991) Age-associated memory impairment diagnoses: problems of reliability and concerns for terminology. Psychol Aging 4: 551–558

Tewes W (1991) HAWIE-R. Hamburg-Wechsler-Intelligenztest für Erwachsene. Revision. Huber, Bern Stuttgart

White L, Katzman R, Losonczy K, Salive M, Wallace R, Berkman L, et al (1994) Association of education with incidence of cognitive impairment in three established populations for epidemiologic studies of the elderly. J Clin Epidemiol 47: 363–374

Wittchen H-U, Zaudig M, Schramm E, Spengler P, Mombour W, Klug J, Horn R (1991) Strukturiertes klinisches Interview für DSM-III-R. Beltz-Test, Göttingen

Zung WWK (1986) Self-rating depression scale. In: Collegium internationale psychiatry (eds) Internationale Skalen für Psychiatrie. Beltz-Test, Göttingen

Authors' address: PD Dr. J. Schröder, Sektion für Gerontopsychiatrie, Psychiatrische Universitätsklinik, Voßstrasse 4, D-69115 Heidelberg, Federal Republic of Germany

Increase of optical illusion in demented patients

B. Weber, L. Frölich, N. Helbing, D. Simminger, J. Fritze, and **K. Maurer**

Department of Psychiatry and Psychotherapy I, Johann Wolfgang Goethe University, Frankfurt / Main, Federal Republic of Germany

Summary. Assuming a particular psychological function of optical gestalt perception, its impairment would lead to a decreasing extent of gestalt related optical illusion. An increase of optical illusion would be expected in the case of a loss of adaptability and cognitive compensation, usually revising the phenomenon of optical illusion. 16 demented out-patients were compared to 16 hospitalized schizophrenics by a 'Computerized Assessment of Change in Optical Illusion' (CACOI), measuring the extent of optical illusion by patient's assessment of 12 variations of the figure of Mueller-Lyer, differing in baseline length. The results showed a significant increase of optical illusion in demented patients compared to the schizophrenic controls (p = 0.019). Taking into account that the extent of optical illusion by the figure of Mueller-Lyer usually is decreasing with age and was found to be increased in schizophrenics, our results support the hypothesis of an early loss of adaptability and cognitive compensation in dementia.

Introduction

Mechanisms underlying optical gestalt perception must be regarded as an important organizing factor, facilitating orientation and comprehension in complex situations and tasks. In the past decades the significance of gestalt perception for the diagnosis of organic brain damage was examined by the Bender (1938) Visual-Motor Gestalt Test (BGT) (Pardue, 1975; Russell, 1976; Holland et al., 1979; Mermelstein, 1983). But studies using the BGT showed a low sensitivity of this method for cortical dysfunction in the elderly (Margolis et al., 1989) and for therapy effects in dementia (Albizzati et al., 1987). A reduced utility in differentiating very mild or mild dementia from normal aging (Storandt, 1990) with false negative results occurring more frequently in individuals with mild neuropsychological impairment (Margolis et al., 1989) was reported.

First studies with the figure of Mueller-Lyer were performed already in the last century by Binet and van Biervliet and the extent of optical illusion usually was found to be decreased with age (Table 1) (Coren and Girgus, 1978). In schizophrenic patients however, the magnitude of illusion was found

Table 1. Age trends in Mueller-Lyer illusion [modified from: Coren S, Girgus JS (1978) Seeing is deceiving: the psychology of visual illusions. Erlbaum, Hillsdale]

Study	Year	Age trend
Barclay and comalli	1970	decreased
Binet	1895	decreased
Gaudreau, Lavoie and Delorme	1963	decreased
Girgus, Coren and Fraenkel	1975	decreased
Murray	1967	decreased
Noelting	1960	decreased
Piaget and von Albertini	1950	decreased
Piaget, Marie and Privat	1954	decreased
Pitner and Anderson	1916	decreased
Pollack	1964	decreased
Segall, Campbell and Herskovits	1966	decreased
Sun	1964	decreased
van Biervliet	1896	decreased
Walters	1942	decreased

to be increased (Rund et al., 1994). Several studies analysed effects of brain damage (Basso et al., 1974; Greene et al., 1979; Mattingley et al., 1995) and psychiatric disorders (Letourneau, 1974; Rund et al., 1994) on the Mueller-Lyer illusion but up to now no results concerning dementia are available.

Assuming the existence of a particular psychological function of optical gestalt perception, a decreasing extent of gestalt effects — as optical illusion — might be expected in the case of an impairment of this function. An increase of optical illusion, however, would be expected in the case of a preserved optical gestalt perception and a loss of adaptability and cognitive compensation, usually revising the phenomenon of optical illusion (Fig. 1).

Material and methods

In the present study 16 demented patients were compared to 16 schizophrenics (DSM-III-R) by a 'Computerized Assessment of Change in Optical Illusion' (CACOI), developed by the authors. The test measures the extent of optical illusion by patients' assessment of 12 variations of the figure of Mueller-Lyer, differing in baseline lengths. Patients were asked to compare baseline length of two figures, presented one on top of the other simultaneously. The figures were presented in a randomised and standardized order with varying baseline in the below wings-in figure. CACOI scores were calculated by addition of the absolute baseline differences between compared figures in case of false assessment, that is illusion. Illusions in the expected direction were calculated with positive signs

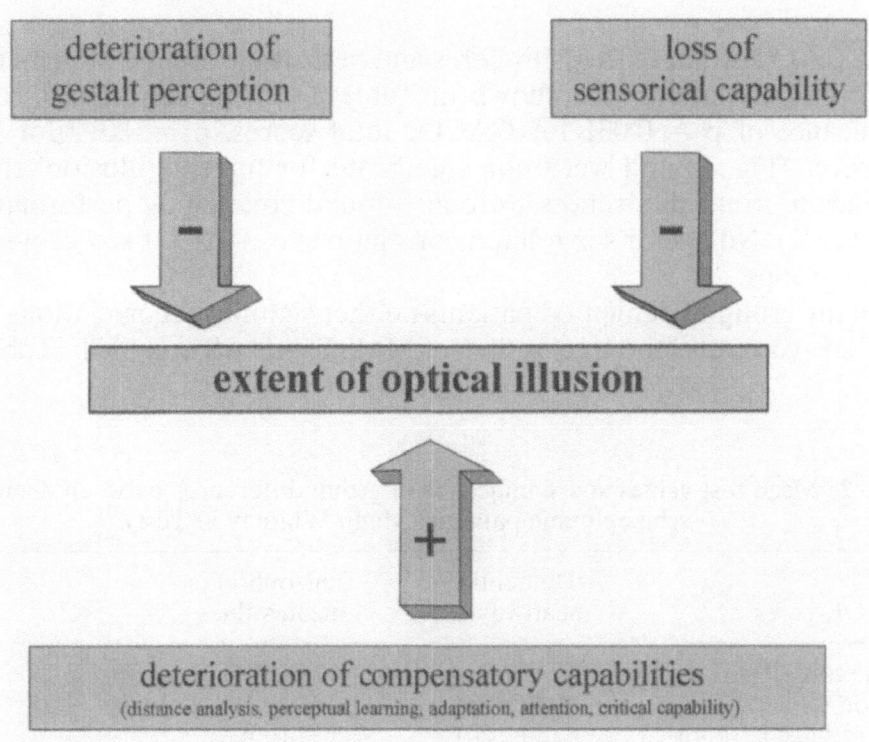

Fig. 1. Model of possible factors involved in changes of optical illusion

('illusion' subscore) and false assessments of unexpected direction with negative signs ('inverse illusion' subscore).

In order to exclude sensoric lesions patients were examined for disorders of sight and vision field. In addition the Alzheimers' Disease Assessment Scale (ADAS), the Syndrome Short Test (SKT) and the Mini Mental State Examination (MMST) were performed for demented patients.

The 16 demented patients consulted our memory out-patients' department, had a mean age of 68.2 ± 8.8 (mean $\pm$ SD) years and nine of them were female. Mean MMST scores were calculated with 22.0 ± 6.2 (range 12–25), mean ADAS scores with 31.3 ± 18.7 (12–74), mean ADAScog scores with 24.3 ± 14.5 (9–55) and mean SKT scores with 14.0 ± 6.6 (10—24). Five patients were classified as dementia of the Alzheimer type, four as dementia of cerebrovascular origin, three as mixed type and four mildly affected patients remained unclassified. The control group of 16 schizophrenic patients had an age of 40.3 ± 11.6 years, six of them were female. According to DSM-III-R 13 patients were classified as chronic and three as subchronic schizophrenia.

The significance of group differences between CACOI scores in demented and schizophrenic patients was tested by the Mann-Whitney U Test. Relations between CACOI, ADAS, SKT and MMST scores were analysed by the Spearman Rank Order Correlation. Owing to inhomogeneity of the dementia scales the relationship between individual ADAS, SKT and MMST subtests and CACOI scores additionally was examined by the Spearman Rank Order Correlation and the Mann-Whitney U Test.

Results

Mean CACOI total scores, subscores and performance time of demented and schizophrenic patients are shown in Table 2. Group differences reached a significance of p = 0.032 for CACOI total scores, p = 0.019 for 'illusion' subscores (Fig. 2) and were non significant for 'inverse illusion' subscores. Significant group differences were also found concerning performance time (p = 0.021). No age or sex related correlations of CACOI scores were found within groups.

In the group of demented patients neither significant correlations between CACOI scores and the total scores of MMST, ADAS and SKT (Table 3) nor

Table 2. Mean test values and significance of group differences between demented and schizophrenic patients (Mann-Whitney U Test)

CACOI scores	Dementia mean values	Schizophrenia mean values	Z	p
Total score	193 (±90)	124 (±110)	−2.15	0.032
Illusion score	198 (±83)	127 (±108)	−2.34	0.019
Inverse illusion score	5 (±20)	3 (±6.8)	—	n.s.
Time (sec.)	208 (±97)	147 (±63)	−2.30	0.021

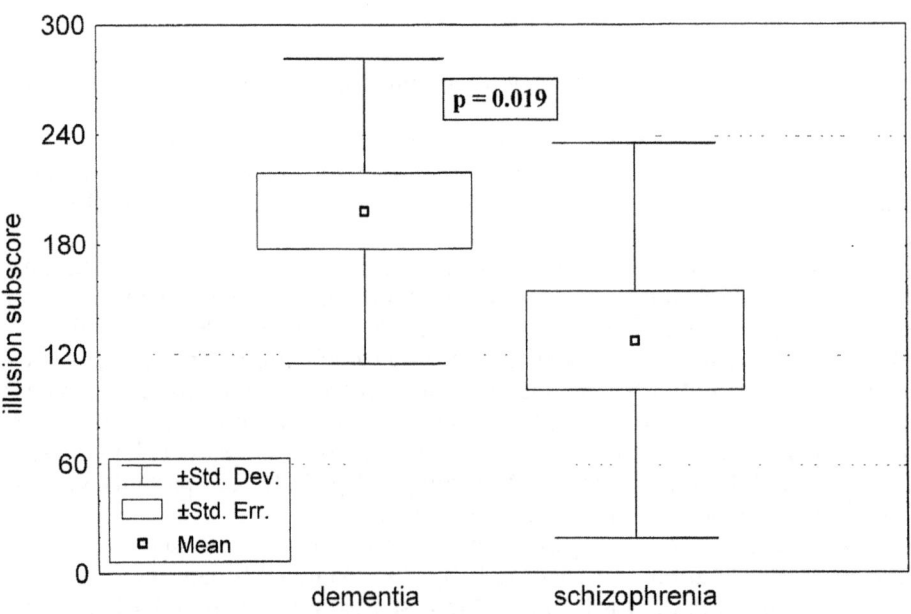

Fig. 2. Group differences between demented and schizophrenic patients in extent of the Mueller-Lyer illusion (CACOI illusion subscore, Mann-Whitney U Test)

Table 3. Relations between CACOI scores and ADAS, SKT and MMST scores in demented patients (Spearman Rank Order Correlation). None of the correlations reaches significance

CACOI scores	ADAS	ADAScog	SKT	MMST
Total score	0.34	0.32	−0.07	0.02
Illusion score	0.32	0.30	−0.09	0.03
Inverse illusion score	0.00	0.00	0.05	−0.20
Time (sec.)	0.28	0.34	0.38	−0.38

Table 4. Significant correlations between CACOI scores and subtests of ADAS, SKT and MMST in demented patients (Spearman Rank Order Correlation and Mann-Whitney U Test). $*p < 0.05$, $^{(*)}p < 0.1$

CACOI scores	ADAS "word recognition"	ADAS "following instructions"	SKT "counting symbols"	MMST "writing"
Total score	R = 0.61*	—	R = −0.60*	Z = 2.13*
Illusion score	—	—	R = 0.53$^{(*)}$	—
Time (sec.)	—	R = 0.70*	—	—

differences between subgroups of dementia were found. But CACOI total scores significantly correlated to the SKT 'counting symbols' task (R = −0.60, p = 0.03), the MMST 'writing' task (Z = 2.13, p = 0.03) and the ADAS 'word recognition' task (R = 0.61, p = 0.03). CACOI 'inverse illusion' subscores showed a trend to a significant correlation to the SKT 'counting symbols' task (R = 0.53, p = 0.06). CACOI performance time showed a significant correlation to the ADAS 'following instructions' task (R = 0.70, p = 0.01) (Table 4).

Discussion

Taking into account that the extent of optical illusion by the figure of Mueller-Lyer usually is decreasing with age (Coren and Girgus, 1978) and was found to be increased in schizophrenics (Rund et al., 1994), it can be concluded, that the magnitude of illusion is distinctly increased in dementia. This result contradicts the hypothesis of an early restriction of optical gestalt perception and rather supports the assumption of a predominating loss of adaptability and cognitive compensation of gestalt effects in demented patients. This finding corresponds to the experience, that the application of gestalt laws is helpful in designing a suitable milieu for demented patients (van der Voordt, 1993).

The detected changes of optical gestalt perception are not correlated to global severity of dementia but to specific sectors of test performance, connected with symbol recognition. The basic optical recognition of simple figures seems to be intensified (SKT 'counting symbols' task) and to predominate the assignment of cognitive meanings to linguistic symbols (letters) with consequences for measurable memory (ADAS 'word recognition' task) and writing (MMST 'writing' task) capability. The phenomenon of 'inverse illusion' — representing a loss of gestalt perception — seems to be connected with a deterioration of simple figure recognition (SKT 'counting symbols' task).

Whether the loss of adaptability and cognitive compensation of gestalt effects precedes or covers a possible impairment of gestalt perception — at least indicated by the observation of 'inverse illusion' — can not be decided by our findings. Possibly gestalt perception itself — as a basic function of information processing — is relativly stable against dementia associated disturbance of brain functions and decreases only just in latest states of dementia. The loss of cognitive compensatory and interpreting functions however seems to be an earlier and stage independent consequence of dementia. Further studies are necessary in order to resolve this question and to evaluate the utility of our test for the early diagnosis of dementia.

References

Albizzati MG, Bassi S, Calloni E, Sbacchi M, Piolti R, Frattola L (1987) Cyclandelate versus flunarizine. A double-blind study in a selected group of patients with dementia. Drugs 33 [Suppl 2]: 90–96

Basso A, Bisiach E, Faglioni P (1974) The Mueller-Lyer illusion in patients with unilateral brain damage. Cortex 10: 26–35

Coren S, Girgus JS (1978) Seeing is deceiving: the psychology of visual illusions. Erlbaum, Hillsdale

Greene E, Tager RM (1979) The influence of stroke on visual illusion magnitude. Neurol Res 1: 169–177

Holland TR, Wadsworth HM (1979) Comparison and combination of recall and Background Interference Procedures for the Bender-Gestalt Test with brain-damaged and schizophrenic patients. J Personality Assessment 43: 123–127

Letourneau JE (1974) The Oppel-Kundt and the Muller-Lyer illusions among schizophrenics. Percept Mot Skills 39: 775–778

Margolis RB, Williger NR, Greenlief CL, Dunn EJ, Gfeller JD (1989) The sensitivity of the Bender-Gestalt Test as a screening instrument for neuropsychological impairment in older adults. J Psychol 123: 179–186

Mattingley JB, Bradshaw JL, Bradshaw JA (1995) The effects of unilateral visuospatial neglect on perception of Muller-Lyer illusory figures. Perception 24: 415–433

Mermelstein JJ (1983) A process approach to the Bender-Gestalt test and its use in differentiating schizophrenic, brain-damaged, and medical patients. J Clin Psychol 39: 173–182

Pardue AM (1975) Bender-Gestalt test and background interference procedure in discernment of organic brain damage. Percept Mot Skills 40: 103–109

Rund BR, Landro NI, Orbeck AL, Nysveen G (1994) Mueller-Lyer illusion and size estimation performance in schizophrenics compared to normal controls. Scand J Psychol 35: 193–197

Russell EW (1976) The Bender-Gestalt and the Halstead-Reitan battery: a case study. J Clin Psychol 32: 355–361

Storandt M (1990) Bender-Gestalt Test performance in senile dementia of the Alzheimer type. Psychol Aging 5: 604–606

van der Voordt DJ (1993) Losing your way in the nursing home: spatial orientation from an architectural viewpoint. A review. Tijdschr Gerontol Geriatr 24: 220–227

Authors' address: Dr. med. Dipl.-Psych. B. Weber, Department of Psychiatry and Psychotherapy I, J. W. Goethe University Frankfurt, Heinrich-Hoffmann-Strasse 10, D-60528 Frankfurt / Main, Federal Republic of Germany

Age and dementia effect on neuropsychological test performance in very old age — influence of risk factors for dementia*

F. M. Reischies[1], D. Felsenberg[3], R. Geßner[2], A. Kage[2], W. Rossius[1], and P. Schlattmann[1]

Departments of [1]Psychiatry and [3]Radiology, Free University Berlin, University Hospital Benjamin Franklin, and [2]Institute of Clinical Chemistry and Biochemistry, Virchow Hospital, Humboldt University of Berlin, Berlin, Federal Republic of Germany

Summary. In old age a large part of the variance in cognitive performance in population samples is explained by normal aging; in addition many subjects over 80 years are demented and therefore dementia also explains a part of cognitive variability. The question is whether the different factors for dementia (such as ApoE4, external atrophy parameter of the cranial computer tomography [cCT], education, sex or serum zinc level) influence the relation between age or dementia and Mini Mental State (MMSE) performance. In an epidemiological study data were analyzed of N = 239 subjects for the above factors. Most statistically significant variables of the MMSE do not change the amount of the partial correlation coefficient between the parameters age or dementia and MMSE. The external atrophy, however, diminishes the magnitude of the partial correlation between age and MMSE. In contrast the dementia-MMSE relation is unchanged. This points to a generally similar factor structure of cognitive aging and dementia in old age, but differences exist with respect to the importance of the external atrophy parameter of the brain. Most factors investigated explain separate parts of variance of cognitive performance in old age.

* The research reported is part of the multidisciplinary Berlin Aging Study (BASE). BASE is conducted by the Committee on Aging and Societal Development of the Berlin-Brandenburg Academy of Sciences and Technology in Berlin in collaboration with the Free University Berlin, the Humboldt University, and the Max Planck Institute for Human Development and Education, Berlin. The project has been supported financially by several organisations including the German Federal Minestry for Research and Technology (1989–91, 13 TA 011 +13 TA 011/A) and the German Federal Ministry for Family, Senior Citizens, Women, and youth (1992–97, 314-1722-102/9 + 314-1722-102/9a). The Berlin Aging study is directed by a steering commitee consisting of P. B. Baltes (chair), K. U. Mayer (vice chair), H. Helmchen, and E. Steinhagen-Thiessen.

Introduction

Age is the most important risk factor of dementia (Jorm et al., 1987). Some of the pathological processes which lead to a clinical dementia syndrome may require many years for development, and this could explain why the demented subjects are old when the clinical syndrome starts. There is an age effect on cognition even within the adult age span which has been demonstrated in longitudinal investigations (Schaie, 1994); cognitive performance is diminished by about one standard deviation of the performance of the young subjects. Thus cognitive performance at an age of about 70 years is already influenced by a certain amount of aging effects. For old age (70 to 100 years) an even stronger age effect has been shown in cross-sectional data (Reischies et al., 1996) i.e. about one to two standard deviations of reduction between 70 to about 100 years. The age effect on cognitive performance may have much in common with the dementia effect, and some researchers assume senile dementia as accelerated aging which is classified as pathological. This argument can be called the continuity position (see Brayne et al., 1988). If this hypothesis is true, then one would expect that age and dementia effects on cognitive performance will be influenced in the same way by variables such as sex or education (Amaducci et al., 1994), and biological variables such as brain atrophy, ApoE4 status or serum zinc level (Reischies et al., submitted).

There are arguments, however, in favor of a distinction of aging processes and dementia diseases, which represents a discontinuity position. It has been shown, that the distribution of neuropsychological dementia scores has bimodal features in a mixture distribution analysis (Reischies et al., 1996). Additionally the speed of deterioration of Mini Mental State Examination Scores (MMSE, Folstein et al., 1975) is much higher than reported for the nondemented elderly (Reischies et al., 1997; Brayne et al., 1995) as well as the speed of the change in mediotemporal CT atrophy (Jobst et al., 1994). Qualitative differences between features of cognitive aging and symptoms of dementia exist: reduction of speed is found in cognitive aging (Salthouse et al., 1994; Lindenberger et al., 1994), but in contrast, learning and fluency deficits are found in early dementia (Grober et al., 1988; Reischies and Lindenberger, 1995; Reischies et al., submitted).

In order to compare the effects of age and dementia we chose the MMSE performance as an appropriate variable, because the MMSE tests the symptoms of the dementia syndrome and has a strong age effect as well (Crum et al., 1993; Reischies et al., 1997). An analysis of the interrelations of risk factors is required, because they may be interrelated and therefore explain the same part of the variance of neuropsychological test performance between subjects of old age. If a variable is related to a depending variable and a third variable is correlated with both the first and the dependent variable, the effect of the first variable is reduced when adjusting for the effect of the third variable. The question was: are risk factors for dementia such as education or ApoE4 etc. related more to the age or more to the dementia effect on the MMSE? If age and dementia explain the same variance of the MMSE performance, all additional risk factors for dementia should affect the age- and dementia effect in a uniform way. The continuity position would claim that the risk factors should change both the age and dementia effect to the same extent, whereas the discontinuity position will predict differences in the relation of risk factors to the age and dementia effect on MMSE performance; especially because of the inclusion of risk factors of dementia in the regression models one would expect that there is a relevant change in the MMSE-variance explained by dementia.

Material and methods

As part of an epidemiological study, the subjects of which were randomly drawn from the Berlin registration office (BASE, Baltes et al., 1993), 239 subjects were investigated by CT scan, ApoE4 genotype determination and for further risk factors for dementia. The average age was 81.46 (sd 7.71) and 44% were females. A research psychiatrist investigated the subjects, applying the Geriatric Mental State-A interview and History and Aetiology Schedule (Copeland et al., 1991), and using the DSM-III-R dementia criteria (290.00). Dementia diagnosis was given according to a clinical evaluation after the interview and a consensus conference together with the geriatric colleagues who performed the somatic investigation. The parameter of the external atrophy was quantitatively determined by a highlighting procedure and relating the area of extracranial CSF at Masui Level 8/15° and Masui Level 9/15° to the respective intracranial area (Matsui et al., 1978). Blood samples were drawn and the apolipoprotein E genotype was determined by restriction isotyping following DNA amplification. Details of the method as well as the frequency of the ApoE4 genotypes are described in detail elsewhere (Geßner et al., 1997). Serum zinc concentration was quantified by absorption spectroscopy (AAS PU 9100X, s. Fimmel et al., 1994). Regression models which explain the variance of MMSE performance were calculated (SPSS), inicially including age and dementia (Table 2, 2-factor solution). The contribution of each individual risk factor is expressed by the partial correlation coefficient (PCC). This parameter is the correlation coefficient of the individual risk factor with the MMSE score after correcting for the linear influence of the other risk factors in the model.

Results

The mean MMSE of the population was 26.82 (sd 3.13, see Fig. 1 for the total population). The dementia rating was $0 = $ no, $1 = $ mild, $2 = $ moderate, and $3 = $ severe (according to the DSM-III-R criteria), 24 subject were demented. Age has been included in the models in 5 years-agegroups in order to have a comparable scale with respect to dementia. For the factor External Atrophy of the brain (CT-EA) the mean parameter was 0.13 (sd 0.06) and formal education 11.07 yrs. (sd 2.42). The mean Zn serum level was 11.85 (sd 2.04) micromol/l. ApoE4 had a mean frequency of 17% (s. Geßner et al., 1997).

The explanation of the variance of the MMSE by age and dementia resulted in a multiple $R = 0.67$, which is high, given an average retest reliability of ca. 0.85. These two variables explain 44.3% of the variance of the MMSE. The individual contribution of the variables was for dementia PCC = 0.55 and for age PCC = 0.41 (see Table 1, Fig. 2).

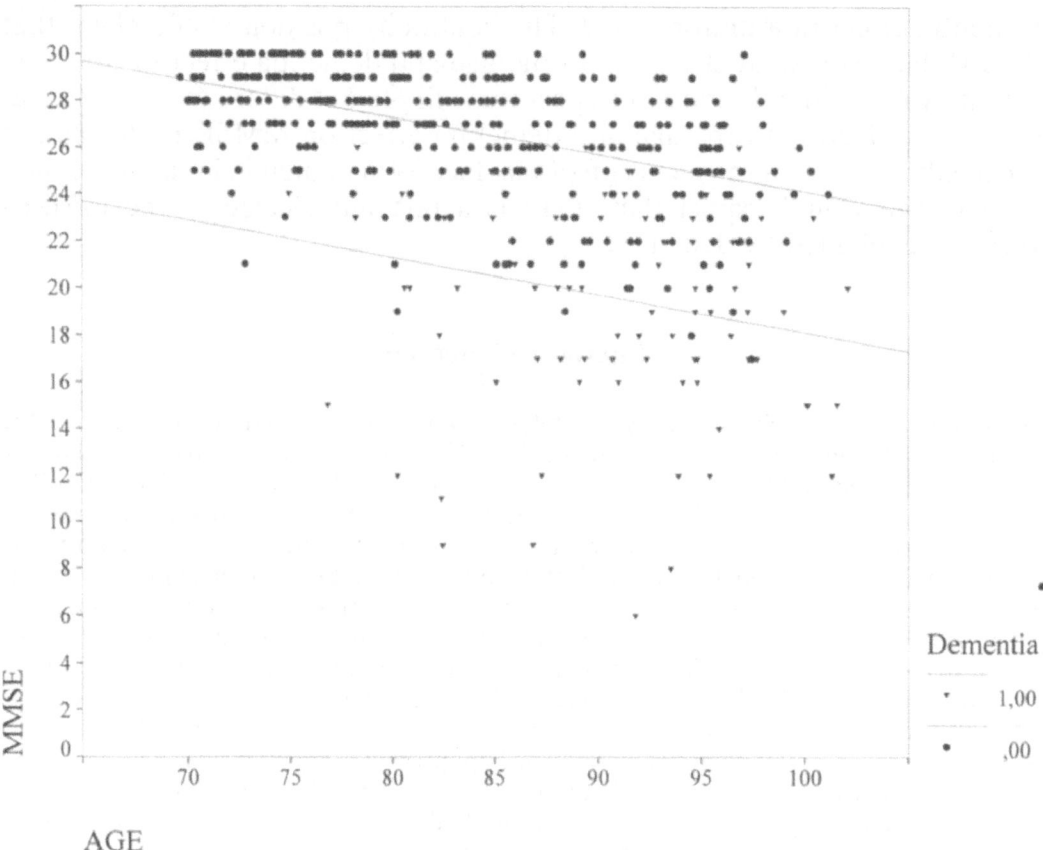

Fig. 1. Age and dementia regression-lines for the MMSE in the total population of the Berlin Aging Study. Age and dementia explain a large part of the variance of cognitive performance in old age

Table 1. Correlation coefficient between dementia factors and MMSE score. Partial correlation coefficient in regression models including either age and dementia (2-factor model) or in 3-factor models each time one of the rest of the factors: external atrophy, Zn, education, ApoE4 or sex

	Single correlation of factor	Partial correlation of factor in the model	Age effect (PCC)	Dementia effect (PCC)
2-factor model (age and dementia)			−.414	−.551
3-factor models				
CT-Ext. Atrophy	−.414	−.234***	−.326	−.533
Zinc	.191	.187**	−.429	−.561
Education	.174	.216**	−.412	−.526
ApoE4	−.063	−.010	−.408	−.568
Sex	.015	−.046	−.416	−.550

T test of the individual factor in the 3-factor models (only for PCC), p level * <0.05 ** <0.01 *** <0.001

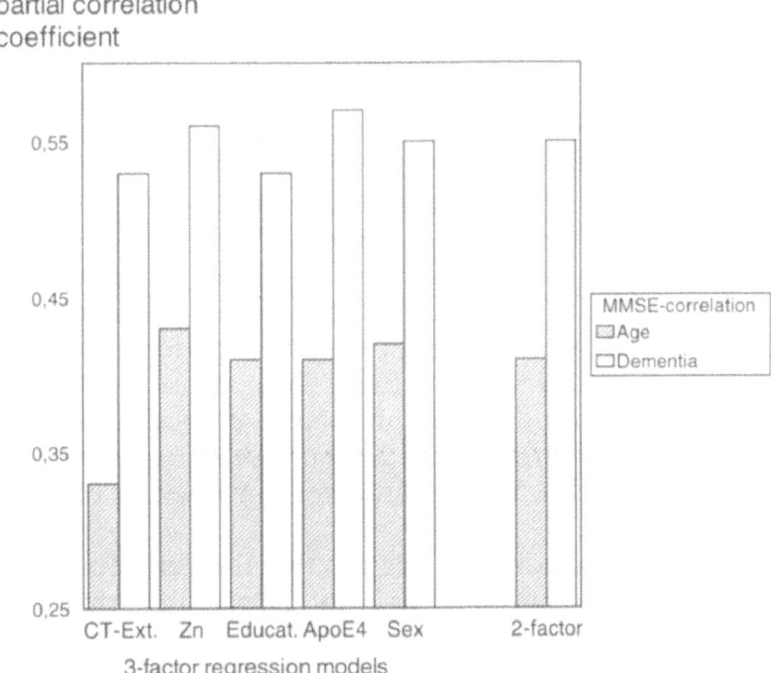

Fig. 2. Change of the partial correlation coefficient between dementia or age and the MMSE-performance, if different factors of dementia are included as third variable in individual 3-factor-regression models. A substantial change is found only for age and external atrophy of the brain

After adding in individual regression models the additional factors for dementia, each time as a third variable, the PCC of dementia was not substantially changed (see Table 1, Fig. 2). This was true also for the age effect with the exception of the CT-EA. After inclusion of CT-EA a substantial reduction was found only of the age effect on MMSE (see Table 1, Fig. 2); the same results were found when the dementia was binary coded (demented vs. nondemented). For statistical comparison, the MMSE-residuals, accounting for dementia and CT-EA, were correlated with age and compared with the models including the other risk factors. For CT-EA the correlation between the residual and age (years) was -0.28, for Zn -0.42 (difference $p < 0.05$). If the age and dementia-interaction is included in the regression models no substantial changes in the pattern of results are found.

Discussion

The results indicate that age and dementia explain a large part of the variance of the MMSE, a test performance which comprises the features of the cognitive dementia syndrome; this holds true in old subjects of a population based sample. One could expect that e.g. education may be either unrelated or more strongly related to the age effect than to the dementia effect. The results indicate, however, that each of the risk factor for dementia explain to a large extent its separate part of the variance of cognitive performance in old age. One exception must be discussed. The CT-EA, which is an indicator of cortical atrophy, obviously explains a part of the variance also explained by age. Because these two variables share the explanation of the same part of the variance of MMSE-performance, the individual PPC decrease (see Table 1).

According to the data it can be postulated that age and dementia have a different factor structure, because in this sample CT-EA alters only the age- but not to the dementia effect. This argues against the continuity hypothesis. It is noteworthy, that the known risk factors for dementia explain a part of the variance in the dementia-related cognitive performance (MMSE) not explained by the age and dementia effect. Thus one can speculate, that these risk factors may influence dementia in a more unspecific way; they may be related to cognitive impairment and an increase of vulnerability but not to the dementia process. The results, however, have yet to be replicated in a larger sample.

One possible explanation of the data is that the dementia disease leads to a very rapid cognitive decline, but this is not the case in normal aging (see Fig. 3). The data confirm the view that some factors may only increase the risk of

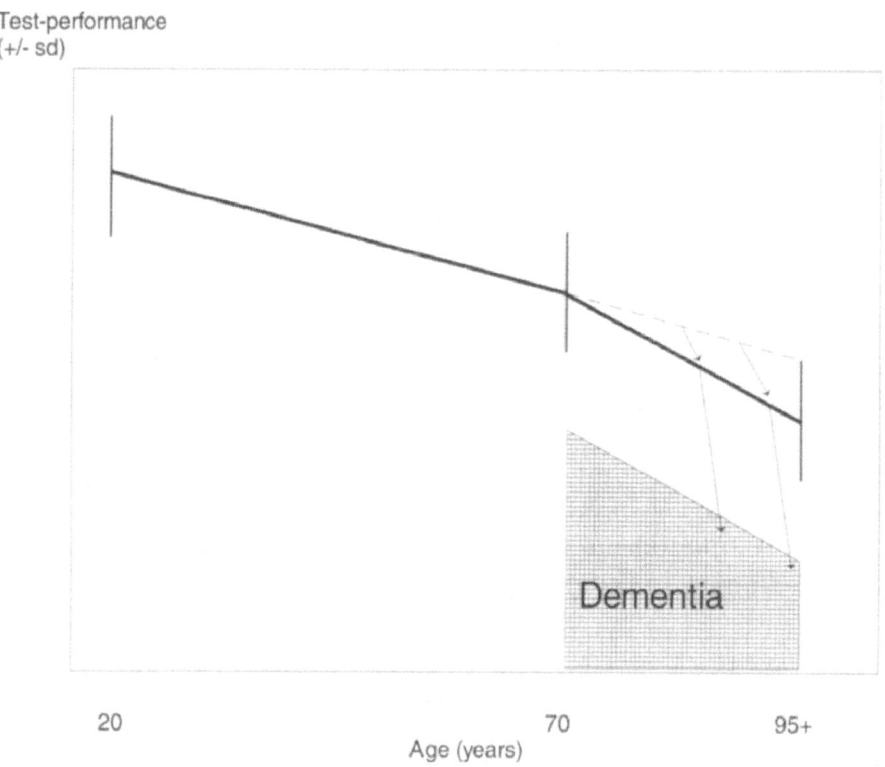

Fig. 3. Lifetime age related-cognitive decline and the acceleration of age related cognitive decline in old age. A mixture of subjects with normal cognitive aging and dementia may explain the accelerated age effect and the dementia effect on the cognitive performance in old age, which is assessed in cross sectional studies. There seem to be a discontinuity between age and dementia-effect, dementia cases show a much more rapid deterioration

the incidence of a dementia disease. The group of diagnosed dementia cases in epidemiological samples mostly comprises the rapid declining subjects in the quick transition period between mild cognitive decline and a terminal state (see Fig. 3). A certain overlap exists because dementia cases are investigated at different stages of the disease and because a part of the dementia in very old age consists of subjects with normal age-related cognitive deterioration but due to various reasons start from a lower cognitive level at adulthood (Reischies, 1998). In old age a part of the age effect can be explained by those incipient dementia cases whose cognitive performance already declined to some extent (Fig. 3).

References

Amaducci L, Lippi A (1994) Risk factors. In: Copeland JRM, Abou-Saleh MT, Blazer DG (eds) Principles and practice of geriatric psychiatry. Wiley, New York, pp 283–292

Baltes PB, Mayer KU, Helmchen H, Steinhagen-Thiessen E (1993) The Berlin Aging Study (BASE): overview and design. Aging and Society 13: 483–515

Braak H, Braak E (1991) Neuropathological stageing of Alzheimer-related changes. Acta Neuropathol 82: 239–259

Brayne C, Calloway P (1988) Normal ageing, impaired cognitive funciton, and senile dementia of the Alzheimer's type: a continuum? Lancet i: 1265–1267

Brayne C, Gill C, Paykel ES, Huppert F, O'Connor DW (1995) Cognitive decline in an elderly population — a two wave study of change. Psychol Med 25: 673–683

Copeland JR, Dewey ME, Saunders P (1991) The epidemiology of dementia: GMS-AGECAT studies of prevalence and incidence, including studies in progress. Eur Arch Psychiatr Clin Neurosci 240: 212–217

Corder EH, Saunders AM, Strittmatter WJ, Schmechel DE, Gaskell PC, Small GW, Roses AD, Haines JL, Pericak-Vance MA (1993) Gene dose of apolipoprotein E type 4 allele and the risk of Alzheimer's disease in late onset families. Science 261: 921–923

Crum RM, Anthony JC, Basset SS, Folstein MF (1993) Population based norms for the mini-mental state examination by age and education level. JAMA 269: 2386–2391

Fimmel S, Borchelt M, Kage A, Köttgen E (1994) Trace elements and carrier proteins in the aged. Arch Geriat Geriatr [Suppl] 4: 67–74

Folstein MF, Folstein SE, McHugh PR (1975) "Mini Mental State": a practical method for grading the cognitive state of patients for the clinician. J Psychiatr Res 12: 189–198

Geßner R, Reischies FM, Kage A, Geiselmann B, Borchelt M, Steinhagen-Thiessen E, Köttgen E (1997) In an epidemiological sample the apolipoprotein E4 allele is associated to dementia and loss of memory only in the very old. Neurosci Lett 222: 29–32

Grober E, Buschke H, Crystal H, Bang S, Dresner R (1988) Screening for dementia by memory testing. Neurol 38: 900–903

Jobst KA, Smith AD, Szatmari M, Esiri MM, Jaskowski A, Hindley N, McDonald B, Molyneux AJ (1994) Rapidly pregressing atrophy of medial temporal lobe in Alzheimer's disease. Lancet 343: 829–830

Jorm AF, Korten AE, Henderson AS (1987) The prevalence of dementia: a quantitative integration of the literature. Acta Psychiatr Scand 76: 465–479

Lindenberger U, Mayr U, Kliegl R (1993) Speed and intelligence in old age. Psychol Aging 8: 207–220

Matsui T, Hirano A (1978) An atlas of the human brain for computerized tomography. G Fischer — Igaku Shoin, Stuttgart

Reischies FM (1998) Age related cognitive decline and the dementia threshold. In: Lomranz J (ed) Handbook of aging and mental health. Plenum, New York (in press)

Reischies FM, Lindenberger U (1995) Discontinuity of dementia and age-related cognitive decline. In: Bergener M, Brocklehurst JC, Finkel SI (eds) Aging, health and healing. Springer, New York, pp 204–211

Reischies FM, Lindenberger U (1996) Grenzen und Potentiale kognitiver Leistungen im hohen Alter. In: Mayer KU, Baltes PB (eds) Die Berliner Altersstudie. Akademie Verlag, Berlin, pp 351–377

Reischies FM, Schaub RT (1997) Epidemiologische Verlaufsuntersuchungen der Demenz. In: Rösler M, Retz W, Thome J (Hrsg) Alzheimer Krankheit. Deutscher Studien Verlag, Weinheim, S 58–66

Reischies FM, Geiselmann B (1997) Age related cognitive decline and vision impairment affecting the detection of dementia syndrome in old age. Br J Psychiatry 171: 449–451

Reischies FM, Kage A Zinc and senile dementia (submitted)

Reischies FM, Schaub RT, Schlattmann P (1996) Normal ageing, impaired cognitive functioning, and senile dementia — a mixture distribution analysis. Psychol Med 26: 785–790

Reischies FM, Geiselmann B, Lindenberger U Recall and learning in non-demented subjects of very old age and mild dementia — qualitative differences. (submitted)

Salthouse TA (1994) The nature of the influence of speed on adult age differences in cognition. Dev Psychol 30: 240–259

Schaie KW (1994) The course of adult intellectual development. Am Psychol 49: 304–313

Authors' address: F. M. Reischies, MD, Psychiatrische Klinik, Freie Universität Berlin, Eschenallee 3, D-14050 Berlin, Federal Republic of Germany

Neuropathology of Alzheimer's disease: a critical update

K. A. Jellinger and **C. Bancher**

L. Boltzmann Institute of Clinical Neurobiology, Vienna, Austria

Summary. The unequivocal diagnosis of Alzheimer's disease (AD) rests on histopathological evidence at brain autopsy or biopsy. The morphology of AD includes cerebral atrophy, deposition of βA4 amyloid (Aβ) (senile plaques and amyloid angiopathy), neuritic changes (neuritic plaques, neurofibrillary tangles (NFT) and neuropil threads) with formation of paired helical filaments (PHF) containing polymerized hyperphosphorylated tau protein triplet, causing disruption of the neuronal cytoskeleton with loss of synapses and neurons, with altered cortico-cortical connectivity, leading to disconnection of the cerebral cortex. Defining criteria for the morphologic diagnosis of AD is difficult due to the phenotypic hetero-geneity of the disease, the absence of specific markers, and overlap of AD morphology with that observed in non-demented elderly individuals. This gray zone between normal to pathologic aging and full-fledged AD represents an important diagnostic problem and should be overcome by better standard-ized criteria that will allow to minimize interrater and interlaboratory variabil-ity in the diagnosis of AD. Current criteria for the morphologic diagnosis of AD are based on (semi)quantitative assessment of diffuse and neuritic plaques (NIA), exclusively neuritic plaques (CERAD), plaques and NFT in neocortex and hippocampus (Tierney et al., 1988), and staging of hierarchic spreading of neuritic AD changes (Braak and Braak, 1991); all of them have weaknesses and need to be revalidated. Multivariant analysis of an autopsy series of elderly subjects revealed significant correlations between psychostatus and both the CERAD criteria and Braak staging. Recent recom-mendations of the NIA-Reagan Institute for the morphologic diagnosis of AD are presented. Although the role of plaques and NFT in the pathogenesis of AD remains undetermined, clinicopathological correlative studies have shown that both lesions, if present in sufficient numbers, particularly in the neocortex, are considered the best morphological signposts for AD. Recent studies on neuron death in AD that, at least in part, appears different from classical apoptosis and may precede the symptomatic stage of AD, have shown varying results indicating only indirect relationship between DNA fragmentation and both Aβ deposition and NFTs. Both these AD-typical markers appear to increase the risk of cells to degenerate, but are not the sole responsibles of the degenerative process in AD, the basic mechanisms of which remain to be elucidated.

Introduction

While the clinical diagnostic accuracy rate of probable Alzheimer's disease (AD) using established criteria and modern neuropsychological and neuroimaging methods is between 87 and 96% (Galasko et al., 1994; Gearing et al., 1995; Klatka et al., 1996; Kosunen et al., 1996) with a diagnostic sensitivity and specifity of 0.81–0.84% (Blacker et al., 1994), the unequivocal diagnosis of AD rests on histopathological evidence at brain autopsy and/or biopsy (Mirra et al., 1993). The morphology of AD includes cerebral atrophy due to selective neuronal loss associated with neuritic changes — neuritic plaques (NP), neurofibrillary tangles (NFT) and neuropil threads (NT) — with formation of paired helical filaments (PHF) comprised mainly of abnormally hyperphosphorylated microtubule-associated tau protein triplet, and extracellular deposition of β-A4 amyloid (Aβ) forming part of diffuse, classical and primitive plaques and amyloid angiopathy (Table 1). Progressive disruption of the neuronal cytoskeleton due to accumulation of PHF leads to loss of neurons and synapses with involvement of specific neuronal populations (Hyman, 1996) with altered cortico-cortical connectivity, leading to specific neuronal system disruption and disconnection of the cerebral cortex as major correlates of dementia (Terry et al., 1991; Hof and Morrison, 1994). The relationship between Aβ deposition and tau pathology to neuronal loss and to each other as well as the relationship of these changes to aging are areas of current scientific interest (Dickson, 1997). In addition, these multiple lesions in Alzheimer brain are not necessarily specific for AD, since Aβ deposits without NFT/PHF occur early in life in Down's syndrome (Leverenz and Raskind, 1998), in normal aging and other conditions and, therefore, may not necessarily induce PHF, while in a variety of other disorders NFT/PHF are present with only few or even no Aβ deposits

Table 1. Histopathology of Alzheimer's disease (diagnostic features)

1. Amyloid (Aβ) deposits: senile plaques
                          amyloid angiopathy
2. Cytoskeletal pathology
   Neurons: Neurofibrillary tangles ⎤
   Dendrites: Neuropil threads   ⎬ PHF
   Neuropil: Neuritic plaques   ⎦
3. Neuron loss ⟹ cerebral atrophy
4. Loss of synapses/synaptic markers
5. Microglial activation (nonspecific; immunologic?)
6. Astroglial proliferation — reactive
7. Strategic spreading of cytoskeletal changes
   Allocortex ⟹ isocortex ⟹ subcortical nuclei
              Diagnostic: 1. Plaques
                          2. Tangles

and thus abnormal tau pathology may not necessarily lead to the formation of amyloid (Table 2).

Morphologic criteria for the diagnosis of Alzheimer's disease

There is not yet a definite set of criteria for the neuropathologic diagnosis of AD. To address this problem, several sets of research criteria have been forward. They are based on age-adjusted numerical assessment of the classical AD markers — SP and NFT:

(1) The most widely used in the past are the NIA criteria (Khachaturian, 1985) based on the age-related minimum number of SP in neocortex with/without additional NFT. These criteria have been criticized because they did not specify a stain or a specific brain region in which quantification should be performed nor the type of plaques (amyloid vs neuritic with tau/PHF positive neurites);

(2) A rarely used set of criteria is based on the semiquantitative assessment of plaques and NFT in neocortex and hippocampus (Tierney et al., 1988) which, at least in part, disregards neocortical AD lesions.

(3) To overcome laboratory to laboratory staining variability and interrater differences in counting, the Consortium to Establish a Registry for Alzheimer's Disease (CERAD) criteria depend on semiquantitative assessment of neuritic plaques using a 4-grade scale (none to frequent) in three neocortical areas and integration of age-related NP scores with clinical history of dementia to determine the level certainty of AD diagnosis (possible, probable, definite) (Mirra et al., 1991,1994). A version of these criteria has been presented as a "primer for practising pathologists" to make the

Table 2. Does the one cause the other? (modified from Terry, 1996; Spillantini et al., 1996; Esiri et al., 1997)

PHF without significant amyloid	β-amyloid without tau pathology
Postencephalitic parkinsonism	"normal" and pathological aging
Guam Parkinson-dementia complex	Plaque-only Alzheimer disease
Progressive supranuclear palsy	
Dementia pugilistica	Lewy body dementia
Gerstmann-Sträußler-Scheinker disease with NFT	
NFT predominant type of dementia Autosomal dominant dementia with NFT	Familial cerebral amyloid angiopathies
Multiple system tauopathy	Cerebral injury
Subacute sclerosing panencephalitis	Cerebral ischemia
Niemann-Pick type C	Arterio-venous malformation
Kuf's disease	Aged primate and dog
Ataxia-telangiectasia	Athena tg mouse
Lead poisoning	APP transgenic mouse[b]

[a]Masliah et al. (1995), [b]Hsiao et al. (1996)

diagnosis of AD (Mirra et al., 1993). However, the CERAD criteria disregard NFT and allocortical AD changes, and give no standardized description of NP which might be helpful in the distinction between normal and pathological aging or early (preclinical) and late stage (definite) AD. In addition, neither of these criteria attempts to differentiate "mild" from "severe" disease, in part because they have not been correlated with the degree of clinical impairment and do not consider the hierarchical distribution of AD lesions.

(4) Independently of the numeric assessment of histologic AD markers a staging of neuritic changes, particularly NFT, according to its hierarchical spreading from the inferotemporal allocortex via hippocampus to neocortical association areas has been proposed by Braak and Braak (1991) which, however, disregards NP and gives no quantification of NFT. In addition, the distribution of NFT is independent of the more general pattern of Aβ deposits throughout the frontal, temporal and parietal lobes for which three spreading stages have been suggested. In general, initial NFT stages I and II develop in the absence of Aβ deposits, while the terminal NFT stages V and VI representing fully developed stages of AD are usually associated with end stages of Aβ deposition involving densely myelinated primary neocortical areas (Braak and Braak, 1996).

(5) Since one may adopt different diagnostic approaches in subjects with clinically manifest dementia and those without cognitive impairment or of unknown psychostatus, we proposed the following criteria for the interpretation of histopathologic findings in patients aged 65 years or older (Table 3):

A) In patients with clinically manifest dementia three morphological constellations allow a diagnosis of *definite AD* independent of age:

1. At least 15 SP (all types except for diffuse Aβ deposits) and/or NP/mm^2 in at least two neocortical areas (frontal, temporal or parietal) and at least 3 NFT/mm^2 in at least one neocortical area. All of these cases will have

Table 3. Recommended histopathologic criteria for the diagnosis of Alzheimer's disease (Jellinger and Bancher, 1997)

A) *Demented subjects*		
a) >15 neocortical SP (all types except diffuse βA4 deposits) and/or NP	and >3 neocortical NFT	
b) >15 neocortical SP (all types except diffuse βA4 deposits) and/or NP	and >10 CA$_1$/subiculum NFT	definite AD
c)	>15 CA$_1$/subiculum NFT	
B) *Non-demented subjects, subjects with unknown psychostatus*		
a) >15 neocortical SP (all types except diffuse βA4 deposits) and/or NP	and >3 neocortical NFT	
b) >20 neocortical SP (all types except diffuse βA4 deposits) and/or >10 neocortical NP	and >10 CA$_1$/subiculum NFT → preclinical AD	

→ Staging of neuritic pathology according to Braak and Braak (1991)

substantial numbers of NFT in allocortical areas that need not to be assessed in detail. This category corresponds to CERAD score C (definite AD) and to Braak stages V and VI.

2. At least 15 SP and/or NP/mm^2 in at least two neocortical areas and at least 10 NFT in subiculum and hippocampal CA 1 sector without neocortical NFT. This category corresponds to CERAD score B (probable AD) and to Braak's limbic stage IV and is comparable to the "plaque-only" type of AD (Terry et al., 1987; Katzman et al., 1988; Corey-Bloom et al., 1997).

3. At least 15 NFT/mm^2 in subiculum and hippocampal sector CA 1, and presence of large numbers of NFT in the parahippocampal cortex, irrespective of the presence of SP or NP. This category correspond, at least in part, to the "NFT-predominant type" of senile dementia (Bancher and Jellinger, 1994; Ulrich et al., 1992; Ikeda et al., 1997; Jellinger and Bancher, 1998). If there is severe neuronal loss in the hippocampus and/or entorhinal region, the number of required NFT may be reduced, but often there are extracellular "ghost" tangles or hippocampal sclerosis (Dickson et al., 1994).

B) In people without dementia or of unknown psychostatus, one histological constellation allows the diagnosis of definite AD and another one suggests preclinical AD.

a) At least 15 SP (all types except diffuse Aβ deposits) and/or NP/mm^2 in at least two neocortical areas and at least 3 NFT/mm^2 in at least one neocortical area. This category corresponding to Braak stages V and VI will only very rarely be found in subjects with unimpaired intellectual functions (Tables 4 and 5).

b) At least 10 NP/mm^2 and/or at least 20 SP/mm^2 in at least two neocortical areas and at least 10 NFT in subiculum and hippocampal sector CA 1 without neocortical NFT. This category corresponding to Braak stage IV, with the presence of either NP or very high numbers of Aβ deposits surpasses age-associated pathology at any age and suggests incipient/preclinical AD or "pathologic aging" (Dickson et al., 1991; Morris et al., 1991, 1996; Troncoso et al., 1996; Gomez et al., 1996). Small numbers of NFT may be present in layers V of the inferior temporal isocortex adjacent to the transentorhinal region, and at least 2–3 NFT may also be seen in frontal, temporal or parietal cortices.

In demented patients under age 65, these criteria may be adjusted downwards, although early onset AD usually is associated with severe histopathology, while the distribution pattern of neuritic AD lesions in very old people over age 90 is distinct from young patients (Ulrich et al., 1992; Giannokopoulos et al., 1995, 1996).

The interlaboratory comparison of neuropathological assessment of AD showed reasonable interrater agreement for semiquantitative analysis but significant differences of SP and NFT counts based on methodological (staining techniques) and interpretation variations (Duyckaerts et al., 1990; Mirra et al., 1994; Bancher et al., 1997) although, under optimal conditions and using standardized criteria, a substantial to almost perfect interrater agreement can be obtained (Paulus et al., 1992; Chui et al., 1993; McKeel et al., 1993).

Table 4. Relationship between psychostatus (MMSE) and morphological Alzheimer disease criteria in 104 consecutive autopsy cases

MMSE Mean age (yrs)	0–10 (n = 66) 86.0	11–22 (n = 29) 88.0	24–30 (n = 9) 77.8
Morphology criteria			
Khachaturian pos.	63	19	5
neg.	3*	10	4
Tierney et al. A2	55	5	0
A1	10	14	
neg.	2*	10*	
CERAD C (definite AD)	49	1	0
B (probable AD)	7	6	
A (possible AD)	6	10	
0 (negative)	4*	12**	9
Braak/Braak stages 5 + 6	50	0	
5	0	2	0
4–5	8	5	0
4	6* (3$^+$)	11	1
3	2$^+$	9*	1
2	0	2	4
0–1	0	0	3

*,** Neurofibrillary predominant type (n = 5*/6**), $^+$ Lewy body dementia (n = 4)

Multiple regression analysis				
Variable	CERAD	Braak	Tierney et al.	NIA
Sig T	.0000	.0003	.2430	.7891

Clinico-pathological correlations

The presence of multiple types of brain lesions makes it difficult to determine exactly which ones are responsible for cognitive dysfunction. While earlier studies have shown positive correlations between the degree of dementia with neocortical SP (Wilcock and Eisiri, 1982), recent studies support the notion that the number of neuritic AD changes, in particular neocortical NFT, more reliably corresponds to the degree of dementia (Morris et al., 1991; Dickson et al., 1991; Arriagada et al., 1992; McKee et al., 1992; Bancher et al., 1993; Bierer et al., 1995a; Nagy et al., 1995). Recent quantitative studies of Aβ deposition in neocortex showed that, although Alzheimer brains contain far more Aβ than controls, the amount does not seem to increase with longer duration of illness (Hyman et al., 1993), is not a predictor of cognitive deterioration, at least during the subsequent few years (Mackenzie et al., 1996), and shows little progression from the time of biopsy to autopsy (Bennett et al., 1993; Gearing et al., 1996). In contrast, large amounts of Aβ-only SP are present in non-demented aged subjects and, in general, neither their regional

Table 5. Relationship between psychostatus (MMSE) and morphological Alzheimer disease criteria in 104 consecutive autopsy cases

MMSE 0–10		(n = 66)	Khachaturian		CERAD			
			pos	neg	C	B	A	0
Braak/Braak	5 + 6	50	50	0	48	2	0	0
	4–5	8	8	0	0	4	4	0
	4	6 (3+)	4	2	0	0	3	3+
	3	2	1	1	0	1+	1	0

MMSE 11–22		(n = 29)	Khachaturian		CERAD			
			pos	neg	C	B	A	0
Braak/Braak	5	2	2	0	1	1	0	0
	4–5	5	5	0	0	3	2	0
	4	11	6	5	0	2	5	4*
	3	9	4	5	0	0	2	7*
	2	2	2	0	0	0	0	1

MMSE 23–30		(n = 9)	Khachaturian		CERAD			
			pos	neg	C	B	A	0
Braak/Braak	4	1	3	1	0	0	0	1
	3	1	1	2	0	0	0	2
	2	4	3	0	0	0	3	
	0–1	3	0	3	0	0	0	3

*NF-dominant type (n = 11). +Lewy body dementia (n = 4)

pattern nor their amount is related to the degree, duration, or type of cognitive impairment (Delaere et al., 1991; Morris et al., 1991; Price et al., 1992; Berg et al., 1993; Crystal et al., 1993; Zhan et al., 1995), except in centennarians (Giannakopoulos et al., 1996). Since the accumulation of diffuse Aβ deposits is not an inevitable consequence of normal aging (Crystal et al., 1989; Kazee et al., 1993; Mackenzie, 1994; Morris et al., 1996) and is associated with cortical cholinergic deficits or fiber loss in non-demented seniors (Katzman et al., 1988; Perry et al., 1996; Beach et al., 1997) in which neuronal degeneration in neocortex and hippocampus have been demonstrated by DNA strand breaks as indicators for cell death (Troncoso et al., 1996b), this condition has been distinguished from AD as "pathological" aging (Dickson et al., 1991) and is now considered a preclinical/inicipient or early "very mild" stage of AD (Morris et al., 1991, 1996; Berg et al., 1993; Wang and Munoz, 1995). While these subjects showing abundant neocortical Aβ deposits with or without entorhinal/hippocampal NFT and rare neocortical NP or even NFT, at least in part, correspond to "possible" AD in the CERAD classification (Mirra et al., 1993), primary motor, sensory, and visual cortices are essentially free of neuritic AD pathology in cognitively intact elderly (Vermersch et al., 1995; Gertz et al., 1996; Esiri et al., 1997).

Statistical evaluation of the relationship between currently used morphologic diagnostic criteria of AD and the staging of neuritic AD lesions (Braak and Braak, 1991) with cognitive dysfunction using Mini-Mental state (MMS) (Folstein et al., 1975) in a consecutive autopsy series of 104 elderly individuals from the Prospective Vienna Dementia Study (Jellinger et al., 1992) with a mean age of 85.3 ± 5.5 years showed highly significant correlations between MMS and both CERAD criteria and Braak staging, less for the criteria by Tierney et al. (1988) and much weaker correlation for NIA criteria (Khachaturian, 1985) (Table 4). The CERAD criteria showed slightly higher correlations with psychostatus than the Braak staging, but less concordance with Tierney criteria, while the NIA criteria are often falsely positive in cognitively intact individuals not fitting into the other diagnostic criteria (Table 5). Positive correlations between cognitive deficit and the density of NFT in frontal and parietal lobes were reported using NIA and CERAD criteria, while these correlations were absent in cases fulfilling the Tierney A 3 criteria for AD (Nagy et al., 1995). Correlative studies of Braak staging with mental status using Blessed test (BTS) and MMS scores in two prospective cohorts of aged individuals showed a highly significant negative correlation between both parameters (Bancher et al., 1993, 1996; Braak et al., 1993). Figure 1 showing these relations in 106 consecutive autopsy cases of eldely patients without parkinsonian symptoms, clearly indicates that Braak stages V and VI featured by abundant NFT in neocortical association areas, are almost exclusively seen in a cluster of severely demented patients (MMS 0-5/30), while the limbic stages III and IV are associated with a wide range of cognitive

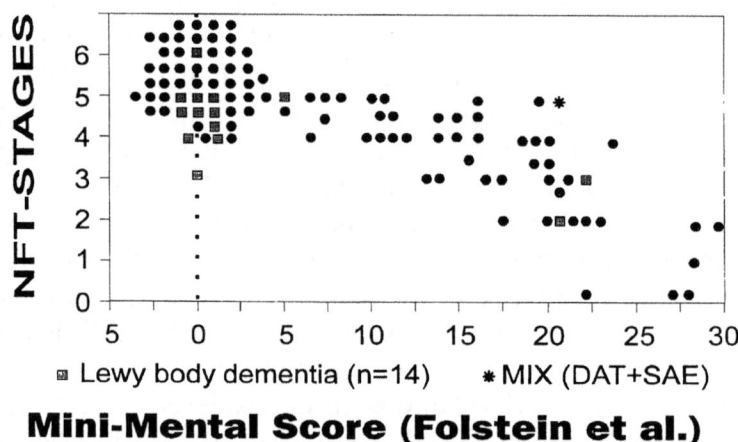

Fig. 1. Correlation between psychostatus (Mini-Mental-State score) and neuropathological stages of neuritic Alzheimer lesions in 106 consecutive elderly subjects (mean age 79.9 years)

performance between mentally almost intact to overt dementia (MMS 26-5/30). These data are in accordance with recent studies showing that the Braak staging does not reliably identify all cases clinically diagnosed as dementia (Xuereb et al., 1995; Gertz et al., 1996). Although the transition from Braak stage III to VI is often associated with the appearance of dementia, there is considerable overlap. The extent of NFT pathology in the allocortex does not provide a quantitative basis for understanding the appearance of dementia in late life, and does not correlate well in elderly subjects with either normal cognitive function or relatively mild levels of mental impairment, thus making the staging model of limited value for clinico-pathological evaluation studies (Gertz et al., 1996; Perl et al., 1997). The only brain region in which NFT counts provide a statistically significant marker for dementia is the association neocortex (Arriagada et al., 1992; Bancher et al., 1993; Bierer et al., 1995b; Nagy et al., 1995; Gertz et al., 1998).

While the majority of AD cases show neocortical "plaque and tangle" type pathology, there are other penotypical variants or subtypes of AD that will not fit into presently conceived diagnostic criteria, e.g. the "plaque-predominant" type (Terry et al., 1987; Corey-Bloom et al., 1997) with very little or no neuritic changes usually restricted to the entorhinal/hippocampal region that may or may not be associated with cortical Lewy bodies (Hansen et al., 1993). These patients may display either dementia or only minimal cognitive changes, with considerable degree of both clinical and morphological overlap and no clear-cut threshold (Bancher et al., 1996; Gertz et al., 1996). Another phenotype referred to as the "tangle predominant variant" of senile dementia (Ulrich et al., 1992; Bancher and Jellinger, 1994; Ikeda et al., 1997) in very old, often demented individuals shows abundant NFT and NT mainly in the allocortex and less in the isocortex, with no or only very few Aβ deposits in the absence of NP. It morphologically resembles some autosomal dominant dementias with NFT related to chromosome 17 (Spillantini et al., 1996, 1998). In contrast to classical AD, this subtype has high incidence of Apoliporotein ε2 or ε3 alleles (Ikeda et al., 1997; Bancher et al., 1997b), absence of Apoliprotein E e4 alleles (Table 6), but its relationship to classical (plaque and tangle) AD is currently unknown.

Other markers of AD severity that parallel well with mental dysfunction are reduced numbers of large and medium-sized neurons in entorhinal/ hippocampal areas (Hyman et al., 1984) and in neocortex (Terry et al., 1981), and synaptic loss in cortex (Scheff et al., 1990; DeKosky et al., 1990; Terry et al., 1991; Masliah, 1995; Heffernan et al., 1998) and in hippocampal areas (Samuel et al., 1994). The loss of synapses is greater than that of neurons and significantly correlates with neuritic AD pathology (Lassmann et al., 1992; Scheff and Price, 1993). It has been related to NFT bearing neurons (Callahan and Coleman, 1995; Gomez-Isla et al., 1997), although, according to some studies, the degree of synapse loss correlates not or only weakly with SP and NFT (Dickson et al., 1995; Heinonen et al., 1995; Blennow et al., 1996) suggesting that synaptic pathology is more closely related to cognitive decline (Terry, 1996). However, significances disappear after the exclusion of non-

Table 6. Tangle predominant senile dementia

a) Clinical features

Incidence:	26/500 autopsy cases of dementia = 4.3%
	26/380 cases with clinical AD diagnosis = 6.8%
	Ulrich et al. (1992): 10/500 demented = 2.0%
	Ikeda et al. (1997): 14/239 demented = 5.9%
Age:	87.0 ± 4.6 yrs (range 80–99 yrs)
Gender:	15/26 females
Duration:	3.7 ± 1.2 yrs (range — 10 yrs)
Clinical diagnosis:	possible AD 16/26
	probable AD 4/26
	mixed/unclear dementia 5/26
Main symptoms:	moderate to severe dementia — MMS 11/30 (range 0–20) (n = 10)
	disorientation 16/26
	paranoid 6/26; depressed 5/26 (n = 44)
Apo E allele frequency:	ε2 0.11; ε3 0.86; ε4 0.03
	Ikeda et al. (1997; n = 28): ε2 0.39; ε3 0.50, ε4 0.11

b) Neuropathology

Cerebral atrophy:	moderate to severe (brain weight 1,091 ± 109 g) (range 890–1,340 g)
NFT:	moderate to severe in allocortex (25/26); mild in isocortex (6/26)
Aβ plaques:	rare: entorhinal 6/26; isocortex 3/26
Neuritic plaques:	none
Amyloid angiopathy:	rare (5/26)
Subcortical NFT:	nucl. basalis 14/26; locus ceruleus 7/26; substantia nigra 2/26; otherwise none
Lacunar state:	microscars 11/26; cerebral infarcts 2/26
Hippocampal sclerosis:	3/26
NIA/Khachaturian:	neg. 25/26
Tierney et al.:	neg. 24/26; A 2/26
Braak staging:	III 2/26; IV 20/26; IV–V 4/26

demented subjects with few or no AD pathology that could have been driving the strong correlations with pathological markers (Dickson et al., 1995), indicating a qualitative rather than a quantitative relation between synapse loss and dementia, since the PHF type neuritic degeneration correlates better with cognitive dysfunction in AD than synapse loss (Dickson et al., 1995; Trojanowski et al., 1995). The mechanism of synaptic pathology and neuronal degeneration that appear to have a central role in the multistep pathogenesis of AD are not yet fully established (Terry, 1996), but recent studies suggest that, although both the local contact with Aβ deposits and the presence of NFT considerably increase the risk of neurons to degenerate, neither lesion may be the sole responsible for programmed cell death in AD (Lassmann et al., 1995; Bancher et al., 1997), while other factors including cell cycle disturbances may trigger neuronal degeneration (Nagy et al., 1997b).

Other studies indicate that neuritic pathology of the cholinergic nucleus basalis of Meynert is a strong predictor of memory deficits in AD (Samuel et al., 1995) reflecting disruption of the basal forebrain cholinergic system confirmed by many morphologic and neurochemical studies (Bierer et al., 1995a; Perry et al., 1996; Poirier et al., 1996; Kasa et al., 1997). Cortical cholinergic denervation in AD is regionally correlated to cytoskeletal pathology, in particular the density of NFT, but not to the density of Aβ deposits (Geula et al., 1998). These and other data strongly suggest that in AD dementia finally results from the breakdown/disconnection of neuronal networks involving both cortical-cortical and cortical-subcortical, limbic, and association circuits (Hof and Morrison, 1994; Hyman, 1996).

Comorbidity and other superimposed pathology may influence the clinical and morphologic features of Alzheimer patients, since a considerable proportion of them shows overlapping or confounding disorders, e.g. cerebrovascular or other cytoskeletal lesions (Jellinger, 1996). A variety of confounding brain lesions can be seen that lead to a diagnosis of subsets of AD, e.g. Lewy body variant of AD (Hansen et al., 1993) or AD with superimposed infarcts or minor cerebrovascular lesions (lacunar state, etc) seen in 20 to 50% of AD brains (Gearing et al., 1995; Kosunen et al., 1995; Jellinger, 1996; Chui et al., 1996), mixed AD and vascular dementia (VaD) with infarcts totalling 50 ml or more or involving strategic brain areas (Pratt and Cervos-Navarro, 1995) ranging in incidence from less than 2 to about 8% (Galasko et al., 1994; Victoroff et al., 1995; Klatka et al., 1996; Giannokopoulos et al., 1996; Sevush et al., 1996). AD with extensive subcortical neuronal and glial tau pathology indicating concomitant progressive supranuclear palsy (PSP) (Hauw et al., 1994; Litvan et al., 1996) or AD with Lewy bodies either in the brainstem (Parkinson's disease with concomitant/superimposed AD) (Jellinger, 1996; Gearing and Mirra, 1997) or fitting the criteria of dementia with Lewy bodies (DLB) (McKeith et al., 1996) are also to be considered.

Conclusions and critical outlook

Recent work has demonstrated that none of the currently used neuropathologic diagnostic protocols or criteria is likely to be satisfactory for both clinical and research purposes in AD. In view of the etiologic, genetical and phenotypical heterogeneity of the disorder, defining appropriate, transferable, versatile and validated diagnostic criteria for AD and its various subtypes has proven difficult. Therefore, a re-evaluation and re-assessment of postmortem diagnostic criteria for AD has been suggested at a recent consensus meeting sponsored by the National Institute of Aging (NIA) and the Reagan Institute of the Alzheimer's Association. These recommendations for improving the neuropathologic criteria for the diagnosis of AD include the following (Hyman and Trojanowski, 1997):

A. Guiding principles for the postmortem diagnosis of AD

1. AD is a heterogeneous clinico-pathological entity. Thus, based on the pathological changes detected in the postmortem brain alone (i.e., Alzheimer

lesions), only probabilistic statements about the presence or absence of dementia can be made in a given patient. Similarly, the presence or amount of Alzheimer lesions in the postmortem brain can only be inferred and not predicted with certainty when a progressive dementia has been documented ante mortem in an elderly individual.

2. Since dementia in an elderly individual may arise from more than one disorder, more than one pathological process (i.e. stroke, Parkinson's disease, PSP, etc.), in addition to Alzheimer lesions, may contribute to the dementia in many patients.

3. Any AD-related changes in the postmortem brain (i.e., diffuse amyloid or neuritic plaques, neurofibrillary tangles) are considered to be abnormal and should be recorded as such. In other words, these changes are considered to be pathological even in instances where they appear to be incidental.

B. Neuropathological assessment

The following categories are recommended to provide an estimate of the likelihood that Alzheimer changes underlie dementia:

1. There is a *high* likelihood that dementia is due to AD lesions, when the postmortem brain shows the presence of both NP and NFT in neocortex (i.e., a frequent NP score according to CERAD for AD and Braak stages V/VI),

2. There is an *intermediate* likelihood that dementia is due to AD lesions, when the postmortem brain shows moderate neocortical NP and NFT in limbic regions (i.e., CERAD moderate, and Braak stages III/VI).

3. There is a *low* likelihood that dementia is due to AD lesions when the postmortem brain shows NP and NFT in a more limited distribution and/or severity (i.e., CERAD infrequent, and Braak stages I/II).

Criteria for the recognition of "incipient" dementia due to AD remain to be determined. Further, it is expected that AD may occur with combinations of NP and NFT in the postmortem brain other than those specified above. Finally, the contribution of diffuse $A\beta$ deposits to cognitive impairments remains uncertain at this time, but the presence of these lesions should be noted.

A recent evaluation of the NIA-Reagan Institute criteria for the neuropathologic diagnosis of AD in 40 patients was able to differentiate between dementia due to AD versus PSP, corticobasal degeneration and found the application of these criteria relatively easy and rapid, while non-demented control patients were found to have a low likelyhood of AD (Newell et al., 1997). Similar results have been achieved in a preliminary evaluation of 114 consecutive autopsy cases with documented cognitive performance using MMS status (Table 7).

To improve upon currently recommended procedures for the postmortem diagnosis of AD, the following goals were suggested:

1. Validate and refine the procedures recommended above.

Table 7. Likelihood of dementia due to AD (NIA-Reagan Institute criteria). Data given in percent

Disorder	Low (CERAD A; Braak 0–II)	Intermediate (CERAD B; Braak III–IV)	High (CERAD C; Braak V–VI)	Mean age (years)
Newell et al. (1997)				
AD (n = 10)	0	20	80	83
DLB (n = 9)	44	56	0	81
PSP (n = 11)	91	9	0	68
Controls (n = 10)	0	0	0	81
Personal series				
AD (n = 58) (MMSE 0–20)	0	14	86	85
DLB (n = 26) (MMSE 0–20)	35	43	22	77
PSP (n = 10)	70	20	10	72
Controls (n = 20) (MMSE 28–39)	100	0	0	81

2. Establish if heterogeneity in AD changes reflect genetic and gender based factors.

3. Investigate well-characterized cohorts of demented patients to determine the effects of age on the clinical and pathological criteria for the diagnosis of AD.

4. Investigate the pathological, cellular and molecular basis for mild cognitive impairment that does not progress to AD in well-characterized cohorts of individuals from age 50 to the end of the human lifespan and contrast this with normal aging as well as AD.

5. Develop biochemical and molecular methods (i.e., soluble assays for hyperphosphorylated tau, Aβ etc.) for the rapid postmortem diagnosis of AD and compare data obtained rising these methods with data obtained from the currently recommended pathological methods.

6. Seek to standardize diagnostic methods and reagents used for the postmortem diagnosis of AD including the establishment of common sources or core facilities for the production and distribution of diagnostic reagents.

7. Seek to develop and standardize quantitative methods including stereology, for application to the postmortem diagnosis of AD.

8. Determine the nature and significance of white matter pathological changes.

It is hoped that these and further molecular genetic and clinicopathological correlation studies will not only improve the diagnosis of AD but also provide better insights into the pathogenic cascade underlying the nature and significance of brain lesions in this disorder that represents one of the most challenging problems of modern neurobiology.

Acknowledgments

Supported by the Austrian Federal Ministry of Science, Arts and Transports and by EBEWE Research Activity.

References

Arriagada PV, Growdon JH, Hedley-Whyte T, Hyman BT (1992) Neurofibrillary tangles but not senile plaques parallel duration and severity of Alzheimer's disease. Neurology 42: 631–639

Bancher C, Jellinger K (1994) Neurofibrillary tangle predominant form of senile dementia of Alzheimer type: a rare subtype in very old subjects. Acta Neuropathol 88: 565–570

Bancher C, Braak H, Fischer P, Jellinger K (1993) Neuropathological staging of Alzheimer lesions and intellectual status in Alzheimer's and Parkinson's disease. Neurosci Lett 162: 179–182

Bancher C, Jellinger K, Lassmann H, Fischer P, Leblhuber F (1996) Correlations between mental state and quantitative neuropathology in the Vienna Prospective Longitudinal Study on Dementia. Eur Arch Psychiatry Clin Neurosci 246: 137–146

Bancher C, Lassmann H, Breitschopf H, Jellinger K (1997) Mechanisms of cell death in Alzheimer's disease. J Neural Transm [Suppl] 50: 141–152

Bancher C, Paulus W, Paukner K, Jellinger K (1997a) Neuropathological diagnosis of Alzheimer's disease: consensus between practicing neuropathologists? Alzheimer Dis Assoc Disord 11: 207–219

Bancher C, Egensperger R, Kösel S, Jellinger K, Graeber MB (1997b) Low prevalence of apolipoprotein E ε4 allele in the neurofibrillary tangle predominant form of senile dementia. Acta Neuropathol 94: 403–409

Beach TG, Honer WG, Hughes LH (1997) Cholinergic fibre loss associated with diffuse plaques in the non-demented elderly: the preclinical stage of Alzheimer's disease? Acta Neuropathol 93: 146–151

Bennett DA, Cochran EJH, Saper CB (1993) Pathological changes in frontal cortex from biopsy to autopsy in Alzheimer's disease. Neurobiol Aging 14: 589–596

Berg L, McKeel DW, Miller JP, Barty J, Morris JC (1993) Neuropathological indexes of Alzheimer's disease in demented and nondemented persons aged 80 years and older. Arch Neurol 50: 349–358

Bierer LM, Haroutunian V, Gabriel S, Knott PJ, Carlin LS, Purohit DP, Perl DP, Schmeidler J, Kanof P, Davis KL (1995a) Neurochemical correlates of dementia severity in Alzheimer's disease: relative importance of the cholinergic deficits. J Neurochem 64: 749–760

Bierer LM, Hof PR, Purohit DP, Carlin L, Schmeidler J, Davis KL, Perl DP (1995b) Neocortical neurofibrillary tangles correlate with dementia severity in Alzheimer's disease. Arch Neurol 52: 81–88

Blacker D, Albert MS, Bassett SS, Go RC, Harrell LE, Folstein MF (1994) Reliability and validity of NINCDS-ADRDA criteria for Alzheimer's disease. The National Institute of Mental Health Genetics Initiative. Arch Neurol 51: 1198–1204

Blennow K, Bogdanovic N, Alafuzoff I, Ekman R, Davidson P (1996) Synaptic pathology in Alzheimer's disease: relation to severity of dementia but not to senile plaques neurofibrillary tangles or the Apo E 4 allele. J Neural Transm 103: 603–618

Bogdanovic N, Morris J (1995) Diagnostic criteria for Alzheimer's disease in multi-centre brain banking. In: Cruz-Sanchez FF, Ravid R, Cuzner M (eds) Neuropathological diagnostic criteria for brain banking. IOS Press, Amsterdam, pp 20–29

Braak H, Braak E (1991) Neuropathological stageing of Alzheimer-related changes. Acta Neuropathol 82: 239–259

Braak H, Braak E (1996) Development of Alzheimer-related neurofibrillary changes in the neocortex inversely recapitulates cortical myelogenesis. Acta Neuropathol 92: 197–201

Braak H, Duyckaerts C, Braak E, Piette F (1993) Neuropathological staging of Alzheimer-related changes correlates with psychometrically assessed intellectual status. In: Corain B, et al (eds) Alzheimer's disease. Advances in clinical and basic research. Wiley, Chichester, pp 131–137

Callahan LM, Coleman PD (1995) Neurons bearing neurofibrillary tangles are responsible for selected synaptic deficits in Alzheimer's disease. Neurobiol Aging 16: 311–314

Chui HC, Tierney M, Zarow C, Lewis A, Sobel E, Perlmutter LS (1993) Neuropathologic diagnosis of Alzheimer disease: interrater reliability in the assessment of senile plaques and neurofibrillary tangles. Alzheimer Dis Assoc Disord 7: 48–54

Chui H, Zhang Q, Victoroff J, Zaias B (1996) Differentiating Alzheimer disease and vascular dementia: reframing the question. In: Becker P, Giacobini F (eds) Alzheimer's disease: from molecular biology to therapy. Birkhäuser, Boston, pp 13–17

Corey-Bloom J, Sabbagh MN, Hansen LA, et al (1997) "Plaque-only" Alzheimer's disease: a clinical and pathologic examination. Neurology 48: A103

Crystal H, Dickson D, Fuld P, Masur D, Scott R, Mehler M, Masdeu J, Kawas C, Aronson M, Wolfson L (1988) Clinico-pathological studies in dementia: nondemented subjects with pathologically confirmed Alzheimer's disease. Neurology 38: 1682–1687

Crystal HA, Dickson DW, Slowinski MJ, Lipton RB, Grober E, Marks-Nelson H, Antis P (1993) Pathological markers associated with normal aging and dementia in the elderly. Ann Neurol 34: 566–573

DeKosky ST, Scheff SW (1990) Synapse loss in frontal cortex biopsies in Alzheimer's disease: correlation with cognitive severity. Ann Neurol 27: 457–464

Delaere P, Duyckaerts C, He Y, Piette F, Hauw JJ (1991) Subtypes and differential laminar distribution of βA4 deposits without neuritic plaques or tangles in Alzheimer's disease: relationship with the intellectual status of 26 cases. Acta Neuropathol 81: 328–338

Dickson DW (1997) The pathogenesis of senile plaques. J Neuropathol Exp Neurol 56: 321–339

Dickson DW, Crystal HA, Mattiace LA, Masur DM, Blau AD, Davies P, Yen SM, Aronson MN (1991) Identification of normal and pathological aging in prospectively studied nondemented elderly humans. Neurobiol Aging 13: 179–189

Dickson DW, Davies P, Bevona C, et al (1994) Hippocampal sclerosis: a common pathological feature of dementia in very old (80 years of age) humans. Acta Neuropathol 88: 212–221

Dickson DW, Crystal HA, Bevona C, Honer W, Vincent I, Davies P (1995) Correlations of synaptic and pathological markers with cognition of the elderly. Neurobiol Aging 16: 285–304

Duyckaerts C, Delaère P, Hauw JJ (1990) Rating of the lesions in senile dementia of the Alzheimer type: concordance between laboratories. J Neurol Sci 97: 295–323

Esiri MM, Hyman BT, Beyreuther K, Masters CL (1997) Ageing and dementia. In: Graham DI, Lantos PL (eds) Greenfield's neuropathology, 6th ed. E Arnold, London Sidney Auckland, pp 152–233

Folstein MF, Folstein SE, McHugh PR (1975) "Mini-Mental State": a practical method for grading the cognitive state of patients for the clinician. J Psychiatry Res 12: 189–198

Galasko D, Hansen LA, Katzman R, Widerholt W, Masliah E, Terry RD, Hill LR, Lessin P, Thal LJ (1994) Clinical-neuropathological correlations in Alzheimer's disease and related dementias. Arch Neurol 51: 888–895

Gearing M, Mirra SS (1997) Alzheimer's disease with concomitant Parkinson's disease changes: two subgroups defined by neurofibrillary pathology (abstr). J Neuropathol Exp Neurol 56: 616

Gearing M, Mirra SS, Hedreen JC, Sumi SM, Hansen LA, Heyman A (1995) The Consortium to Establish a Registry for Alzheimer's Disease (CERAD). Part X. Neuropathology confirmation of the clinical diagnosis of Alzheimer's disease. Neurology 45: 461–461

Gearing M, Schneider LA, Mori H, Mirra SS (1996) Progression of Alzheimer's disease pathology from biopsy to autopsy (abstr). J Neuropathol Exp Neurol 62: 64

Gertz HJ, Xuereb JH, Huppert FA, et al (1996) The relationship between clinical dementia and neuropathological staging (Braak) in a very elderly community sample. Eur Arch Psychiatry Clin Neurosci 246: 152–156

Gertz HJ, Xuereb J, Huppert F, Brayne C, McGee MA, Paykel E, Harrington C, Mukaetova-Ladinska E, Arend T, Wischik CM (1998) Examination of the validity of the hierarchical model of neuropathological staging in normal aging and Alzheimer's disease. Acta Neuropathol 95: 154–158

Geula C, Mesulam MM, Saroff DM, Wu C-K (1998) Relationship between plaques, tangles, and loss of cortical cholinergic fibers in Alzheimer's disease. J Neuropathol Exp Neurol 57: 63–75

Giannakopoulos P, Hof PR, Giannakopoulos A-S, Herrmann FR, Michel J-P, Bouras C (1995) Regional distribution of neurofibrillary tangles and senile plaques in the cerebral cortex of very old patients. Arch Neurol 52: 1150–1159

Giannakopoulos P, Hof PR, Kovari E, Vallet P, Hermann FR, Bouras C (1996) Distinct patterns of neuronal loss and Alzheimer's disease lesion distribution in elderly individuals older than 90 years. J Neuropathol Exp Neurol 55: 1210–1220

Gomez-Igla T, Price T, Hyman BT, Morris DW, Growdon JH, Hyman BT (1996) Profound loss of layer II of entorhinal cortex neurons in very mild Alzheimer's disease. J Neurosci 16: 4491–4500

Gomez-Isla T, Hollister R, West H, et al (1997) Neuronal loss correlates with but exceeds neurofibrillary tangles in Alzheimer's disease. Ann Neurol 41: 17–24

Hansen LA, Masliah E, Galasko D, Terry RD (1993) Plaque-only Alzheimer disease is usually the Lewy body variant and vice versa. J Neuropathol Exp Neurol 52: 648–654

Heinonen O, Soininen H, Sorvari H, Kosunen O, Paljärvi I, Koivisto E, Riekkienen PJ (1995) Loss of synaptophysin-like immunoreactivity in the hippocampal formation as an early phenomenon in Alzheimer's disease. Neuroscience 64: 375–384

Heffernan M, Eastwood JS, Nagy Z, Sanders MW, McDonald B, Harrison PG (1998) Temporal cortex synaptophysin mRNA is reduced in Alzheimer's disease and is negatively correlated with the severity of dementia. Exp Neurol 150: 235–239

Hof PR, Morrison JH (1994) The cellular basis of cortical disconnection in Alzheimer disease and related dementing conditions. In: Terry RD, Katzman R, Bick KL (eds) Alzheimer disease. Raven Press, New York, pp 197–229

Hsiao K, Chapman P, Nilsen S, et al (1996) Correlative memory deficits, Aβ elevation, and amyloid plaques in transgenic mice. Science 274: 99–102

Hyman BT (1996) Anatomy of pathological alterations in Alzheimer's disease. In: Wlasco W, Tanzi E (eds) Molecular mechanisms of dementia. Humana Press, Totowa NJ, pp 219–223

Hyman BT, Trojanowski JQ (1997) Editorial on Consensus recommendations for the postmortem diagnosis of Alzheimer disease from the National Institute on Aging and the Reagan Institute Working group on diagnostic criteria for the neuropathological assessment of Alzheimer disease. J Neuropathol Exp Neurol 56: 1095–1097

Hyman BT, Marzloff K, Arriagada PV (1993) The lack of accumulation of senile plaques or amyloid burden in Alzheimer's disease suggests a dynamic balance between amyloid deposition and resolution. J Neuropathol Exp Neurol 52: 594–600

Ikeda K, Akiyama H, Arai T, Sahara N, Mori H, Usami M, Sakata M, Mizutani T, Wakabayashi K, Takahashi H (1997) A subset of senile dementia high incidence of the ApoE ε2 allele. Ann Neurol 41: 693–695

Jellinger KA (1996) Structural basis of dementia in neurodegenerative disorders Neuropathological overview. J Neural Transm [suppl] 47: 1–29

Jellinger KA, Bancher C (1997) Proposals for re-evaluation of current autopsy criteria for the diagnosis of Alzheimer's disease. Neurobiol Aging 18/S4: S55–S65

Jellinger KA, Bancher C (1998) Senile dementia with tangles (tangle predominant form of senile dementia). Brain Pathol 8: 367–376

Jellinger K, Bancher C, Fischer P, Lassmann H (1992) Quantitative histopathologic validation of senile dementia of the Alzheimer type. Eur J Gerontol 3: 146–156

Kasa P, Rakonczay Z, Gulyai K (1997) The cholinergic system in Alzheimer's disease. Progr Neurobiol 52: 511–535

Katzman R, Terry R, DeTeresa R, Brown T, Davies P, Fuld P, Renbig X, Peck A (1988) Clinical pathological and neurochemical changes in dementia: a subgroup with preserved mental status and numerous neocortical plaques. Ann Neurol 23: 138–144

Kazee AM, Eskin TA, Lapham LW, Gabriel RR, McDaniel RD, Hamill RW (1993) Clinicopathologic correlates in Alzheimer's disease — assessment of clinical and pathologic diagnostic criteria. Alzheimer Dis Assoc Disord 7: 152–164

Khachaturian ZS (1985) Diagnosis of Alzheimer's disease. Arch Neurol 42: 1097–1105

Klatka LA, Schiffer RB, Powers JM, Kazee AM (1996) Incorrect diagnosis of Alzheimer's disease A clinicopathological study. Arch Neurol 53: 35–42

Kosunen O, Soininen H, Paljarvi L, Heinonen O, Talasniemi S, Riekkinen S (1996) Diagnostic accuracy of Alzheimer's disease: a neuropathologic study. Acta Neuropathol 91: 185–193

Lassmann H, Weiler R, Fischer P, Bancher C, Jellinger K (1992) Synaptic pathology in Alzheimer's disease: immunological data for markers of synaptic and large dense core vesicles. Neuroscience 46: 1–8

Lassmann H, Bancher C, Breitschopf H, Wegiel F, Bobinski M, Jellinger K, Wisniewski HM (1995) Cell death in Alzheimer's disease evaluated by DNA fragmentation in situ. Acta Neuropathol 89: 35–41

Leverenz JB, Raskind MA (1998) Early amyloid deposition in medial temporal lobe of young Down syndrome patients: a regional quantitative analysis. Exp Neurol 150: 296–304

Litvan I, Hauw JJ, Bartko JJ, et al (1996) Validity and reliability of the preliminary NINDS neuropathological criteria for progressive supranuclear palsy and related disorders. J Neuropathol Exp Neurol 55: 97–105

Mackenzie IRA (1994) Senile plaques do not progressively accumulate with normal aging. Acta Neuropathol 87: 520–525

Mackenzie IRA, McLachlan RS, Kubu CS, Miller LA (1996) Prospective neuropsychological assessment of nondemented patients with biopsy proven senile plaques. Neurology 46: 425–429

Masliah E, Mallory M, Alford M, Ge N, Mucke L (1995) Abnormal synaptoc regeneration in hAPP695 transgenic and APOE knockout mice. In: Iqbal K, Mortimer JA, Winblad B, Wisniewski HM (eds) Research advances in Alzheimer's disease and related disorders. Wiley, London, pp 405–414

McKee AC, Kosik KS, Kowall NW (1992) Neuritic pathology and dementia in Alzheimer's disease. Ann Neurol 30: 156–165

McKeel DW Jr, Ball MJ, Price JL, Smith DS, Miller JP, Berg L (1993) Interlaboratory histopathologic assessment of Alzheimer's neuropathology: different methodologies yield comparable diagnostic results. Alzheimer Dis Assoc Disord 7: 136–153

McKeith IG, Galasko D, Kosaka K, Perry EK, Dickson DW, Hansen LA, Salmon DP, Lowe J, Mirra SS, Byrne EJ, Quinn NP, Edwardson JA, Ince PG, Bergeron C, Burns A, Miller BL, Loverstone S, Collerton D, Jansen ENH, de Vos RAI, Wilcock GK, Jellinger KA, Perry RH (1996) Clinical and pathological diagnosis of dementia with Lewy bodies (DLB): report of the CDLB International Workshop. Neurology 47: 1113–1124

Mirra SS, Heyman A McKeel D, Sumi SM, Crain BJ, Brownlee LM, Vogel FS, Hughes JP, Van Belle G, Berg L (1991) The Consortium to establish a registry for Alzheimer's disease (CERAD) II. Standardization of the neuropathologic assessment of Alzheimer's disease. Neurology 41: 479–486

Mirra SS, Hart MN, Terry RD (1993) Making the diagnosis of Alzheimer's disease. Arch Pathol Lab Med 117: 132–144

Mirra SS, Gearing M, McKeel D, Crain BJ, Hughes JP, Van Belle G, Heyman A (1994) Interlaboratory comparison of neuropathology assessments in Alzheimer's disease: a study of the Consortium to Establish a Registry for Alzheimer's disease (CERAD). J Neuropathol Exp Neurol 53: 303–315

Mirra SS, Gearing M, Heyman A (1994) CERAD guide to the neuropathological assessment of Alzheimer's disease and other dementias. CERAD, Durham NC

Morris JC, McKeel DW Jr, Storandt M, Rubin EM, Price JL, Grant EA, Ball MJ, Berg L (1991) Very mild Alzheimer's disease: informant-based clinical psychometric and pathological distinction from normal aging. Neurology 41: 469–478

Morris JC, Storandt M, McKeel DW, Rubin EH, Price JL, Grant EA, Berg L (1996) Cerebral amyloid deposition and diffuse plaques in "normal" aging: evidence for presymptomatic and very mild Alzheimer's disease. Neurology 46: 707–719

Nagy Z, Esiri MM, Cate AM, Smith AD (1997b) Cell cycle markers in the hippocampus in Alzheimer's disease. Acta Neuropathol 94: 6–15

Nagy Z, Esiri MM, Jobst KA, et al (1997b) The effects of additional pathology on the cognitive deficit in Alzheimer disease. J Neuropathol Exp Neurol 56: 165–170

Newell K, Hyman B, Growdon J, Hedley-Whyte ET (1997) Evaluation of NIA-Reagan institute criteria for the neuropathological diagnosis of Alzheimer's disease (abstr). J Neuropathol Exp Neurol 56: 593

Paulus W, Bancher C, Jellinger K (1992) Interrater reliability in the neuropathologic diagnosis of Alzheimer's disease. Neurology 42: 329–332

Perl DP, Purohit DP, Haroutunian V (1997) Clinicopathologic correlations of the Alzheimer's disease staging system introduced by Braak and Braak (abstr). J Neuropathol Exp Neurol 56: 577

Perry EK, Court JA, Lloyd S, Johnson M, Griffiths MH, Spurden D, Piggott MA, Turner J, Perry RH (1996) β-amyloidosis in normal aging and transmitter signaling in human temporal lobe. Ann NY Acad Sci 777: 388–392

Poirier J, Aubert I, Quirion R, Gauthier S, et al (1996) Apolipoprotein E4 and cholinergic activity in Alzheimer's brains. In: Becker R, Giacobini E (eds) Alzheimer disease: from molecular biology to therapy. Birkhäuser, Boston, pp 55–60

Pratt S, Prinz M, Mitrovic T, Cervos-Navarro J (1995) Neuropathological diagnostic criteria for vascular dementia. In: Cruz-Sanchez FF, Ravid R, Cuzner M (eds) Neuropathological diagnostic criteria for brain banking. IOS Press, Amsterdam, pp 55–64

Price JL, Davis PB, Morris JC, White DL (1992) The distribution of tangles plaques and related immunohistochemical markers in healthy aging and Alzheimer's disease. Neurobiol Aging 12: 295–312

Samuel W, Masliah E, Hill R, Butters N, Terry R (1994) Hippocampal connectivity and Alzheimer's dementia: effects of synapse loss and tangle frequency in a two-component model. Neurology 44: 2081–2088

Samuel W, Terry RD, DeTeresa R, Butters N, Masliah E (1994) Clinical correlates of cortical and nucleus basalis pathology in Alzheimer dementia. Arch Neurol 51: 772–778

Scheff SW, Price DA (1993) Synapse loss in the temporal lobe in Alzheimer's disease. Ann Neurol 33: 190–199

Spillantini MG, Crowther RA, Goedert M (1996) Comparison of the neurofibrillary pathology in Alzheimer's disease and familial presenile dementia with tangles. Acta Neuropathol 92: 42–48

Spillantini MG, Bird TD, Ghetti B (1998) Frontotemporal dementia and parkinonism linked to chromosome 17: a new group of tauopathies. Brain Pathol 8: 387–402

Terry RD, Hansen LA, DeTeresa R, Davies P, Tobias H, Katzman R (1987) Senile dementia of the Alzheimer type without neocortical neurofibrillary tangles. J Neuropathol Exp Neurol 46: 262–268

Terry RD, Masliah E, Salmon DP (1991) Physical basis of cognitive alterations in Alzheimer's disease: synapse loss is the major correlate of cognitive impairment. Ann Neurol 30: 572–580

Terry RT (1996) Basis of structural Alzheimer disease and some pathogenic concepts. In: Becker P, Giacobini F (eds) Alzheimer's disease: from molecular biology to therapy. Birkhäuser, Boston, pp 19–23

Tierney MC, Fischer H, Lewis AJ, Zorzitto ML, Snow WG, Reid DW, Nieuwstraten P (1988) The NINCDS-ADRDA Work Group criteria for the clinical diagnosis of probable Alzheimer's disease: clinicopathological study of 57 cases. Neurology 38: 356–364

Trojanowski JQ, Shin RW, Schmidt ML, Lee VMY (1995) Relationship between plaques tangles and dystrophic processes in Alzheimers disease. Neurobiol Aging 16: 335–340

Troncoso JC, Suknov RR, Kawas CH, Koliatsos VE (1996a) In situ labelling of dying cortical neurons in normal aging and in Alzheimer's disease: correlations with senile plaques and disease progression. J Neuropathol Exp Neurol 55: 1134–1142

Troncoso JC, Margin LJ, Dal Forno G, Kawas CH (1996b) Neuropathology in controls and demented subjects from the Baltimore Longitudinal Study of Aging. Neurobiol Aging 17: 365–371

Ulrich J, Spillantini MG, Goedert M, Dukas L, Stähelin HB (1992) Abundant neurofibrillary tangles without senile plaques in a subset of patients with senile dementia. Neurodegeneration 1: 257–284

Vermersch P, David JP, Frigard B, Falletbianco C, Wattez A, Petit H, Delacourte A (1995) Cortical mapping of Alzheimer pathology in brains of aged non-demented subjects. Prog Neuropsychopharmacol Biol Psychiatry 19: 1035–1047

Victoroff J, Mack WJ, Lyness SA, Chui HC (1995) Multicenter clinicopathological correlation in dementia. Am J Psychiatry 152: 1476–1484

Wang D, Munoz DG (1995) Qualitative and quantitative differences in senile plaque dystrophic neurites of Alzheimer's disease and normal aged brain. J Neuropathol Exp Neurol 54: 548–556

Wilcock GK, Esiri MM (1982) Plaques tangles and dementia. A quantitative study. J Neurol Sci 56: 343–356

Xuereb JH, Gertz HJ, Huppert F, Brayne C, Wischik CM, Mukaetova-Ladinska E (1995) The application of Braak's staging model of Alzheimer-type pathology to neuropathological diagnosis of dementia (abstr). Neuropathol Appl Neurobiol 21: 44

Zhan S-S, Veerhuis R, Kamphorst W, Eikelenboom P (1995) Distribution of beta amyloid associated proteins in plaques in Alzheimer's disease and in the non-demented elderly. Neurodegeneration 4: 291–297

Authors' address: Prof. Dr. K. Jellinger, Ludwig Boltzmann Institute of Clinical Neurobiology, PKH/B-Gebäude, Baumgartner Höhe 1, A-1140 Vienna, Austria

Evolution of Alzheimer's disease related cortical lesions

H. Braak[1], E. Braak[1], J. Bohl[2], and H. Bratzke[3]

Departments of [1]Anatomy and [3]Forensic Medicine, J.W.Goethe University, Frankfurt, and [2]Department of Neuropathology, J.Gutenberg University, Mainz, Federal Republic of Germany

Summary. Alzheimer's disease is an immutably progressing dementing disorder. Its major pathologic hallmark is the gradual development of neurofibrillary changes in a few susceptible nerve cell types. The cortical changes do not occur inevitably with advancing age. Once the disease has begun, spontaneous recovery or remissions are not observed. The initial changes develop in poorly myelinated areas of the temporal lobe. The destructive process then follows a predictable pattern as it extends into other cortical areas. Advanced age is not a prerequisite for the evolution of the lesions. Alzheimer's disease is thus an age-related, but not an age-dependent disease. The spread of the neurofibrillary changes resembles the process of cortical myelination, however in reverse order.

The human cerebral cortex consists of a small allocortex and an extensive neocortex. The allocortex is located chiefly in the anteromedial portions of the temporal lobe and includes the hippocampal formation and the entorhinal region. The subcortical amygdala is closely related. The parietal, occipital, and temporal neocortices are each comprised of a primary core field, a secondary belt region, and related association areas. Sensory data proceeds through the core and belt fields to the respective association areas, and is then conveyed to the frontal association cortex (prefrontal cortex). Tracts generated in this highest organisational level of the human brain guide the data through the frontal belt (premotor areas) to the primary motor area. The striatal loop and the cerebellar loop provide the major routes for this transport. Part of the stream of data from the sensory association areas branches off and converges upon the entorhinal region and the amygdala (afferent leg of the limbic loop). The information is processed in the entorhinal region, amygdala, and hippocampal formation, and projections from all these areas contribute to the efferent leg of the limbic loop, which heads toward the prefrontal cortex (Fig. 1). All components of the limbic loop play a significant role in the maintenance of memory functions. Precisely these areas are susceptible to early and grave pathologic changes in Alzheimer's disease (AD) (Kemper, 1978).

The destructive process underlying AD is by no means diffuse. On the contrary, the cortical changes exhibit an area-specific, lamina-specific, and even cell-type-specific distribution pattern (Hyman et al., 1990; Arnold et al.,

98   H. Braak et al.

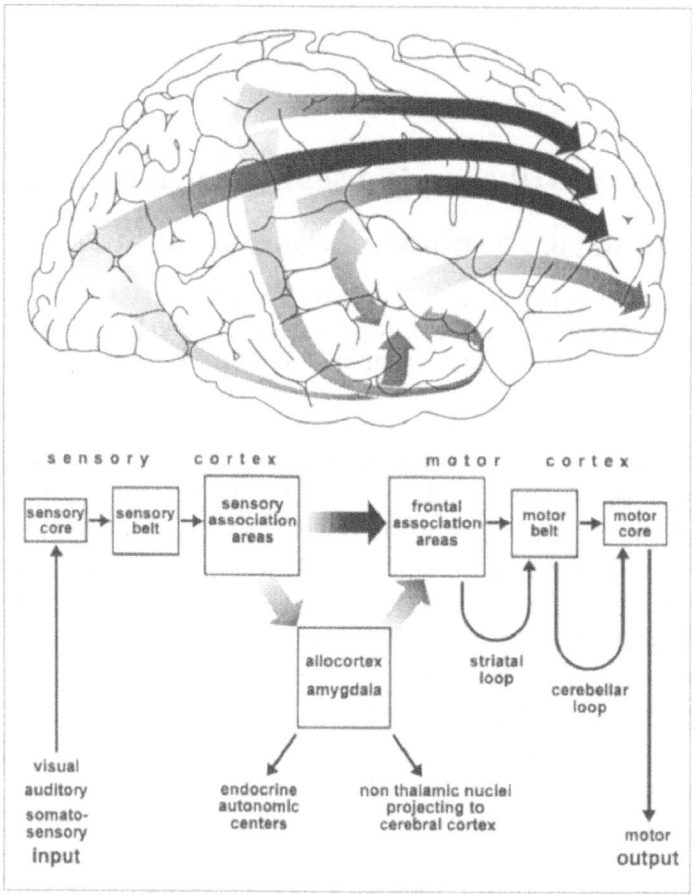

Fig. 1. Somato-sensory, visual, and auditory information proceeds through core and belt fields of the neocortex to a variety of related association areas. The data is then transported via long cortico-cortical pathways to the frontal association cortex (prefrontal areas). From there, the data is transferred — preferably by way of the striatal and cerebellar loops — to the motor belt and motor core field. Part of the stream of data from the sensory association areas to the prefrontal cortex branches off and converges upon the entorhinal region and the amygdala (afferent leg of the limbic loop). Projections from the entorhinal region, the amygdala, and the hippocampus (efferent leg of the limbic loop) exert important influence upon the prefrontal cortex (lower part with permission from Braak et al., 1995)

1991; Braak and Braak, 1991, 1994; Price et al., 1991; van Hoesen et al., 1991; Hyman and Gomez-Isla, 1994). Most conspicuous is the deposition of abnormally phosphorylated and cross-linked tau protein in a few susceptible types of nerve cells. The changes appear in the form of neurofibrillary tangles (NFTs), neuropil threads (NTs), and argyrophilic components of neuritic plaques (NPs) (Goedert, 1993; Duyckaerts et al., 1995; Iqbal et al., 1994; Trojanowski et al., 1995). After deterioration of NFT-bearing cells, the remnants of the pathologic material turn into extraneuronal "ghost" tangles (Bancher et al., 1989; Braak et al., 1994). Fresh NFTs and variable numbers of "ghost" tangles usually co-occur in cases with intraneuronal pathology. The presence of fresh NFTs in every case indicates that the pathologic process continued up to the time of death. Once the destructive process has begun, it relentlessly progresses. Spontaneous remission does not occur in AD. NFTs and NTs develop selectively in specific cortical predilection sites (Figs. 2, 3). The lesions then spread in a predictable manner across other areas of the cortex. This sequence of changes provides a basis for distinguishing six stages in the evolution of the changes (Fig. 3; Braak and Braak, 1991, 1994). Early stages occur predominantly in relatively young individuals, while the more advanced stages gradually appear with increasing age (Ohm et al., 1995). Many cases exhibit no neurofibrillary changes at all, even at an advanced age (Fig. 4, first line). There is a continuum of the intraneuronal changes starting with the first NFTs (stage I) and extending to the destruction seen in fully developed AD (Fig. 3, stages V/VI). No single feature permits definition of a specific form of the neurofibrillary changes exclusively related to age.

Specific projection cells in the entorhinal territory are the first cortical neurons to show NFTs and NTs (stage I). In stage II, additional mild changes are seen in the hippocampal formation and amygdala. The initial lesions can very well develop in young and otherwise healthy individuals (Fig. 4, second line). Further advance of the disease leads to limbic stages III and IV with severe involvement of the entorhinal territory, the amygdala, and the hippocampal formation (Fig. 4, third line). Data transfer through the limbic loop is impaired in these stages (Fig. 2, upper half). The final stages show high densities of neurofibrillary changes in virtually every sub-division of the cerebral cortex (Fig. 2, lower half, Fig. 3). A key feature of stage V is the destruction of neocortical association areas, leaving only the core areas and belt regions uninvolved or mildly affected. At stage VI, the pathologic process extends into the primary areas. There is a marked rise in prevalence of fully developed AD (stages V/VI) as a function of age (Fig. 4, fourth line).

The pattern of cortical lesions gradually developing in the course of AD is strikingly reminiscent of the progress of cortical myelination in early ontogenesis, but in reverse order. Poorly myelinated areas develop NFTs/NTs earlier in the course of AD and at higher density than richly myelinated fields (Braak and Braak, 1996). The human cortex exhibits particularly late and prolonged myelination (Flechsig, 1920; Yakovlev and Lecours, 1967). The first traces of myelin appear in the neocortical core areas. The process then spreads through the border fields into the association areas (Figs. 5 and 6). The result is a dense myelination of the core fields in the adult and a decrease in cortical myelin with increasing distance from these areas. The site of the first neurofibrillary changes (entorhinal territory and the adjoining temporal proneocortex) is particularly sparsely myelinated. From here, the changes proceed into the adjoining neocortical association areas. Involvement of the more densely myelinated belt and core fields is observed only in the late stages of the disease (Figs. 5 and 6). Regressive changes in components of the brain often repeat the process of their maturation, but in reverse order

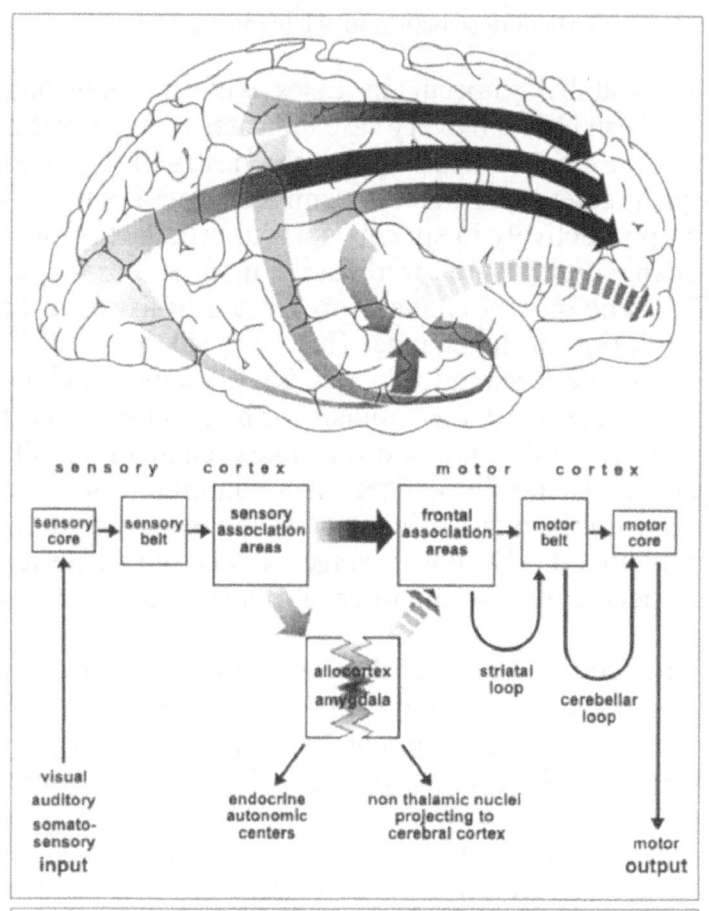

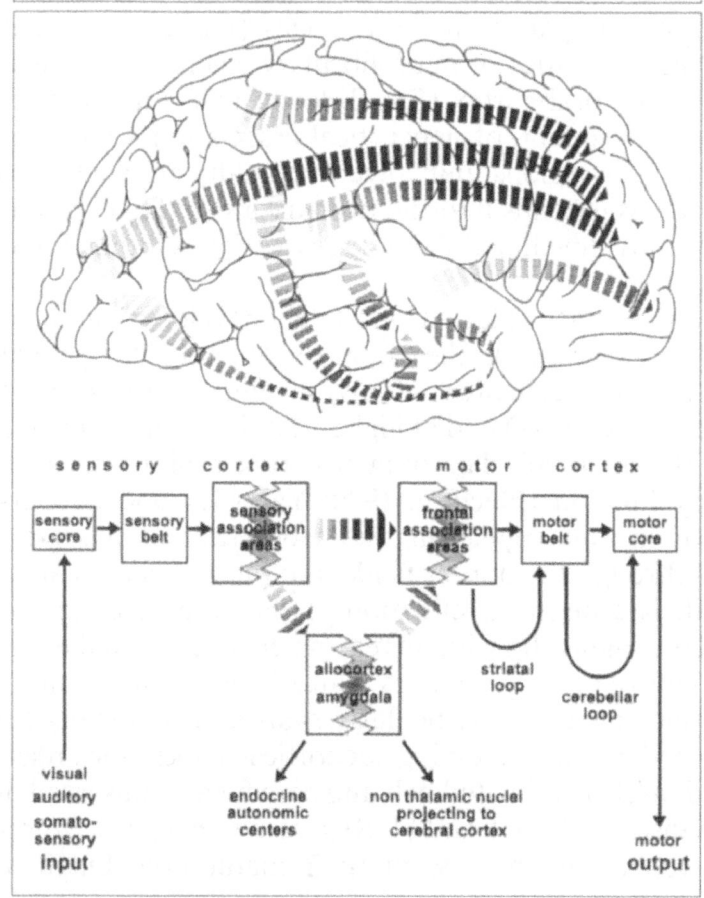

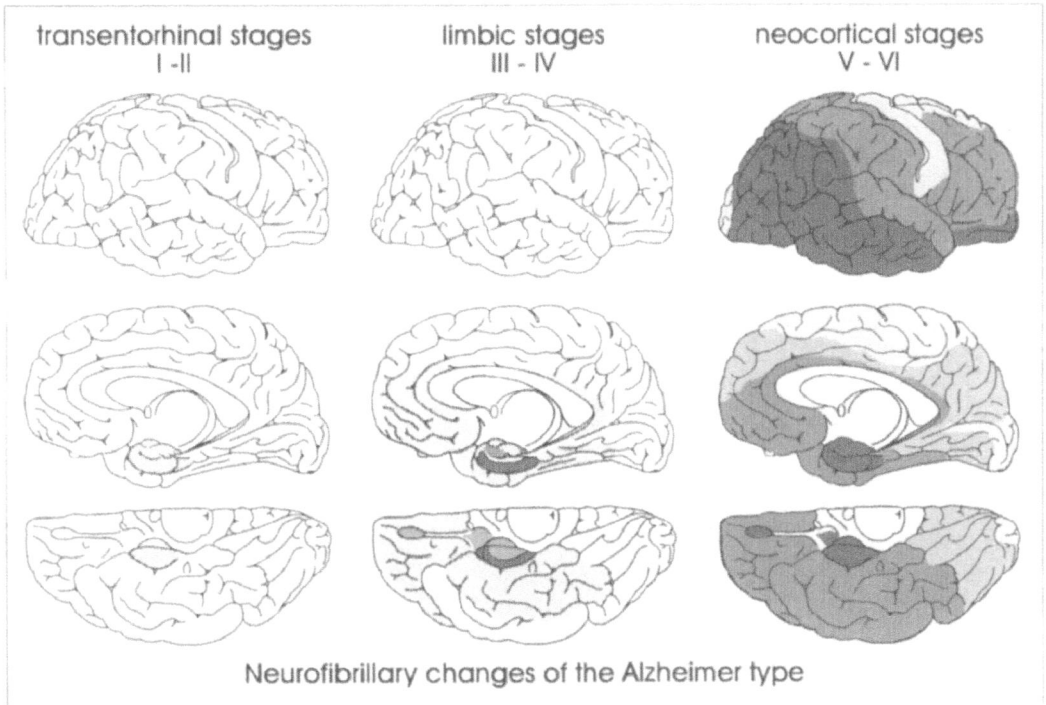

Neurofibrillary changes of the Alzheimer type

Fig. 3. Changes in the pattern of neurofibrillary tangles and neuropil threads in different stages of disease progression. Stages I–II show subtle alterations virtually confined to a single layer of the transentorhinal region (transentorhinal I–II). The key characteristic of stages III–IV is the severe involvement of the entorhinal and transentorhinal regions (limbic III–IV). End stages V–VI are marked by neocortical destruction (isocortical V–VI). Increasing shading indicates growing density of the changes (with permission from Braak and Braak, 1991)

(Reisberg et al., 1992; McGeer et al., 1990). The similarities between myelination and development of AD-related neurofibrillary changes can be explained by postulating dysfunction in late maturing cortical oligodendrocytes. Factors released by oligodendrocytes influence associated neurons and suppress neuritic outgrowth (Schwab, 1990; Kapfhammer and Schwab, 1994). Stability of nerve cells increases with myelination of their axons. Age-related instability may thus be the result of premature dysfunction in oligodendro-

◀——————————————————————————————————————

Fig. 2. *Upper half*: Components of the limbic loop play a significant role in the maintenance of memory functions. Precisely these areas are susceptible to initial pathologic changes. Transfer of data from neocortical sensory association areas through the limbic loop to the prefrontal cortex is impaired early in the course of Alzheimer's disease. *Lower half*: Further advance of the disease leads to severe destruction of the neocortical association areas. Transfer of data from neocortical sensory association areas through long cortico-cortical pathways to the prefrontal cortex is impaired late in the course of Alzheimer's disease

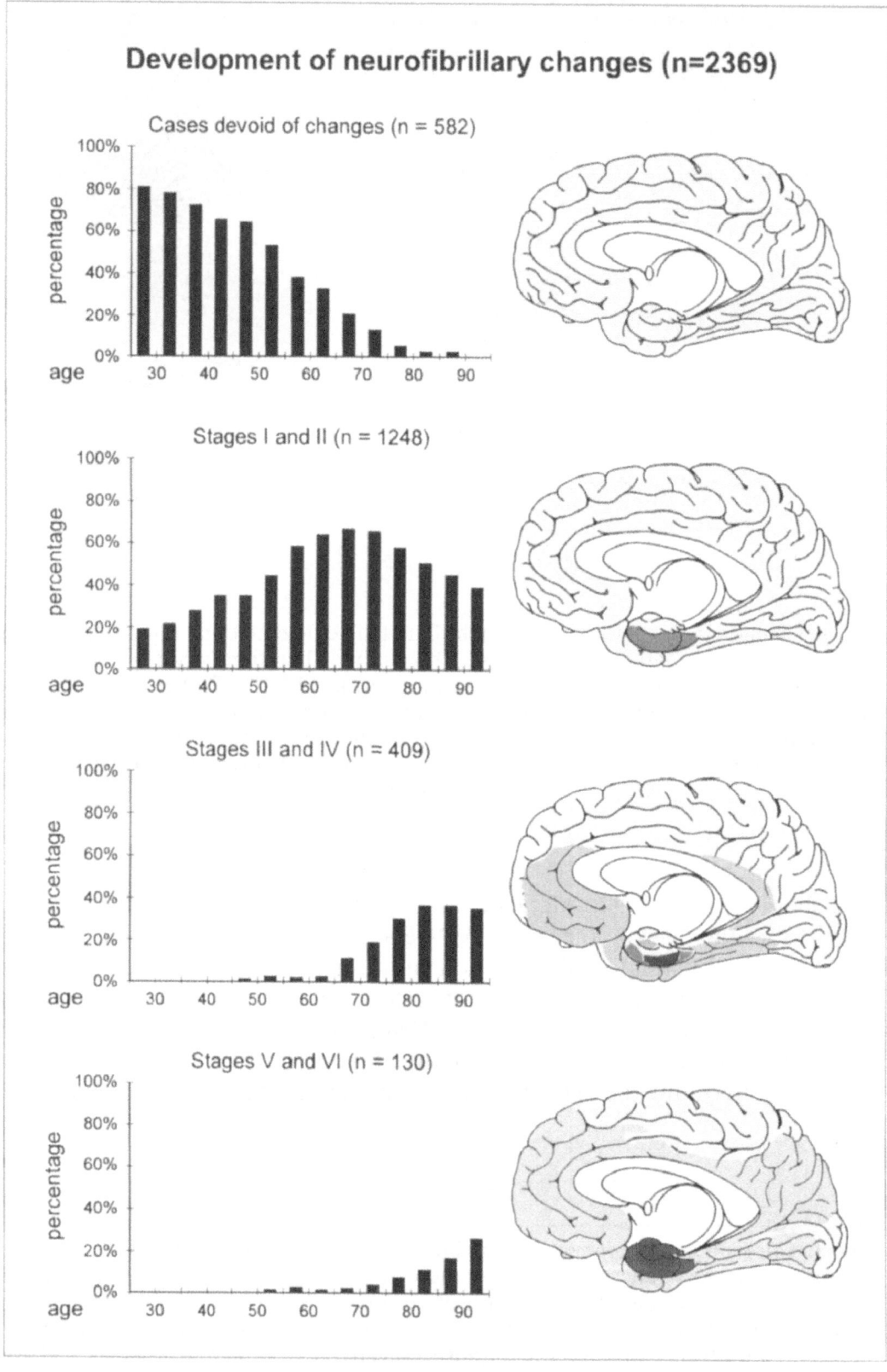

Development of neurofibrillary changes (n=2369)

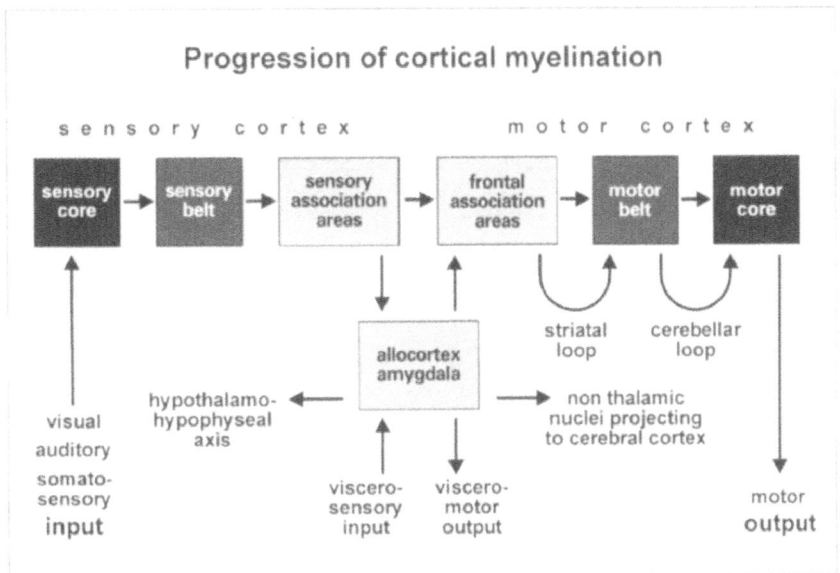

Progression of cortical myelination

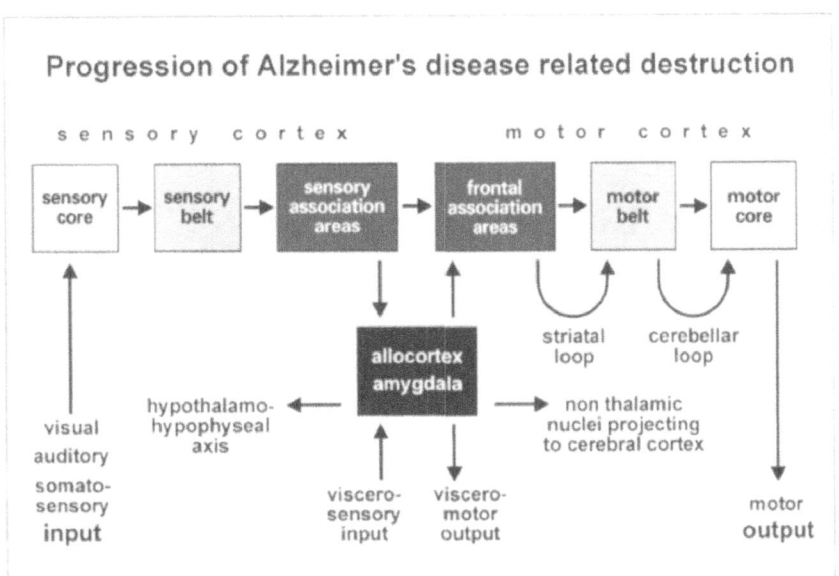

Progression of Alzheimer's disease related destruction

Fig. 5. *Upper half*: Cortical myelination begins in neocortical core fields and progresses via belt areas to the related association areas (increasing shading indicates growing density of cortical myelin). *Lower half*: Alzheimer's disease-related cortical destruction begins in the entorhinal territory, from which the changes extend into adjoining areas, eventually reaching the neocortical core fields. Note that the sequence of destruction inversely recapitulates that of cortical myelination (with permission from Braak and Braak, 1996)

◄───

Fig. 4. Evolution of the neurofibrillary changes in a total number of 2369 non-selected autopsy cases. The first line displays the percentage of cases devoid of neurofibrillary changes to the total number of cases within each age category. The brains of some elderly individuals are free of neurofibrillary changes. The 2nd, 3rd, and 4th lines are similarly designed. Some individuals develop lesions corresponding to stage I or II surprisingly early in life. Thus, old age is not an indispensible prerequisite for the evolution of the changes. Since spontaneous remissions are not observed, stage I lesions mark the beginning of the disease. The third line represents cases of the limbic stages III/IV and the fourth line those with fully developed Alzheimer's disease (stages V/VI). Note that early stages occur preferably in younger age categories, while more advanced stages gradually appear with increasing age (with permission from Braak and Braak, 1997)

Progression of
cortical myelination

Progression of Alzheimer's
disease related destruction

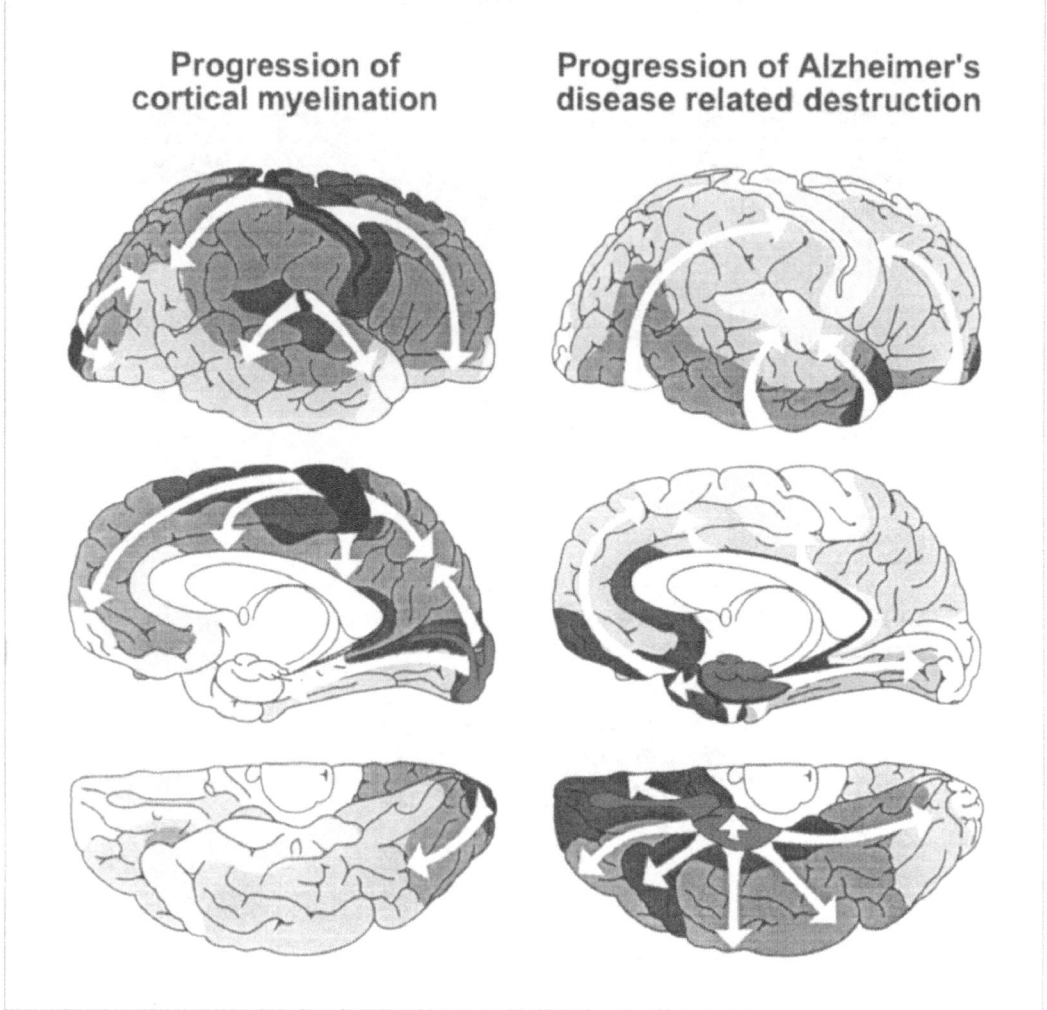

Fig. 6. Drawings of a right hemisphere showing the outward progression of myelination from the neocortical core fields into the association areas on the left side, and the progression of Alzheimer's disease-related neurofibrillary changes from the entorhinal territory via neocortical association fields and belt areas into the core fields on the right. Note the inverse pattern of the two processes (with permission from Braak and Braak, 1996)

cytes. One speculative scenario is that a lack of factors produced by oligodendrocytes results in alterations of the neuronal cytoskeleton and eventually in the induction of neurofibrillary changes of the Alzheimer type (Braak and Braak, 1996).

Acknowledgements

This study was supported by grants from the Deutsche Forschungsgemeinschaft, the Bundesministerium für Bildung, Wissenschaft, Forschung und Technologie, and Degussa, Hanau. The skilful assistance of Ms. Szasz (drawings) is gratefully acknowledged.

References

Arnold SE, Hyman BT, Flory J, Damasio AR, van Hoesen GW (1991) The topographical and neuroanatomical distribution of neurofibrillary tangles and neuritic plaques in the cerebral cortex of patients with Alzheimer's disease. Cerebral Cortex 1: 103–116

Bancher C, Brunner C, Lassmann H, Budka H, Jellinger K, Wiche G, Seitelberger F, Grundke-Iqbal I, Wisniewski HM (1989) Accumulation of abnormally phosphorylated τ precedes the formation of neurofibrillary tangles in Alzheimer's disease. Brain Res 477: 90–99

Braak E, Braak H, Mandelkow EM (1994) A sequence of cytoskeleton changes related to the formation of neurofibrillary tangles and neuropil threads. Acta Neuropathol 87: 554–567

Braak H, Braak E (1991) Neuropathological stageing of Alzheimer-related changes. Acta Neuropathol 82: 239–259

Braak H, Braak E (1994) Pathology of Alzheimer's disease. In: Calne DB (ed) Neurodegenerative diseases. Saunders, Philadelphia, pp 585–613

Braak H, Braak E (1996) Development of Alzheimer-related neurofibrillary changes in the neocortex inversely recapitulates cortical myelogenesis. Acta Neuropathol 92: 197–201

Braak H, Braak E (1997) Aspects of cortical destruction in Alzheimer's disease. In: Hyman BT, Duyckaerts, Christen Y (eds) Connections, cognition and Alzheimer's disease. Springer, Berlin Heidelberg New York Tokyo, pp 1–16

Braak H, Braak E, Yilmazer D, Schultz C, DeVos RAI, Jansen ENH (1995) Nigral and extranigral pathology in Parkinson's disease. J Neural Transm [Suppl] 46: 15–31

Duyckaerts C, Delaère P, He Y, Camilleri S, Braak H, Piette F, Hauw JJ (1995) The relative merits of tau- and amyloid markers in the neuropathology of Alzheimer's disease. In: Bergener M, Finkel SI (eds) Treating Alzheimer's and other dementias. Springer, New York, pp 81–89

Flechsig P (1920) Anatomie des menschlichen Gehirns und Rückenmarks auf myelogenetischer Grundlage. Thieme, Leipzig

Goedert M (1993) Tau protein and the neurofibrillary pathology of Alzheimer's disease. Trends Neurosci 16: 460–465

Hyman BT, Gomez-Isla T (1994) Alzheimer's disease is a laminar, regional, and neural system specific diasease, not a global brain disease. Neurobiol Aging 15: 353–354

Hyman BT, van Hoesen GW, Damasio AR (1990) Memory-related neural systems in Alzheimer's disease: an anatomic study. Neurology 40: 1721–1730

Iqbal K, Alonso AC, Gong CX, Khatoon S, Singh TJ, Grundke-Iqbal I (1994) Mechanism of neurofibrillary degeneration in Alzheimer's disease. Mol Neurobiol 9: 119–123

Kapfhammer JP, Schwab ME (1994) Inverse patterns of myelination and GAP-43 expression in the adult CNS: neurite growth inhibitors as regulators of neuronal plasticity. J Comp Neurol 340: 194–206

Kemper TL (1978) Senile dementia: a focal disease in the temporal lobe. In: Nandy E (ed) Senile dementia: a biomedical approach. Elsevier, Amsterdam, pp 105–113

McGeer PL, McGeer EG, Akiyama H, Itagaki S, Harrop R, Peppard R (1990) Neuronal degeneration and memory loss in Alzheimer's disease and aging. Exp Brain Res [Suppl]21: 411–426

Ohm TG, Müller H, Braak H, Bohl J (1995) Close-meshed prevalence rates of different stages as a tool to uncover the rate of Alzheimer's disease-related neurofibrillary changes. Neuroscience 64: 209–217

Price JL, Davis PB, Morris JC, White DL (1991) The distribution of tangles, plaques and related immunohistochemical markers in healthy aging and Alzheimer's disease. Neurobiol Aging 12: 295–312

Reisberg B, Pattschull-Furlan A, Franssen E, Sclan SG, Kluger A, Dingcong L, Ferris SH (1992) Dementia of the Alzheimer type recapitulates ontogeny inversely on specific ordinal and temporal parameters. In: Kostovic I, Knezevic S, Wisniewski HM,

Spillich GJ (eds) Neurodevelopment, aging and cognition. Birkhäuser, Boston, pp 345–369

Schwab ME (1990) Myelin-associated inhibitors of neurite growth and regeneration in the CNS. Trends Neurosci 13: 452–456

Trojanowski JQ, Shin RW, Schmidt ML, Lee VMY (1995) Relationship between plaques, tangles, and dystrophic processes in Alzheimer's disease. Neurobiol Aging 16: 335–340

van Hoesen GW, Hyman BT, Damasio AR (1991) Entorhinal cortex pathology in Alzheimer's disease. Hippocampus 1: 1–8

Yakovlev PI, Lecours AR (1967) The myelogenetic cycles of regional maturation of the brain. In: Minkowksi A (ed) Regional development of the brain in early life. Blackwell, Oxford, pp 3–70

Authors' address: Prof. Dr. med. H. Braak, Department of Anatomy, J.W.Goethe-University, Theodor Stern Kai 7, D-60590 Frankfurt, Federal Republic of Germany

What are the relations between Lewy body disease and AD?

I. G. McKeith[1], P. Ince[2], E. B. Jaros[3], A. Fairbairn[1], C. Ballard[2], J. Grace[1], C. M. Morris[2], and R. H. Perry[3]

[1]Department of Old Age Psychiatry, [2]MRC Neurochemical Pathology Unit, and [3]Department of Neuropathology, Institute for the Health of the Elderly, University of Newcastle upon Tyne, Newcastle General Hospital, Newcastle upon Tyne, United Kingdom

Summary. Several hospital based autopsy series indicate dementia with Lewy bodies (DLB) to be the second most common pathological subtype of degenerative dementia in elderly subjects. The majority of DLB cases have high densities of β amyloid senile plaques, whereas neocortical neurofibrillary tangle density is only slightly increased above age-matched normal control values and over tenfold lower than the average in Alzheimer's disease. The interpretation of this Alzheimer type pathology is problematic, reflecting in part changing views about the neuropathological diagnosis of AD itself. AD is characterised by hyperphosphorylation of the microtubular associated protein tau, and DLB by neurofilament abnormalities including phosphorylation, ubiquitination, proteolysis, and cross-linking of constituent proteins. The two diseases appear therefore to be distinct at an ultrastructural and molecular level, a conclusion which is consistent with the fact that the clinical syndromes associated with DLB and AD are sufficiently differentiated to allow for accurate antemortem diagnosis.

Introduction

Several hospital based autopsy series (Ala et al., 1997; Jellinger, 1996; Hansen et al., 1990; Perry et al., 1990a) indicate dementia with Lewy bodies (DLB) to be the second most common pathological subtype of degenerative dementia in elderly subjects, accounting for 12–36% of all cases. In a recent series (Perry et al., 1990a) of 83 dementia autopsies in Newcastle upon Tyne, (Fig. 1), 18% were identified as having DLB compared with Alzheimer's disease (AD) in 60% (54% "pure" and 6% with additional vascular pathology) (Perry et al., 1990a). This paper addresses the extent to which DLB can be regarded as a disorder separate from AD and considers also it's relationship with Parkinson's disease (PD). The interpretation of Alzheimer type pathology in DLB cases is particularly problematic reflecting in part, changing views about levels of certainty in the neuropathological diagnosis of AD itself (Trojanowski et al., 1998).

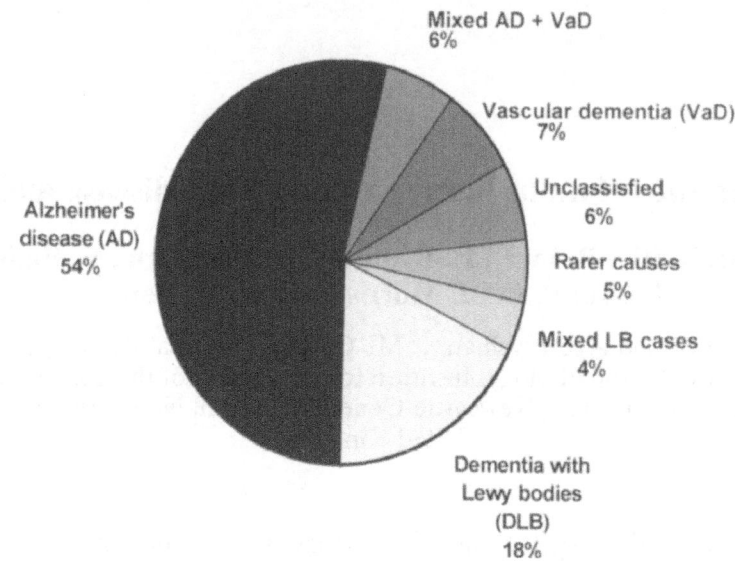

Fig. 1. Causes of dementia in the elderly (Newcastle Neuropathology Analysis 1982–87,
number of cases — 83, age 70+ years)

The pathological diagnosis of DLB

Lewy bodies and Lewy neurites

Consensus criteria for methods of pathological assessment and diagnosis of
DLB have recently been agreed (McKeith et al., 1996) — the key features are
listed in Table 1.

Although the distribution of subcortical LB in DLB cases cannot be
distinguished from that seen in idiopathic motor PD, the extent of associated
neuronal loss is typically less. In the substantia nigra (SN) for example, an
average of 40% reduction in numbers of neurones occurs in DLB (Perry et al.,
1990a), a decrement which is significantly less than that typically seen in PD
(70%). The profile of SN loss in DLB is consistent with clinical observations
that most patients have either no or only mild spontaneous extrapyramidal
features (McKeith et al., 1996; Galasko et al., 1996; McKeith et al., 1992; Perry
et al., 1989), but that they are unduly sensitive to the effects of medications
which acutely block nigro-striatal dopaminergic neurotransmission (Piggott
et al., 1994; McKeith et al., 1992).

Cortical LB are by contrast rather poorly defined spherical inclusions
usually lacking the characteristic core and halo appearance which facilitates
recognition of their brainstem counterparts. Although cortical LB may be
identified by an experienced eye using conventional H&E staining, they are
more readily visualised (see McKeith et al., 1996 for references) by anti-
ubiquitin immunocytochemistry. Cortical LB are found throughout the
cerebral cortex (except occipital lobes) but are preferentially found in limbic

Table 1. Pathologic features associated with DLB

Essential for diagnosis of DLB
— Lewy bodies

Associated but not essential
— Lewy-related neurites
— Plaques (all morphologic types)
— Neurofibrillary tangles
— Regional neuronal loss — especially brainstem (substantia nigra and locus coeruleus) and nucleus basalis of Meynert
— Microvacuolation (spongiform change) and synapse loss
— Neurochemical abnormalities and neurotransmitter deficits

cortex (including cingulate, parahippocampal gyrus and insula) and in neocortex (including frontal, parietal and temporal regions) where they are usually present in small nerve cells in deeper cortical layers (Perry et al., 1990a; Kosaka et al., 1984). LB are also present in the amygdala, the medial accessory basal and basal nuclei, and the cortico-amygdaloid transition area according to Kosaka and Iseki (1996). These nuclei are known to be associated with limbic and hippocampal circuitry and their involvement may contribute to the memory disturbance of DLB. Hippocampal LB are rare, although ubiquitin positive (Lewy) neurites are found in hippocampal areas CA2-3 (Dickson et al., 1991) and the extent of this neuritic degeneration has been reported to be correlated with the density of cortical LB (Pollanen et al., 1993). Lewy neurites have also been described in other brain regions including the amygdala (Braak et al., 1994), basal forebrain, substantia nigra, pedunculo-pontine nuclei, raphe nuclei and dorsal motor nucleus of the vagus (Dickson et al., 1996).

Alzheimer pathology in DLB

A variety of additional pathological findings (Table 1) are also seen in addition to LB (McKeith et al., 1996), and in particular the majority of DLB cases have β amyloid senile plaques (SP) sufficient to qualify for a diagnosis of "plaque predominant" (Terry et al., 1987) or "CERAD probable" AD (Mirra et al., 1991). Neocortical NFT density is by contrast only slightly increased above age-matched normal control values and over tenfold lower than the average in Alzheimer's disease (Perry et al., 1990a, 1989). The precise interpretation of these observations remains contentious. Some authorities (Hansen et al., 1990) have regarded them as evidence of coexistent Alzheimer's disease, which has an earlier clinical presentation than pure AD as a consequence of the additional burden of LB formation and associated neuronal loss. Others (Dickson et al., 1996, 1991) regard the Alzheimer pathology in most cases merely to constitute "pathological ageing" rather than evidence of concomitant AD. This debate about the interpretation of

Alzheimer pathology in DLB revolves around long-standing, unresolved issues in the pathological definition of AD itself, in particular the relative significance of plaques versus tangles, and plaque type (neuritic versus non-neuritic)

The Lewy body variant of AD

The San Diego group originally coined the term, "Lewy body variant of AD" (Hansen et al., 1990) which was derived from their use of the NIA and CERAD (Mirra et al., 1991) criteria which allow probable AD to be diagnosed on the basis of neocortical plaque-only or plaque predominant Alzheimer pathology. The majority (89%) of their LB dementia brains met NIA criteria for concomitant AD (diffuse and neuritic plaques), 68% were CERAD probable AD (neuritic plaques only) and only 32% had CERAD definite AD (neocortical plaques and tangles) (Hansen, 1996). They proposed that since AD itself does not suddenly appear full blown, but rather, progresses insidiously, it is possible that DLB cases represent a "brought forward" presentation of AD, the additional LB formation and associated neuronal loss leading to cognitive impairment approaching that seen in classical AD despite a lighter burden of AD pathology (Hansen et al., 1993; Hansen and Galasko, 1992). In a slightly modified formulation, the San Diego group have also conceptualised the LB variant of AD as "a neurodegenerative hybrid separate and distinct from AD and PD but with clinical and neuropathological features of both. By analogy, just as a mule is neither a horse nor a donkey, despite being composed of nothing other than horse or donkey, so too is LBV a "different animal" than AD or PD, despite sharing features with both" (Samuel et al., 1996). Genetic data lends some support to this model — DLB has a raised apolipoprotein-E ε4 allele frequency similar to that seen in AD but not observed in PD (Galasko et al., 1994; Benjamin et al., 1994). A converse relationship has been reported for the cytochrome p450 CYP2D6 debrisoquine-4 hydroxylase gene on chromosome 22, with the inactive mutant B allele frequency being increased in LBV and PD but not in AD (Saitoh et al., 1995). Most recently, Samuel et al. (1997) have reported that 52% of neuritic plaques in AD are anti-PHF positive, but only 12% of LBV cases which lack NFT in midfrontal cortex have anti-PHF positive neuritic plaques ($p < 0.05$). They conclude on the basis of all of the clinical, neuropathological and neurochemical data now available, that LBV is a distinct category of dementia not properly described as a subtype either of LB disease or of AD.

Others have challenged these interpretations of the neuropathological findings. Dickson et al. find the plaques in most DLB cases to be diffuse deposits of β-protein (Aβ) with few or no neuritic components (Dickson et al., 1996, 1989). These plaques are similar to those seen in elderly individuals without cognitive decline or dementia, and therefore designated as "pathological ageing". By contrast the minority of DLB cases with concomitant AD defined by neocortical SP and NFT, have plaques of the neuritic type with tau-positive, argyrophilic and thioflavin-S fluorescent neurites. Even in these cases the CA1 region of the hippocampus tends to be relatively preserved. Dickson concludes that it is currently untenable to consider most DLB cases to be variants of AD. McKenzie et al. (1996) however found no differences in either the density or relative proportions of classic and diffuse plaques in their DLB and AD cases using $\beta A4$ immunoctyochemistry only. This method does not however allow investigation of neuritic components in plaques.

Cytoskeletal abnormalities in DLB and AD

Given these difficulties in resolving the extent and significance of neuropathological lesions in DLB and AD at the microscopic level, differences have also been sought in discrete profiles of cytoskeletal derangement using ultrastructural, immunocytochemical and direct biochemical methods. Altered processing of the microtubule associated protein tau is a characteristic feature of AD which is not seen to any significant extent in DLB cases. Harrington et al. (1994) found no evidence that the accumulation of either protease resistant paired helical filaments (PHF) or of hyperphosphorylated tau could distinguish DLB patients from age-matched controls or PD cases. The mean level of either PHF or NFT was no greater than 5% of that found in AD, suggesting the abundant PHF in neurites does not provide an adequate explanation for dementia in DLB. The levels of PHF were by contrast increased in AD by more than twenty-fold.

Detailed ultrastructural examination of sub-cortical and cortical LB reveals them to consist of neurofilament-like fibrils, an observation supported by immunological techniques, although not yet confirmed by direct protein chemical analysis of the isolated proteins (Carter et al., 1996). Using the Mallory body of the liver as a dynamic model of intermediate filament inclusion formation, Bergeron and Pollanen (1996) have proposed a speculative model of LB pathogenesis in which neurofilaments are assembled normally and subsequently undergo phosphorylation, proteolysis and cross-linking at a post-translational post-assembly stage. These changes are not seen in AD.

In summary, both AD and DLB are characterised by dysregulation and hyperphosphorylation of cytoskeletal proteins. DLB appears primarily to be a disorder of neurofilament proteins in contrast to AD in which the major cytoskeletal abnormalities involve microtubule associated PHF tau. The two diseases thus appear to be distinct at a molecular level although clearly there are considerable areas of overlap. The complete inter-relationships between them can probably only be further resolved when more has been learned about the pathogenesis of LB and NFT and the relationship of each inclusion with β amyloid deposition.

Are Lewy bodies "incidental" or "additional" lesions in DLB?

An influential earlier interpretation of the occurrence of cortical LB in demented patients (Quinn et al., 1986) was that they might be coincidentally present in patients who had, or were in the early stages of developing dementia due to Alzheimer pathology. This formulation was based upon the view, originally proposed by Forno (1969) and still prevailing at the time, that "incidental" LB formation commonly occurs as a part of normal ageing, with a reported prevalence of 4.5–10.3%. This hypothesis was based upon three major hospital based neuropathological surveys (Forno, 1969; Woodard, 1962; Lipkin, 1959) The cases were however drawn from populations with acknowledged biases towards psychiatric cases and non-PD neurological disorders and cannot therefore be regarded as representative of normal ageing. More recently Perry et al. (1990b) reported upon 131 cases collected from general medical and surgical sources after exclusion of those with evidence of cognitive decline, psychiatric illness or diagnosed neurological disorder. LB were seen in no cases under the age of 70 years, in 2.8% aged 71–80 years, in 3.6% aged 81–90 years and 7.1% aged 91–100 years. The prevalence rate in the whole group aged over 50 years was therefore only 2.3%. This is compatible with the known prevalence of PD in the elderly (1–2%) and the estimated prevalence of dementia associated with LB (1.5–2.5%) (Perry et al., 1990b), supporting a view that LB are associated with specific central nervous system disease rather than occurring as a non-specific age-associated change. The incidental LB hypothesis of DLB is also weakened by the pathoplastic effect of cortical LB upon the clinical presentation. Compared with AD cases which show no cortical LB, DLB cases characteristically have prominent attentional

Table 2. Consensus criteria for the clinical diagnosis of *probable* and *possible* dementia with Lewy bodies (DLB)

1. The central feature required for a diagnosis of DLB is progressive cognitive decline of sufficient magnitude to interfere with normal social or occupational function. Prominent or persistent memory impairment may not necessarily occur in the early stages but is usually evident with progression. Deficits on tests of attention and of frontal-subcortical skills and visuospatial ability may be especially prominent.

2. *Two* of the following core features are *essential* for a diagnosis of *probable* DLB, *one* is *essential* for *possible* DLB.
   (a) Fluctuating cognition with pronounced variations in attention and alterness
   (b) Recurrent visual hallucinations which are typically well formed and detailed
   (c) Spontaneous motor features of parkinsonism

3. Features *supportive* of the diagnosis are
   (a) Repeated falls
   (b) Syncope
   (c) Transient loss of consciousness
   (d) Neuroleptic sensitivity
   (e) Systematised delusions
   (f) Hallucinations in other modalities

4. A diagnosis of DLB is *less likely* in the presence of
   (a) Stroke disease, evident as focal neurological signs or on brain imaging
   (b) Evidence on physical examination and investigation of any physical illness, or other brain disorder, sufficient to account for the clinical picture

deficits and visuospatial dysfunction, fluctuating cognition, visual hallucinations and mild parkinsonism (Table 2). This syndrome is so characteristic that DLB patients can be identified from clinical records with autopsy confirmed sensitivity (75%) and specificity (79%) (Mega et al., 1996) which is similar to that achieved for AD (Kukull et al., 1990) and PD (Hughes et al., 1993).

What "causes" the dementia in DLB?

The extent to which different pathological lesions contribute to the cognitive impairment and other neuropsychiatric features of DLB is uncertain. The degenerative process associated with cortical LB pathology [designated as "pure" diffuse LB disease (Kosaka et al., 1984)] appears to be sufficient in itself to produce a primary dementia in the absence of any SP or NFT (Hely et al., 1996). In more typical or Kosaka "common" cases, Samuel et al. (1996) found LB concentrations in the cingulate and superior temporal cortex to correlate with the severity of dementia assessed using the Mini-Mental State Examination (MMSE). Significant clinicopathological correlations were not found in mid-frontal or inferior parietal regions. Neocortical plaque and tangle counts were not associated with mental status. Lennox et al. (1989) had previously reported similar findings. Perry et al. (1990a) were however unable to find a direct relationship between LB density in the limbic cortex and severity of dementia, nor between cortical LB densities and other key clinical variables such as the presence or absence of hallucinations. This lack of consistent correlation between LB density and clinical parameters may reflect the methodological problems inherent in comparing lifetime clinical measures with pathological data which may reflect an "end stage" of disease months or even years later, or the limited applicability of existing measures of cognitive function to a disease with fluctuating symptomatology. Perry et al. (1996) have also suggested that the presence of LB in the cortex may represent a "tip of the iceberg" phenomenon — the remainder of the iceberg consisting of as yet unidentified cell loss in a select but critical population of cortical neurones. Quantitative assessments of neuronal populations and synaptic connectivity in key cortical areas need to address this issue.

References

Ala TA, Yang K-H, Sung JH, Frey WHI (1997) Hallucinations and signs of Parkinsonism help distinguish patients with dementia and cortical Lewy bodies from patients with Alzheimer's disease. J Neurol Neurosurg Psychiatry 62: 16–21

Benjamin R, Leake A, Edwardson JA, McKeith IG, Ince PG, Perry RH, Morris CM (1994) Apolipoprotein E genes in Lewy body and Parkinson's disease. Lancet 343: 1565

Bergeron C, Pollanen MS (1996) Pathogenesis of the Lewy body. In: Perry R, McKeith I, Perry E (eds) Dementia with Lewy bodies. Cambridge University Press, New York, pp 302–307

Braak H, Braak E, Yilmazer D, de Vos RA, Jansen EN, Bohl J, Jellinger K (1994) Amygdala pathology in Parkinson's disease. Acta Neuropathol 88: 493–500

Carter J, Hanger D, Lovestone S (1996) Cytoskeletal pathology in Alzheimer's disease and Lewy body dementia — an epiphenomenon? In: Perry R, McKeith I, Perry E (eds) Dementia with Lewy bodies. Cambridge University Press, New York, pp 324–335

Dickson DW, Crystal H, Mattiace LA, Kress Y, Schwagerl A, Ksiezak-Reding H, Davies P, Yen S-HC (1989) Diffuse Lewy body disease: light and electron microscopic immunocytochemistry of senile plaques. Acta Neuropathol 78: 572–584

Dickson DW, Ruan D, Crystal H, Mark MH, Davies P, Kress Y, Yen S-H (1991) Hippocampal degeneration differentiates diffuse Lewy body disease (DLBD) from Alzheimer's disease: light and electron microscopic immunocytochemistry of CA2–3 neurites specific to DLBD. Neurology 41: 1402–1409

Dickson DW, Crystal HA, Davies P, Hardy J (1996) Cytoskeletal and Alzheimer-type pathology in Lewy body disease. In: Perry R, McKeith I, Perry E (eds) Dementia with Lewy bodies. Cambridge University Press, New York, pp 224–237

Forno LS (1969) Concentric hyalin intraneuronal inclusions of Lewy type in the brains of elderly persons (50 incidental cases): relationship to parkinsonism. J Am Geriatr Soc 17: 557–575

Galasko D, Saitoh T, Xia Y, Thal LJ, Katzman R, Hill LR, Hansen L (1994) The apolipoprotein E allele ε4 is overrepresented in patients with the Lewy body variant of Alzheimer's disease. Neurology 44: 1950–1951

Galasko D, Salmon DF, Thal LJ (1996) The nosological status of Lewy body dementia. In: Perry R, McKeith I, Perry E (eds) Dementia with Lewy bodies. Cambridge University Press, New York, pp 21–33

Hansen L, Salmon D, Galasko D, Masliah E, Katzman R, DeTeresa R, Thal L, Pay MM, Hofstetter R, Klauber M, Rice V, Butters N, Alford M (1990) The Lewy body variant of Alzheimer's disease: a clinical and pathologic entity. Neurology 40: 1–8

Hansen LA (1996) Tautological tangles in neuropathologic criteria for dementias associated with Lewy bodies. In: Perry R, McKeith I, Perry E (eds) Dementia with Lewy bodies. Cambridge University Press, New York, pp 204–212

Hansen LA, Galasko D (1992) Lewy body disease. Curr Opin Neurol Neurosurg 5: 889–894

Hansen LA, Masliah E, Galasko D, Terry RD (1993) Plaque-only Alzheimer disease is usually the Lewy body variant, and vice versa. J Neuropathol Exp Neurol 52: 648–654

Harrington CR, Perry RH, Perry EK, Hurt J, McKeith IG, Roth M, Wischik CM (1994) Senile dementia of Lewy body type and Alzheimer type are biochemically distinct in terms of paired helical filaments and hyperphosphorylated tau protein. Dementia 5: 215–228

Hely MA, Reid WGJ, Halliday GM, McRitchie DA, Leicester J, Joffe R, Brooks W, Broe GA, Morris JGL (1996) Diffuse Lewy body disease: clinical features in nine cases without coexistent Alzheimer's disease. J Neurol Neurosurg Psychiatry 60: 531–538

Hughes AJ, Daniel SE, Kilford L, Less AJ (1993) Accuracy of clinical diagnosis of Parkinson's disease. A clinicopathological study of 100 cases. J Neurol Neurosurg Psychiatry 55: 181–184

Jellinger KA (1996) Structural basis of dementia in neurodegenerative disorders. J Neural Transm 47: 1–29

Kosaka K, Iseki E (1996) Diffuse Lewy body disease within the spectrum of Lewy body disease. In: Perry R, McKeith I, Perry E (eds) Dementia with lewy bodies. Cambridge University Press, New York, pp 238–247

Kosaka K, Yoshimura M, Ikeda K, Budka H (1984) Diffuse type of Lewy body disease: progressive dementia with abundant cortical Lewy bodies and senile changes of varying degree — A new disease? Clin Neuropathol 3: 185–192

Kukull WA, Larson EB, Reifler BV, Lampe TH, Yerby MS, Hughes JP (1990) The validity of 3 diagnostic criteria for Alzheimer's disease. Neurology 40: 1364–1369

Lennox G, Lowe J, Landon M, Byrne EJ, Mayer RJ, Godwin-Austen RB (1989) Diffuse Lewy body disease: correlative neuropathology using anti-ubiquitin immunocytochemistry. J Neurol Neurosurg Psychiatry 52: 1236–1247

Lipkin LE (1959) Cytoplasmic inclusions of ganglion cells associated with parkinsonian states. A neurocellular change studied in 53 cases and 206 controls. Am J Pathol 35: 1117–1133

McKeith I, Fairbairn A, Perry R, Thompson P, Perry E (1992) Neuroleptic sensitivity in patients with senile dementia of Lewy body type. Br Med J 305: 673–678

McKeith IG, Perry RH, Fairbairn AF, Jabeen S, Perry EK (1992) Operational criteria for senile dementia of Lewy body type (SDLT). Psychol Med 22: 911–922

McKeith IG, Galasko D, Kosaka K, Perry EK, Dickson DW, Hansen LA, Salmon DP, Lowe J, Mirra SS, Byrne EJ, Lennox G, Quinn NP, Edwardson JA, Ince PG, Bergeron D, Burns A, Miller BL, Lovestone S, Collerton D, Jansen ENH, Ballard C, de Vos RAI, Wilcock GK, Jellinger KA, Perry RH (1996) Consensus guidelines for the clinical and pathologic diagnosis of dementia with Lewy bodies (DLB): report of the consortium on DLB international workshop. Neurology 47: 1113–1124

McKenzie JE, Edwards RJ, Gentleman SM, Ince PG, Royston MC, Roberts GW (1996) A quantitative comparison of plaque types in Alzheimer's disease and senile dementia of the Lewy body type. Acta Neuropathol 91(5): 526–529

Mega MS, Masterman DL, Benson F, Vinters HV, Tomiyasu U, Craig AH, Foti DJ, Kaufer D, Scharne DW, Fairbanks L, Cummings JL (1996) Dementia with Lewy bodies: reliability and validity of clinical and pathologic criteria. Neurology 47: 1403–1409

Mirra SS, Heyman A, McKeel D, Sumi SM, Crain BJ, Brownlee LM, Vogel FS, Hughes JP, Van Belle G, Berg L, and participating CERAD neuropathologists (1991) The Consortium to Establish a Registry for Alzheimer's Disease (CERAD) II. Standardisation of the neuropathological assessment of Alzheimer's disease. Neurology 41: 479–486

Perry RH, Irving D, Blessed G, Perry EK, Fairbairn AF (1989) Clinically and neuropathologically distinct form of dementia in the elderly. Lancet: 166

Perry RH, Irving D, Blessed G, Fairbairn A, Perry EK (1990a) Senile dementia of Lewy body type. A clinically and neuropathologicall distinct form of Lewy body dementia in the elderly. J Neurol Sci 95: 119–139

Perry RH, Irving D, Tomlinson BE (1990b) Lewy body prevalence in the aging brain: relationship to neuropsychiatric disorders, Alzheimer-type pathology and catecholaminergic nuclei. J Neurol Sci 100: 223–233

Perry RH, Jaros EB, Irving D, Scoones DJ, Brown A, McMeekin WM, Perry EK, Morris CM, Kelly PJ, Ince PG (1996) What is the neuropathological basis of dementia associated with Lewy bodies? In: Perry R, McKeith I, Perry E (eds) Dementia with Lewy bodies. Cambridge University Press, New York, pp 212–224

Piggott MA, Perry EK, McKeith IG, Marshall E, Perry RH (1994) Dopamine D2 receptors in demented patients with severe neuroleptic sensitivity. Lancet 343: 1044–1045

Pollanen MS, Dickson DW, Bergeron C (1993) Pathology and biology of the Lewy body. J Neuropathol Exp Neurol 52: 183–191

Quinn NP, Rossor MN, Marsden CD (1986) Dementia and Parkinson's disease: pathological and neurochemical considerations. Br Med Bull 42: 86–90

Saitoh T, Xia Y, Chen X, Masliah E, Galasko D, Shults C, Thal LJ, Hansen LA, Katzman R (1995) The CYP2D6B mutant allele is overrepresented in the Lewy body variant of Alzheimer's disease. Am Neurol Assoc 110–112

Samuel W, Galasko D, Masliah E, Hansen LA (1996) Neocortical Lewy body counts correlate with dementia in the Lewy body variant of Alzheimer's disease. J Neuropathol Exp Neurol 55: 44–52

Samuel W, Crowder R, Hofstetter CR, Hansen LA (1997) Neuritic plaques in the Lewy body variant of Alzheimer disease lack paired helical filaments. Neurosci Lett 223: 73–76

Terry RD, Hansen LA, DeTeresa R, Davies P, Tobias H, Katzman R (1987) Senile dementia of the Alzheimer type without neocortical neurofibrillary tangles. J Neuropathol Exp Neurol 46: 262–268

Trojanowski TJ, et al (National Institute on Aging and Reagan Institute Working Group on Diagnostic Criteria for the Neuropathological Assessment of Alzheimer's Disease (1998) Neurobiol Aging (in preparation)

Woodard JS (1962) Concentric hyaline inclusion body formation in mental disease: analysis of twenty-seven cases. J Neuropathol Exp Neurol 21: 442–449

Authors' address: Prof. I. G. McKeith, Department of Old Age Psychiatry, Institute for the Health of the Elderly, Newcastle General Hospital, Westgate Road, Newcastle upon Tyne NE4 6BE, United Kingdom

The influence of coincidental vascular pathology on symptomatology and course of Alzheimer's disease

F. Pasquier[1], **D. Leys**[2], and **P. Scheltens**[3]

[1] Memory and [2] Stroke Units, Department of Neurology, University of Lille, France
[3] Department of Neurology, Academisch Ziekenhuis Vrije Universiteit, Amsterdam,
The Netherlands

Summary. The aim of this review is to determine the influence of coincidental cerebrovascular pathology on the symptomatology and course of Alzheimer's disease (AD). The link between stroke and AD is probably higher than expected by chance for the following reasons: (i) both pathologies share genetic risk factors such as the ε4 allele of the apolipoprotein E gene; (ii) AD patients have changes in the brain vessels that may lead to either ischemic or hemorrhagic stroke or white matter changes or both; (iii) there is evidence of an increased risk of stroke in AD patients; (iv) there is evidence of a frequent association of AD and stroke at autopsy. Because of the summation of the various types of lesions, stroke lesions may lead to an increase progression of cognitive decline in AD patients. Recognition of a vascular component in a dementia syndrome is therefore useful for the management of AD patients. Whether an optimal management of risk factors for stroke may delay the clinical expression of dementia in patients with preclinical Alzheimer pathology should be evaluated.

Introduction

Alzheimer's disease (AD) is the most frequent degenerative dementia. Strict diagnostic criteria require exclusion of stroke (McKhann et al., 1984): therefore, possible relations between AD and stroke or risk factors for stroke may have been underestimated in the past. There is now compelling evidence that a link does exist between AD and stroke (Pasquier and Leys, 1997). The aim of this review is to determine the influence of coincidental cerebrovascular pathology on the symptomatology and course of AD. We will not evaluate the influence of isolated risk factors for stroke on the symptomatology and course of AD unless they are associated with stroke.

Are stroke and Alzheimer pathology associated by chance?

The incidence of both AD and stroke increases with age (Rocca et al., 1990; Alperovitch et al., 1986). Therefore, their association is likely to be frequent.

However, the link between stroke and AD is probably higher than expected by chance (Pasquier and Leys, 1997).

Stroke and AD share genetic risk factors

The ε4 allele of the apolipoprotein E gene (APOE) has been firmly established to be associated with an increased risk of late-onset AD (Saunders et al., 1993; Frisoni et al., 1994): the odds ratio is 4 for the ε3/ε4 genotype and 16 for the ε4/ε4 genotype. The APOE ε4 allele is also associated with a higher risk of ischemic events, such as coronary heart disease [odds ratio: 1.5, without evidence of a gene dose effect (Gerdes et al., 1994)], ischemic stroke and vascular dementia (Frisoni et al., 1994; Shimano et al., 1989). Besides, amyloid precursor protein accumulates in regions of neurodegeneration following focal cerebral ischemia in the rat (Stephenson et al., 1992). A unifying explanation for the association of the ε4 allele with both stroke and AD might involve the role of apoE isoforms in the repair processes in the nervous system and in normal brain lipid metabolism (Rubinsztein et al., 1995). Moreover, Albert et al., (1996) showed a strong association between the ε4 genotype and a poor neurological outcome after intracerebral hemorrhage. It can therefore be hypothesized that different aggressions of the brain, either degenerative or vascular in origin, might result in greater damage in patients with the ε4 genotype (Frisoni et al., 1994). A synergistic relationship between stroke and a marker of genetic susceptibility to AD may therefore exist.

Evidence of vascular changes in AD patients

Several studies have shown that AD patients have some degree of changes in cerebral arteries. These changes may occur in the deep perforators, with non-specific fibrohyaline thickening of their wall, in cortical vessels, with amyloid, and in cervical arteries with atherosclerotic changes. Non-specific fibrohyaline thickening of the wall of the small perforating intracerebral arteries is a frequent finding in AD patients (Rezek et al., 1987), even in those who are free of any vascular risk factor (Leys et al., 1991); this kind of small-vessel disease may lead to lacunes (Fisher, 1969) and may be associated with white matter changes in patients with stroke (Hijdra et al., 1990; Leys et al., 1992) or AD (Leys et al., 1992; Rezek et al., 1987). Cerebral amyloid angiopathy, a frequent factor of non-hypertensive intracerebral hemorrhage (Vinters, 1987), is more frequent in AD than in controls (Yamada et al., 1987). It may lead to cerebral hemorrhages (Ellis et al., 1996; Lucas et al., 1992) and to cerebral infarcts (Ellis et al., 1996) in AD as well. Thus, amyloid angiopathy is a vascular component frequently associated with Alzheimer pathology. Moreover, the dementia syndrome occurring in the course of hereditary cerebral hemorrhages with amyloidosis of the Dutch type is a combination of vascular and Alzheimer lesions (Haan et al., 1994a,b). Cervical arteries may show significant changes in AD patients: in the Rotterdam study, AD patients had an increased intima-media thickness in the common carotid artery (Hofman et al., 1997) which is an indicator of increased risk of stroke in the community (Blots et al., 1996). Therefore, AD patients have changes in the brain vessels that may lead to ischemic or hemorrhagic stroke, white matter changes or both (Pasquier and Leys, 1997).

Evidence of stroke in AD patients

A way to address the question whether AD patients have more stroke is to determine whether stroke lesions are more frequent in AD patients than in age- and sex- matched controls after adjustment for risk factors for stroke. However, this question can hardly be solved because the presence of a stroke is an exclusion criteria for probable AD anytime the clinician thinks that this stroke lesion may contribute to the cognitive decline (McKhann et al., 1984). Therefore, such studies would underestimate the frequency of stroke lesions in AD patients.

Evidence of an increased risk of stroke in AD patients

Another way to address the question of increased incidence of stroke in AD patients is to determine, by means of epidemiological studies, whether AD patients have an increased risk of stroke. In an Italian community-based study, Ferrucci et al. (1996) found a higher risk of stroke in stroke-free elderly subjects with dementia than in the remainders. Although the presumed cause of dementia was not detailed in this large epidemiological study, one may presumed that the majority was due to AD, because AD is the main cause of dementia in this age-category, as already shown in an Italian population (Rocca et al., 1990) and because patients with a clinical history of stroke were excluded from the study, leading to an underrepresentation of vascular dementia, the second most frequent cause of dementia. These findings support the hypothesis that AD is associated with an increased risk of stroke.

Evidence of a frequent association of AD and stroke at autopsy

In a study performed before the NINDS-AIREN criteria for vascular dementia were established, approximately 20% of patients with clinically diagnosed "multi-infarct dementia" and 14% of patients classified as having "mixed dementia" fulfilled histopathological criteria for AD (Jellinger et al., 1990). On the other hand 10 to 18% of histological confirmed AD patients had associated cerebrovascular lesions (Ince et al., 1995; Victoroff et al., 1995). In addition, Alzheimer-type pathology is often associated with cerebral amyloid angiopathy (Yoshimura et al., 1992) and with infarcts (Ince et al., 1995). These neuropathological findings also provide strong arguments for a link between AD and vascular pathology.

Does the white matter matter?

White matter abnormalities are often associated with stroke (Hijdra et al., 1990; Inzitari et al., 1987; Leys et al., 1992) and with risk factors for stroke such as age (Inzitari et al., 1987), arterial hypertension (Breteler et al., 1994a; Schmidt et al., 1991), cardiac diseases (Hénon et al., 1996) and diabetes mellitus (Hijdra et al., 1990; Schmidt et al., 1992). They are also associated with late- (Scheltens et al., 1992) but not with early- (Leys et al., 1990) onset AD. They are associated with subtle neuropsychological and behavioral changes (Ellis et al., 1996; Schmidt et al., 1991). Moreover, white matter changes are associated with an increased risk of post-stroke dementia (Liu et al., 1992, 58, Tatemichi et al., 1994). Therefore, the contribution of white matter changes to the symptomatology and course of AD should be considered.

White matter changes and dementia

White matter changes are more frequent in so-called "vascular dementia" than in other types of dementia and normal elderly (Aharon-Peretz et al., 1988; Erkinjuntti et al., 1987; Inzitari et al., 1987; Schmidt, 1992). However, most studies (Aharon-Peretz et al., 1988; Erkinjuntti et al., 1987; Inzitari et al., 1987; Schmidt, 1992) were conducted before the NINDS-AIREN criteria for "vascular dementia" (Roman et al., 1993) were established. Large coalescent hyperintense areas extending from the periventricular region far into the deep white matter in demented patients are one of the imaging hallmarks of a cerebrovascular disease associated with dementia (Erkinjuntti et al., 1987; Kinkel et al., 1985; Liu et al., 1992; Schmidt, 1992). Less frequently, white matter changes are also found in AD patients (Erkinjuntti et al., 1994; Leys et al., 1992; Rezek et al., 1987), especially with late-onset (Brun and Englund, 1986; Scheltens et al., 1992), even after exclusion of risk factors for stroke (Leys et al., 1992; Scheltens et al., 1992). The mechanisms leading to white matter changes in late-onset AD may be multiple: lipohyalinosis of the deep perforators (Rezek et al., 1987), amyloid angiopathy (Bogucki et al., 1987), associated risk factors for stroke (Skoog et al., 1996) and Wallerian degeneration (Leys et al., 1992).

In stroke patients, white matter changes are more frequent in those with lacunes (Cadelo et al., 1991; Hijdra et al., 1990; Leys et al., 1992) or deep hemorrhages (Cadelo et al., 1991; Hijdra et al., 1990; Inzitari et al., 1987; Leys et al., 1992). The relationship between white matter changes and lacunes or deep cerebral hemorrhages is stronger than the relationship between white matter changes and arterial hypertension (Cadelo et al., 1991; Hijdra et al., 1990; Leys et al., 1992): this finding suggests that arterial hypertension leads to leuko-araiosis only after having caused small-vessel disease to such a degree that lacunes or deep cerebral hemorrhages are almost always present (Hijdra et al., 1990; Leys et al., 1992). Thus, among AD patients, those who have the highest risk of coincidental brain infarcts are those with lacunes and white matter changes, a view supported by the Nun Study (Snowden et al., 1997).

White matter changes may induce specific cognitive decline

In AD patients, the contribution of white matter changes is usually masked by the cause of dementia (Hachinski et al., 1987). The severity of white matter changes is correlated with the severity of dementia (Steingart et al., 1989) but brain atrophy may be a confounding factor because of a strong correlation between cerebral atrophy and white matter changes (Hijdra et al., 1990). The location of white matter changes may influence cognitive functions: patients with lacunes and dementia have more white matter lesions in the frontal lobes and their severity correlates with the cognitive decline (Fukuda et al., 1990; Ishii et al., 1986).

In studies performed in large groups of healthy individuals, white matter hyperintensities are associated with subtle neuropsychological deficits especially in memory (DeCarli et al., 1995; Schmidt et al., 1991), attention capacities (Van Swieten et al., 1991), and frontal lobe cognitive function (DeCarli et al., 1995). A threshold of severity of white matter changes is required before cognitive deficits occur in healthy elderly individuals (Boone et al., 1992). In non-demented stroke-free subjects who where randomly selected from the Rotterdam cohort, those who had white matter hyperintensities performed worse in tests measuring executive control functions, mental speed and delayed verbal recall (Breteler et al., 1994b). Mild disturbances in attention and increased perseverations may be the earliest signs of cognitive decline associated with white matter hyperintensities (Blots et al., 1996; Schmidt et al., 1993; Van Swieten et al., 1991; Ylilosky et al., 1993). These findings suggest that white matter hyperintensities are primarily related to subcortical frontal dysfunction. However, again, cerebral atrophy may be a confounding factor (Hijdra et al., 1991; Leys and Bogousslavsky, 1994).

Influence of stroke lesions in patients with preclinical Alzheimer pathology

Stroke patients are at risk for dementia: the prevalence of dementia 3 months after an ischemic stroke, in patients over 60 years of age is 26.3%, i.e. 9 fold higher than in controls (Tatemichi et al., 1992). One year after stroke, the probability of new-onset dementia is 5.4% in patients aged 60 years or more and 10.4% in patients over 90 years (Tatemichi et al., 1990). Four years after a first small infarct, presumably of lacunar type, 23.1% of patients develop dementia i.e. 4 to 12 times more than controls (Loeb et al., 1992). After exclusion of patients who are demented 3 months after an ischemic stroke, the relative risk of dementia within 4 years is 5.5 (Tatemichi et al., 1994). Previous stroke and cortical atrophy are associated with a higher risk of post-stroke dementia (Liu et al., 1992; Loeb et al., 1992; Tatemichi et al., 1990). Stroke is considered as the direct cause of only one half of post-stroke dementia (Tatemichi et al., 1992). In some stroke patients, dementia has a progressive onset and course suggesting a degenerative rather than a vascular process (Pasquier et al., 1994; Pasquier et al., 1995; Tatemichi et al., 1994). As previously mentioned, white matter changes, often associated with stroke and AD, might also contribute to cognitive decline (Hachinski et al., 1987; Hijdra et al., 1990; Leys et al., 1992). Therefore, there is evidence that even a small ischemic lesion, such as a lacunar infarct, increases the risk of developing new-onset dementia during the next few years, and that some of these dementia may be AD cases revealed by a coincidental stroke (Hénon et al., 1996). Pasquier and Leys (1997) suggested the following mechanisms, based upon the effects of the summation of various lesion types. In normal aging, the cognitive decline remains moderate and will never reach the threshold of dementia; in patients with "pure" Alzheimer pathology, the slope of the cognitive decline is dramatically modified and the threshold of dementia is reached after a period of preclinical AD; in "pure" vascular dementia, each stroke is associated with a sudden cognitive impairment leading to dementia in a stepwise fashion; when a stroke occurs in a patient with preclinical Alzheimer pathology, the period of preclinical AD is shortened by the summation of vascular and Alzheimer lesions and the threshold of dementia is reached earlier than in patients with "pure" Alzheimer pathology: these patients develop progressive dementia with a time-course suggestive of AD. In all circumstances, white matter changes lead to a moderate increase in the loss of cognitive functions due to aging, AD or stroke, and probably contribute independently to dementia. Therefore, dementia may be the consequence of the additive effect of the cerebrovascular lesions, Alzheimer pathology, white matter changes and aging. Even when these changes by their own, do not lead to dementia, their summation may reach the threshold of lesions required to induce dementia (Boone et al., 1992; Erkinjuntti et al., 1993; Pasquier and Leys, 1997).

Influence of stroke lesions on the course of Alzheimer's disease

Mild progressive dementia may be present before stroke and unrecognized by the family: in community studies, the prevalence of all types of dementia is of 2% in the age category of 65 to 74 years and above 10% in the age category of 75 to 84 years (Rocca et al., 1990); therefore, similar figures are expected in stroke patients. As suggested by Hénon et al. (1996) unrecognized pre-stroke dementia may contribute to the increased incidence rate of dementia (Tatemichi et al., 1994) and of AD (Kokmen et al., 1996) 1 year after a first ischemic stroke. The prevalence of pre-stroke dementia has been estimated at 18% (95% confidence interval: 11–25%) in patients with a mean age of 73 years (Hénon et al., 1996); most pre-existing dementia may be due to AD (Leys et al., 1997). The contribution of vascular pathology on the symptomatology and course of clinically patent AD remains almost unsettled. The results of the Nun study (Snowdon et al., 1997) suggest that cerebrovascular disorders may play an important role in determining the presence and the severity of the clinical symptoms of AD: among 61 patients who met neuropathological criteria for AD, those with brain infarcts had poorer cognitive function and were more often demented than those without infarcts. In contrast, among 41 patients who did not meet neuropathological criteria for AD, brain infarcts were only weakly associated with dementia and poor cognitive functions (Snowdon et al., 1997). Because of the summation of the various types of lesions, stroke probably leads to a worsening of the cognitive status of an AD patient. Moreover, stroke patients with pre-existing dementia, irrespective of its cause, have a worse prognosis at the acute stage, with a higher mortality rate (Hénon et al., 1996). Therefore, stroke may be associated with an increased mortality rate in AD patients.

Is stroke prevention an effective prevention of Alzheimer's disease in some patients?

It has been shown that most factors associated with an increased risk of stroke are also associated with an increased risk of AD (Skoog et al., 1996). Whether risk factors for stroke increase the risk of AD because they increase the risk of stroke which may sum up with the Alzheimer pathology remains unsettled. From a theoretical point of view, an optimal management of risk factors for stroke should decrease the incidence rate of AD. However, one cannot exclude that the reverse situation may also be true, because an optimal management of risk factors for stroke increases the life expectancy and may, therefore, increase the risk of AD. Moreover, treatments may also have direct side effects. In addition, drugs trials dealing with primary or secondary prevention of stroke should also include cognitive evaluation.

Conclusion

This review provides evidence that stroke and AD occur in the same patient more frequently than expected by chance, and that stroke, even with minor physical consequences, may lead to an increase progression of cognitive decline in AD patients. Recognition of a vascular component in a dementia syndrome is therefore useful for the management of AD patients. Whether an optimal management of risk factors for stroke may delay the clinical expression of dementia in patients with preclinical Alzheimer pathology should be evaluated.

References

Aharon-Peretz J, Cummings JL, Hill MA (1988) Vascular dementia and dementia of the Alzheimer type. Cognition, ventricular size and leuko-araiosis. Arch Neurol 45: 719–721

Albert MJ, Graffagnino C, McClenny C, DeLong D, Strittmatter W, Saunders AM, Roses AD (1995) ApoE genotype and survival from intracerebral haemorrhage. Lancet 346: 575

Alperovitch A, Mas JL, Doyon B, Myquel P (1986) Mortality from stroke in France 1968–1982. Neuroepidemiology 5: 80–87

Blots ML, Hoes AW, Koudstaal PJ, Hofman A, Grobbee DE (1996) Common carotid intima media thickness predicts stroke in the Rotterdam study. J Neurol 243: 6

Bogucki A, Papierz W, Szymanska R, Staniaszczyk R (1988) Cerebral amyloïd angiopathy with attenuation of the white matter on CT-scans: subcortical arteriosclerotic encephalopathy (Binswanger) in a normotensive patient. J Neurol 235: 435–437

Boone KB, Miller BL, Mehringer CM, Hill-Gutierrez E, Goldberg MA, Berman NG (1992) Neuropsychological correlates of white-matter lesions in healty elderly subject. A threshold effect. Arch Neurol 49: 549–554

Breteler MMB, Van Swieten JC, Bots ML, Grobbee DE, Claus JJ, van den Hout JHW, van Harskamp F, Tanghe HLJ, de Jong PRVM, van Gijn J, Hofman A (1994a) Cerebral white matter lesions, vascular risk factors, and cognitive function in a population-based study: The Rotterdam Study. Neurology 44: 1246–1252

Breteler MMB, Claus JJ, Grobbee DE, Hofman A (1994b) Cardiovascular disease and distribution of cognitive function in elderly people: the Rotterdam study. Br Med J 308: 1604–1608

Brun A, Englund E (1986) A white matter disorder in dementia of the Alzheimer type: a pathoanatomical study. Ann Neurol 19: 253–262

Cadelo M, Inzitari D, Pracucci G, Mascalchi M (1991) Predictors of leukoaraiosis in elderly neurological patients. Cerebrovasc Dis 1: 345–351

DeCarli C, Murphy DGM, Tranh M, Grady CL, Haxby JV, Gilette JA, Salerno JA, Gonzales-Aviles A, Horwitz B, Rapoport SI, Schapiro MB (1995) The effect of white matter hyperintensity volume on brain structure, cognitive performance, and cerebral metabolism of glucose in 51 healthy adults. Neurology 45: 2077–2084

Ellis RJ, Olichney JM, Thal LJ, Mirra SS, Morris JC, Beekly D, Heyman A (1996) Cerebral amyloid angiopathy in the brains of patients with Alzheimer's disease: the CERAD experience, part XV. Neurology 46: 1592–1596

Erkinjuntti T, Hachinski VC (1993) Rethinking vascular dementia. Cerebrovasc Dis 3: 3–23

Erkinjuntti T, Ketonen L, Sulkava R, Sipponen J, Vuorialho M, Iivanainen M (1987) Do white matter changes on MRI and CT differentiate vascular dementia from Alzheimer's disease? J Neurol Neurosurg Psychiatry 50: 37–42

Erkinjuntti T, Gao F, Lee DH, Eliasziw M, Merskey H, Hachinski VC (1994) Lack of difference in brain hyperintensities between patients with early Alzheimer's disease and control subjects. Arch Neurol 51: 260–268

Ferrucci L, Guralnik JM, Salive ME, Pahor M, Corti MC, Baroni A, Havlik RJ (1996) Cognitive impairment and risk of stroke in the older population. J Am Geriatr Soc 44: 237–241

Fisher MC (1969) The arterial lesions underlying lacunes. Acta Neuropathol (Berl) 12: 1–15

Frisoni G, Geroldi C, Blanquetti A, Trabucchi M, Govoni S, Franceschini G, Calabresi L (1994) Apolipoprotein e4 allele frequency in vascular dementia and Alzheimer's disease (letter). Stroke 25: 1703

Fukuda H, Kobayaski S, Okada K, Tsunematsu T (1990) Frontal white matter lesions and dementia in lacunar infarction. Stroke 21: 1143–1149

Gerdes LU (1994) Apolipoprotein E genotypes and cardiovascular disease: a quantitative overview of 42 studies. Genet Epidemiol 11: 294

Haan J, Maat-Schieman MLC, Roos RAC (1994a) Clinical effects of cerebral amyloid angiopathy. Dementia 5: 210–213

Haan J, Maat-Schieman MLC, Van Duinen SG, Jensson O, Thorsteinsson L, Roos RAC (1994b) Co-localization of βA4 and cystatin C in cortical blood vessels in Dutch, but not in Icelandic hereditary cerebral hemorrhage with amyloidosis. Acta Neurol Scand 89: 367–371

Hachinski VC, Potter P, Merskey H (1987) Leuko-Araiosis. Arch Neurol 44: 21–23

Hénon H, Durieu I, Lucas C, Godefroy O, Pasquier F, Leys D (1996) Prevalence of preexisting dementia in consecutive stroke patients. Neurology 47: 852–853

Hénon H, Godefroy O, Lucas Ch, Pruvo JP, Leys D (1996) Risk factors for leuko-araiosis in stroke patients. Acta Neurol Scand 94: 137–144

Hijdra A, Verbeeten B Jr (1991) Leuko-araiosis and ventricular enlargement in patients with ischemic stroke. Stroke 22: 447–450

Hijdra A, Verbeeten B Jr, Verhulst JAPM (1990) Relation of Leukoaraiosis to lesion type in stroke patients. Stroke 21: 890–894

Hofman A, Ott A, Breteler MMB, Bots ML, Slooter AJC, Van Harskamp F, Van Duijn CN, Van Broeckhoven C, Grobbee DE (1997) Atherosclerosis, apolopoprotein E and prevalence of dementia and Alzheimer's disease in the Rotterdam study. Lancet 349: 151–154

Ince PG, McArthur FK, Bjertness E, Torvik A, Candy JM, Edwardson JA (1995) Neuropathological diagnoses in elderly patients in Oslo: Alzheimer's disease, Lewy body disease, vascular lesions. Dementia 6: 162–168

Inzitari D, Diaz F, Fox A, Hachinski VC, Steingart A, Lau C, Donald A, Wade J, Mulic H, Merskey H (1987) Vascular risk factors and Leuko-Araiosis. Arch Neurol 44: 42–47

Inzitari D, Giordano GP, Ancona AL, Pracucci G, Mascalchi M, Amaducci L (1990) Leuko-araiosis, intracerebral hemorrhage and arterial hypertension. Stroke 21: 1419–1423

Ishii N, Nishihara Y, Imamura T (1986) Why do frontal lobe symptoms predominate in vascular dementia with lacunes? Neurology 36: 340–345

Jellinger K, Danielczyk W, Fischer P, Gabriel E (1990) Clinico-pathological analysis of dementia disorders in the elderly. J Neurol Sci 95: 239–258

Kinkel WR, Jacobs L, Polachini I, Bates V, Heffner RR Jr (1995) Subcortical arteriosclerotic encephalopathy (Binswanger's disease). Computer tomographic nuclear magnetic resonance and clinical correlations. Arch Neurol 42: 951–959

Kokmen E, Whisnant JP, O'Fallon WN, Chu CP, Beard CM (1996) Dementia after ischemic stroke: a population-based study in Rochester, Minnesota (1960–1984). Neurology 46: 154–159

Leys D, Bogousslavsky J (1994) Mechanisms of vascular dementia. In: Leys D, Scheltens P (eds) Vascular dementia. ICG Publications, Dordrecht, pp 121–132

Leys D, Pruvo JP, Parent M, Vermersch P, Soetaert G, Steinling M, Delacourte A, Defossez A, Rapoport A, Clarisse J, Petit H (1991) Could Wallerian degeneration contribute to "Leuko-Araïosis" in subjects free of any vascular disorder? J Neurol Neurosurg Psychiatry 54: 46–50.

Leys D, Pruvo JP, Scheltens Ph, Rondepierre Ph, Godefroy O, Leclerc X, De Reuck J (1992) Leuko-araiosis. Relationship with the types of focal lesions occurring in acute cerebrovascular disorders. Cerebrovasc Disord 2: 169–176

Leys D, Hénon H, Pasquier F, Durieu I, Pruvo JP (1997) Medial temporal lobe atrophy in stroke patients: relationship with pre-stroke dementia. Neurology 48: A206

Liu CK, Miller BL, Cummings JL, Mehringer CM, Goldberg MA, Howng SL, Benson DF (1992) A quantitative MRI study of vascular dementia. Neurology 42: 138–143

Loeb C, Gandolfo C, Croce R, Conti M (1992) Dementia associated with lacunar infarction. Stroke 23: 1225–1229

Lucas C, Parent M, Delandsheer E, Delacourte A, Fournier Y, Defossez A, Leys D (1992) Hémorragies cér'brales multiples et angiopathie amyloide de la substance blanche dans un cas de maladie d'Alzheimer. Rev Neurol (Paris) 148: 218–220

McKhann G, Drachman D, Folstein M, Katzman R, Price D, Stadlan EM (1984) Clinical diagnosis of Alzheimer's disease: report of the NINCDS-ADRDA work group under the auspices of department of health and human services task force on Alzheimer's disease. Neurology 34: 939–944

Pasquier F, Leys D (1997) Why are stroke patients prone to develop dementia? J Neurol 244: 135–142

Pasquier F, Lebert F, Petit H (1994) Pseudo progressive dementia and "strategic" infarcts. In: Leys D, Scheltens P (eds) Vascular dementia. ICG Publications, Dordrecht, pp 47–54

Pasquier F, Lebert F, Petit H (1995) Dementia, apathy and thalamic infarcts. Neuropsychiat Neuropsychol Behav Neurol 8: 208–214

Rezek DL, Morris JC, Fulling KH, Gado MH (1987) Periventricular white matter lucencies in senile dementia of the Alzheimer type and in normal ageing. Neurology 37: 1365–1368

Rocca WA, Bonaiuto S, Lippi A, Luciani P, Turtù F, Cavarzeran F, Amaducci L (1990) Prevalence of clinically diagnosed Alzheimer's disease and other dementing disorders: a door-to-door survey in Appignano, Macerata Province, Italy. Neurology 40: 626–631

Roman GC, Tatemichi TK, Erkinjuntti T, Cummings JL, Masdeu JC, Garcia JH, Amaducci L, Orgogozo JM, Brun A, Hofman A, Moody DM, O'Brien MD, Yamaguchi T, Grafman J, Drayer BP, Bennett DA, Fisher M, Ogata J, Kokmen E, Bermejo F, Wolf PA, Gorelick PB, Bick KL, Pajeau AK, Bell MA, DeCarli C, Culebras A, Korczyn AD, Bogousslavsky J, Hartmann A, Scheinberg P (1993) Vascular dementia: diagnostic criteria for research studies. Neurology 43: 250–260

Rubinsztein DC (1995) Apolipoprotein E: a review of its roles in lipoprotein metabolism, neuronal growth and repair and as a risk factor for Alzheimer's disease. Psychol Med 25: 223–229

Saunders AM, Roses AD (1993) Apolipoprotein E allele frequency, ischemic cerebrovascular disease, and Alzheimer's disease (letter). Stroke 24: 1416

Scheltens Ph, Barkhof F, Valk J, Algra PR, Gerritsen Van Der Hoop R, Nauta J, Wolters E Ch (1992) White matter lesions on magnetic resonance imaging in Alzheimer's disease: evidence for heterogeneity. Brain 115: 735–743

Schmidt R (1992) Comparison of magnetic resonance imaging in Alzheimer's disease, vascular dementia and normal aging. Eur Neurol 32: 164–169

Schmidt R, Fazekas F, Offenbacher H, Lytwyn H, Blematl B, Niederkorn K, Horner S, Payer F, Freidl W (1991) Magnetic resonance imaging white matter lesions and cognitive impairment in hypertensive individuals. Arch Neurol 48: 417–420

Schmidt R, Fazekas F, Kleinert G, Offenbacher H, Gindl K, Payer F, Friedl W, Niderkorn K, Lechner H (1992) Magnetic resonance imaging signal hyperintensities in the deep and subcortical white matter. A comparative study between stroke patients and normal volunteers. Arch Neurol 49: 825–827

Schmidt R, Fazekas F, Offenbacher H, Dusek T, Zach E, Reinhart B, Grieshofer P, Freidl W, Eber B, Schumacher M, Koch M, Lechner H (1993) Neuropsychologic correlates of MRI white matter hyperintensities: a study of 150 normal volunteers. Neurology 43: 2490–2494

Shimano H, Ishibashi S, Murase T (1989) Plasma apolipoproteins in patients with multi-infarct dementia. Atherosclerosis 79: 257–260

Skoog I, Lernfelt B, Landahl S, Palmertz B, Andreasson LA, Nilsson L, Persson G, Odén A, Svanborg A (1996) 15-year longitudinal study of blood pressure and dementia. Lancet 347: 1141–1145

Snowdon DA, Greiner LH, Mortimer JA, Riley KP, Greiner PA, Markesbery WR (1997) Brain infarction and the clinical expression of Alzheimer disease. The nun study. JAMA 277: 813–817

Steingart A, Hachinski VC, Lau C, Fox AJ, Fox H, Lee D, Inzitari D, Merskey H (1987) Cognitive and neurologic findings in demented patients with diffuse white matter lucencies on computed tomographic scan (Leuko-Araiosis). Arch Neurol 44: 36–39

Stephenson DT, Rash K, Clemens JA (1992) Amyloid precursor protein accumulates in regions of neurodegeneration following focal cerebral ischemia in the rat. Brain Res 593: 128–135

Tatemichi TK, Foulkes MA, Mohr JP, Hewitt JR, Hier DB, Price TR, Wolf PA (1990) Dementia in stroke survivors in the stroke data bank cohort. Prevalence, incidence, risk factors, and computed tomographic findings. Stroke 21: 858–866

Tatemichi TK, Desmond DW, Mayeux R Paik M, Stern Y, Sano M, Remien RH, Williams JBW, Mohr JP, Hauser WA, Figueroa M (1992) Dementia after stroke: baseline frequency, risks, and clinical features in a hospitalized cohort. Neurology 42: 1185–1193

Tatemichi TK, Paik M, Bagiella E, Desmond DW, Stern Y, Sano M, Hauser WA, Mayeux R (1994) Risk of dementia after stroke in a hospitalized cohort: results of a longitudinal study. Neurology 44: 1885–1891

Terayama, Meyer JS, Kawamura J, Weathers S, Mortel KF (1992) Patterns of cerebral hypoperfusion compared among demented and nondemented patients with stroke. Stroke 23: 686–692

van Swieten JC, Geyskes GG, Derix MMA, Peeck BM, Ramos LMP, van Latum JC, van Gijn J (1991) Hypertension in the elderly is associated with white matter lesions and cognitive decline. Ann Neurol 30: 825–830

Victoroff J, Mack WJ, Lyness SC, Chui HC (1995) Multicenter clinicopathological correlation in dementia. Am J Psychiatry 152: 1476–1484

Vinters HV (1987) Cerebral amyloid angiopathy. A critical review. Stroke 18: 311–324

Yamada M, Tsukagoshi H, Otomo E, Hayakawa M (1987) Cerebral amyloid angiopathy in the aged. J Neurol 234: 371–376

Ylikoski R, Ylikoski A, Erkinjuntti T, Sulkava R, Raininko R, Tilvis R (1993) White matter changes in healthy elderly persons correlate with attention and speed of mental processing. Arch Neurol 50: 818–824

Yoshimura M, Yamanouchi H, Kuzuhara S, Mori H, Sugiura S, Mizutani T, Shimada H, Tomonaga M, Toyokura Y (1992) Dementia in cerebral amyloid angiopathy: a clinicopathological study. J Neurol 239: 441–450

Authors' address: P. Scheltens, MD, PhD, Department of Neurology, Academisch Ziekenhuis VU, PO Box 7057, 1007 MB Amsterdam, The Netherlands

Corpus callosum in Alzheimer's disease and vascular dementia — a quantitative magnetic resonance study

J. Pantel[1], J. Schröder[1], M. Essig[2], R. Minakaran[1], L. R. Schad[2], M. Friedlinger[2], M. Jauss[1], and M. V. Knopp[2]

[1] Section of Geriatric Psychiatry, University of Heidelberg, and
[2] German Center of Cancer Research (DKFZ), INF 280, Heidelberg,
Federal Republic of Germany

Summary. We investigated atrophic alterations in different regions of the corpus callosum in Alzheimer's disease (AD) and vascular dementia (VD) with respect to clinical changes. 32 patients with AD (NINCDS-ADRDA criteria), 17 patients with VD (NINDS-AIREN criteria) and 13 healthy control subjects were included. 3-D MRI sequences were acquired using a 1.5 T MRI scanner. The size of the corpus callosum and its subdivisions was sampled on 5 mid-saggital slices using a personal computer-based software. Total callosal size was significantly reduced in AD but not in VD. Furthermore, the most rostral parts of the corpus callosum were significantly smaller in AD when compared to controls. Again, these changes were not found in patients with VD. Severity of dementia was significantly correlated with the size of the midbody of the corpus callosum in AD. Callosal atrophy in AD may reflect the severity and pattern of cortical neuronal damage occurring mostly in the inferior frontal, anterior parietal and midtemporal regions. Correlations between regional callosal atrophy and severity of dementia indicate that interhemispheric cortico-cortical disconnections may contribute to the dementia syndrome.

Introduction

The corpus callosum is the most important structure involved in the transmission of interhemispheric information. Changes of the corpus callosum associated with brain disorders may therefore reflect changes in the functional integrity of inter-hemispheric association fibres. Since the corpus callosum is organized topographically (Fig. 1), regional differences in atrophy within the corpus callosum may provide information on the functional integrity of different cortical regions. According to a pathological study of De Lacoste et al. (1985) fibres from the inferior frontal and anterior parietal regions course through the rostrum and genu of the corpus callosum, fibres deriving from the mid-temporal regions cross through the mid-body, whereas connections from the parieto-occipital regions course through the splenium and caudal portions

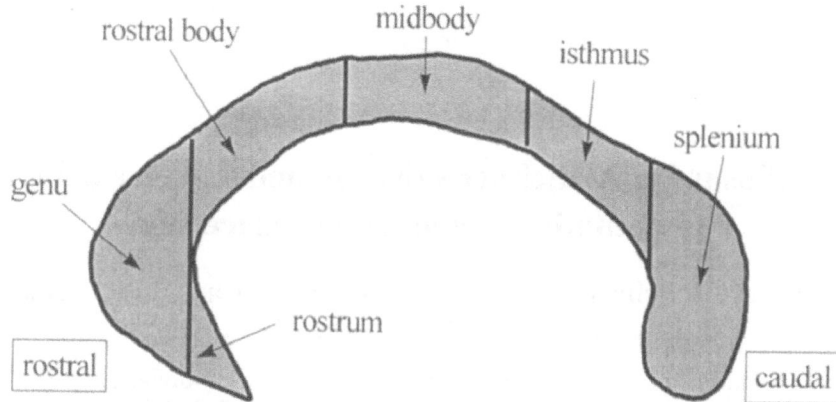

Fig. 1. Anatomical subdivisions of the human corpus callosum. Subdivisions approximately correspond to the measured subsections as described in the text (genu and rostrum = CC1; rostral body = CC2; midbody = CC3; isthmus = CC4; splenium = CC5)

of the body. Only few studies investigated regional changes of the corpus callosum in different dementing diseases in vivo (Vermesch et al., 1993; Yamauchi et al., 1993; Biegon et al., 1994; Janowsky et al., 1996; Kaufer et al., 1997). However, there is no study comparing alterations of the corpus callosum in the most common forms of dementia — Alzheimer's disease and vascular dementia. Aims of our study were therefore:

1. To investigate global and regional changes in the size of the corpus callosum in Alzheimer's disease and vascular dementia
2. To establish the relationship between regional alterations in the corpus callosum and clinical changes such as the severity of dementia

Patients and methods

The study was approved by the local ethical committee. Patients were consecutively admitted inpatients under the care of the Section of Geriatric Psychiatry of the University of Heidelberg. Patients with a history of head trauma, birth injury, electroconvulsive therapy and a significant substance abuse were excluded. All patients underwent thorough standardized general and neurological examinations as well as a CT scan and laboratory studies in order to exclude metabolic, toxic and inflammatory causes of their dementia syndrome. CT scans were carefully screened for the presence and types of cerebrovascular lesions. An extensive neuropsychological investigation was performed using a test battery which has been described in detail elsewhere (Pantel et al., 1997). Severity of cognitive impairment was established on the Mini Mental State Examination (MMSE/ Folstein et al., 1975) and the Brief Cognitive Rating Scale (BCRS/ Reisberg and Ferris, 1988).

Diagnosis of Alzheimer's disease and vascular dementia was strictly based on the criteria of the NINDS-AIREN work group (Roman et al., 1993) and the NINCDS-ADRDA work group (McKhann et al., 1984) using all relevant informations concerning history, clinical, neuropsychological, and neuroradiological findings. The control subjects were volunteers from the local community and were all in a good mental and physical state of health with no history of hypertension, diabetes, neurological or psychiatric diseases. In order to exclude any latent brain disorders control subjects were investigated using the same neuropsychological and clinical measures. In total, 32 patients with Alzheimer's disease, 17 patients with vascular dementia and 13 healthy control subjects were investigated.

MR Image acquisition and image processing

For each patient and control subject a set of T1-weighted images, providing good differentiation between corpus callosum and the adjacent brain tissue were acquired. All measurements were performed on a 1.5 T MAGNETOM 63/84 SP Siemens scanner using a 3D MPRAGE sequence (TR: 10 ms, TE: 4 ms). MR images were taken at 15 degree cranial to the orbito-meatal line. The total measurement time was about 10 minutes per patient. The 3D image data cube with a slab thickness of 160 mm consisted of 128 sagittal image slices, resulting in a slice thickness of 1.25 mm. There was no interslice gap. The slices had an in-plane field of view of 260 mm, the volume pixels were of the size $1.02 \times 1.02 \times 1.25\,mm^3$.

Image data processing was performed on a conventional 80486/66 MHz personal computer using the software NMRWin. Detailed structure and function of this software is described elsewhere (Friedlinger et al., 1995). Size of the corpus callosum was sampled on 5 midsagittal slices using the manual segmentation function of NMRWin. We used those 5 slices on which the corpus callosum could be clearly demarcated from the adjacent brain tissue. Corpus callosum and its subsections was manually traced on each of the 5 slices following a modified protocol described by Weiß et al. (1991): A horizontal line was drawn from the most anterior to the most posterior point of the corpus callosum. Subsequently, 6 vertical lines were constructed perpendicular to the horizontal line. These lines dissected the corpus callosum into 5 subsections called CC1 to CC2 where CC1 represents the most rostral part and CC5 the most caudal part of the structure. The resulting subsections correspond approximately to the 5 anatomical subdivisions shown in Fig. 1. In order to achieve a measure of test-retest reliability each measurement was performed twice by the same rater (R.M.). The rater was blind to the diagnosis. The resulting areas were multiplied by the slice thickness, summed up and documented in a protocol file.

To address potential inter-individual differences in head size, all morphometric data were corrected for the subject's intracranial area measured on the midsagittal slice. For statistical comparison between groups we performed a Wilcoxon rank sum test for independent samples. Correlations between the clinical variables and volumetric data were calculated for each group separately by Spearman rank correlation.

Results

Patient groups did not differ with respect to age and severity of dementia (Table 1). Test-retest reliability was 0.96 for CC1, 0.89 for CC2, and 0.95 for CC3, CC4 and CC5 ($p < 0.0001$). Total callosal size was significantly reduced in Alzheimer's disease when compared to controls. There was also a certain amount of callosal size reduction in vascular dementia. However, these differences did not reach significance (Fig. 2). Furthermore, the most rostral parts of the corpus callosum (CC1 and CC2) were significantly ($p < 0.05$) reduced in Alzheimer's disease when compared to controls (Fig. 3). Again, these changes were not found in patients with vascular dementia. Severity of dementia as expressed by the scores of the MMSE and the BCRS were significantly correlated with the size of the rostral body and the midbody of

Wilcoxon rank sum test for independent samples

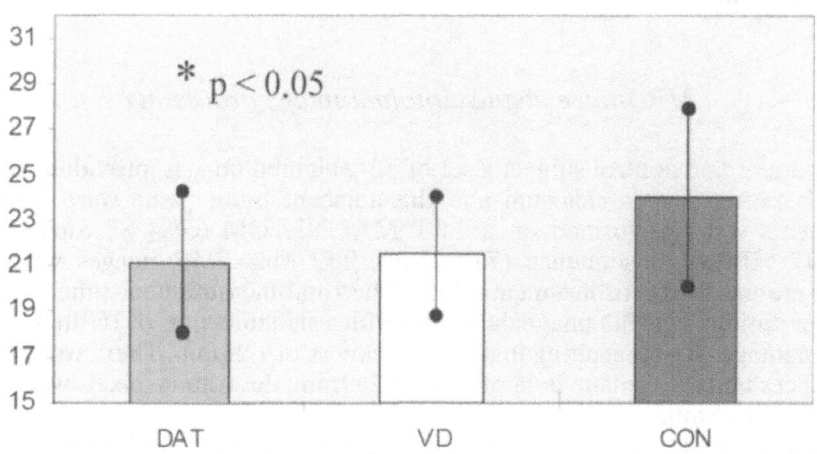

Fig. 2. Comparison of total callosal size normalized to the midsagittal intracranial area in Alzheimer's disease, vascular dementia and healthy ageing. Vertical bars indicate standard deviations. (*significant differences in comparison to controls; *DAT* Alzheimer's disease; *VD* vascular dementia; *CON* control subjects)

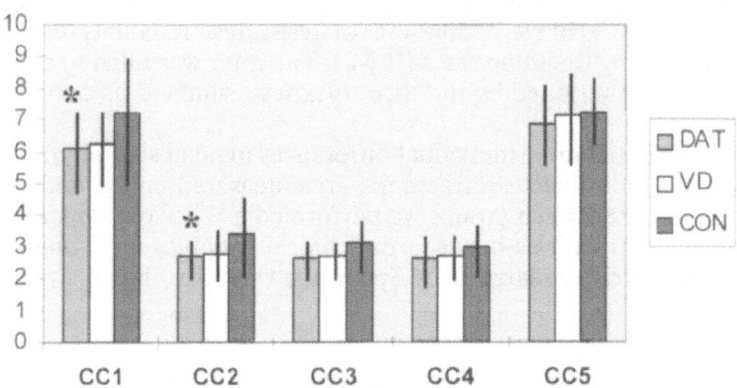

Fig. 3. Comparison of regional callosal size normalized to the midsagittal intracranial area in Alzheimer's disease, vascular dementia and healthy ageing. Vertical bars indicate standard deviations (*significant differences in comparison to controls; *DAT* Alzheimer's disease; *VD* vascular dementia; *CON* control subjects; *CC1* to *CC5* subsections of the corpus callosum)

the corpus callosum (CC2 and CC3) in Alzheimer's disease (Table 2). Additionally, total callosal size was significantly correlated with age. However, there was no correlation with duration of disease. Similar relationships between global and regional callosal size and clinical variables were found in vascular dementia (Table 3).

Table 1. Clinical characteristics of the investigated samples

	Alzheimer's disease	Vascular dementia	Controls	
n	32	17	13	
Age (years)	72.5 (±8.5)	76.6 (±6.6)	68.2 (±5.3)	n.sig.
Duration of illness (month)	45.0 (±31.8)	44.8 (±64.1)	n.a	n.sig.
MMSE	16.3 (±6.4)	18.4 (±5.4)	29.3 (±0.8)	n.sig.
BCRS (I–V)	4.15 (±1.1)	3.8 (±1)	n.d.	n.sig.

MMSE mini mental state examination; *BCRS (I–V)* brief cognitive rating scale, axis I–V; *n.sig.* not significant; *n.a.* not applicable; *n.d.* not done

Table 2. Correlations between clinical data and corpus callosum size in Alzheimer's disease

	CC Sum	CC1	CC2	CC3	CC4	CC5
Duration of illness	0.03	0.16	0.05	0.05	0.03	−0.04
MMSE	0.24	0.3	0.36*	0.38*	0.23	−0.06
BCRS (I–V)	−0.36	−0.34	−0.46*	−0.47*	−0.37	−0.06
Age	−0.44*	−0.43*	−0.38*	−0.23	−0.21	−0.35

*p < 0.05; *MMSE* min mental state examination; *BCRS (I–V)* brief cognitive rating scale, axis I–V; *CC Sum* total callosal size; *CC1* to *CC5* subsections of the corpus callosum

Table 3. Correlations between clinical data and corpus callosum size in vascular dementia

	CC Sum	CC1	CC2	CC3	CC4	CC5
Duration of illness	−0.44	−0.12	−0.4	−0.58*	−0.4	−0.32
MMSE	0.46	0.2	0.56*	0.51*	0.5	0.24
BCRS (I–V)	−0.63*	−0.23	−0.65*	−0.63*	−0.56	−0.65*
Age	0.23	0.22	−0.24	−0.14	−0.17	0.46

*p < 0.05; *MMSE* min mental state examination; *BCRS (I–V)* brief cognitive rating scale, axis I–V; *CC Sum* total callosal size; *CC1* to *CC5* subsections of the corpus callosum

Discussion

The main results of our study include the finding that in moderate to severe Alzheimer's disease, atrophy of the corpus callosum occurs mainly in its anterior parts (genu, rostrum, rostral body). This finding confirms results from previous studies using MRI-based morphometry (Yoshii and Duara, 1989;

Biegon et al., 1994; Janowsky et al., 1996). Janowsky et al. (1996) demonstrated that in Alzheimer's disease all sectors of the corpus callosum show a certain degree of atrophic changes. However, the size reduction in the anterior sector of the corpus callosum best distinguished Alzheimer's disease from healthy aging. Our results are further supported by a a study conducted by Biegon et al. (1993) who reported that Alzheimer's disease was associated by a large and statistically significant reduction in the genu area in comparison to both young and old control subjects. These and our results are in accordance with a post mortem study by Yamanouchi et al. (1989) who found the corpus callosum to be smaller in a sample of male Alzheimer patients in comparison with age matched controls. There were fewer callosal fibres, and their diameter was smaller in the anterior parts of the structure when compared to the control subjects.

The most likely explanation for callosal atrophy in Alzheimer's disease is that changes in the callosal thickness reflect degeneration of axons of cortical neurons lost during the disease process. The observed alterations may therefore reflect a strong involvement of inferior frontal, anterior parietal and mid-temporal cortical neurons in AD (De Lacoste et al., 1985). Another important finding of our study involves a significant correlation between regional size in the middle parts of the corpus callosum and severity of dementia. Similar results have been reported previously (Janowsky et al., 1996). This relationship suggests that in AD interhemispheric cortico-cortical disconnections contribute to the dementia syndrome and that corpus callosum atrophy may be used as a morphological index of disease progression. However, regional callosal size was not only correlated with the disease severity but also with age. This was particularly true for the anterior parts of the corpus callosum which is in accordance with the findings of Kaufer et al. (1997). Weis et al. (1993) showed that the anterior parts of the corpus callosum (genu and anterior parts of the trunk) are significantly decreased during normal ageing. These and our results emphasize that age is another important factor contributing to callosal atrophy.

We did not find significant global and regional callosal size reduction in patients with vascular dementia. However, recent studies suggest that callosal atrophy is probably not specific for Alzheimer's disease and may also occur in patients affected with cerebrovascular disease (Yamauchi et al., 1994, 1995). Using MRI and PET Yamauchi et al. (1994, 1995) showed that atrophy of the corpus callosum progresses with deterioration of cerebral cortical oxygen metabolism in patients with carotid artery occlusion. They also reported that callosal atrophy may be used as an indicator of cognitive impairment in patients with lacunar infarctions and extensive leukoaraiosis. In these patients callosal atrophy may be the expression of white matter damage with involvement of inter-hemispheric fibre systems, which may determine the severity of intellectual decline. This hypothesis is in accordance with our finding that size of the corpus callosum is significantly correlated with the severity of cognitive impairment not only in Alzheimer's disease but also in patients with vascular dementia. Our failure to demonstrate significant differences between vascular dementia and controls with respect to global and regional callosal size may be explained by a greater heterogeneity of the vascular dementia sample which not only included patients with extensive white matter disease but also some patients with territorial infarctions.

In summary, our findings suggest that callosal atrophy might be used as morphological index reflecting the severity and the pattern of destruction of interhemispheric association neurons. This may be true in both, Alzheimer's disease and vascular dementia. However, since Alzheimer's disease preferably affects cortical neurons and subcortical vascular dementia involves mostly severe white matter lesions, callosal atrophy in both dementia syndroms is probably caused by different mechanisms. In order to investigate this further future research should include studies on the association between callosal atrophy and specific neuropsychological functions (memory, language etc.). Similarly, the relationship between callosal atrophy and region-specific volume reduction of the grey and white matter determined by quantitative MRI should be adressed. Furthermore, it might be necessary to perform follow-up investigations in order to study the relationship between morphological changes of the corpus callosum and clinical changes longitudinally.

References

Biegon A, Eberling JL, Richardson BC, Roos MS, Wong STS, Reed BR, Jagust J (1994) Human corpus callosum in aging and Alzheimer's disease: a magnetic resonance imaging study. Neurobiol Aging 15: 393–397

De Lacoste MC, Kirkpatrick JB, Ross ED (1985) Topography of the human corpus callosum. J Neuropathol Exp Neurol 44: 578–591

Folstein MF, Folstein SE, McHugh PR (1975) "Mini-mental-state": a practical method for grading the cognitive state of patients for the clinician. J Psychiatr Res 12: 189–198

Friedlinger M, Schad LR, Blüml S, Tritsch B, Lorenz WJ (1995) Rapid automatic brain volumetry on the basis of multispectral 3D MR imaging data on personal computers. Comput Med Imaging Graph 19(2): 185–205

Janowsky JS, Jeffrey AK, Carper RA (1996) Atrophy of the corpus callosum in Alzheimer's disease versus healthy aging. J Am Geriatr Soc 44: 798–803

Kaufer DI, Miller BL, Itti L, Fairbanks LA, Li J, Fishman J, Kushi J, Cummings JL (1997) Midline cerebral morphometry distinguishes frontotemporal dementia and Alzheimer's disease. Neurology 48: 978–985

McKhann G, Drachman D, Folstein M, Katzman R, Price D, Stadlan EM (1984) Clinical diagnosis of Alzheimer's disease: Report of the NINCDS-ADRDA work group under the auspices of department of health an human services task force on Alzheimer's disease. Neurology 34: 939–965

Pantel J, Schröder J, Schad LR, Friedlinger M, Knopp MV, Schmitt R, Geißler M, Blüml S, Essig M, Sauer H (1997) Quantitative magnetic resonance imaging and neuropsychological functions in dementia of the Alzheimer type. Psychol Med 27: 221–229

Reisberg B, Ferris SH (1988) The brief cognitive rating scale (BCRS). Psychopharmacol Bull 24: 629–636

Roman GC, Tatemichi TK, Erkinjuntti T, Cummings JL, Masdeu JC, Garcia JH, Amaducci L, Orgogozo JM, Brun A, et al (1993) Vascular dementia: diagnostic criteria for research studies. Report of the NINDS-AIREN International Workshop. Neurology 43: 250–260

Vermesch P, Sheltens P, Barkhof F, Steinling M, Leys D (1993) Evidence for atrophy of the corpus callosum in Alzheimer's disease. Eur Neurol 34: 83–86

Weis S, Jellinger K, Wenger E (1991) Morphometry of the corpus callosum in normal aging and Alzheimer's disease. J Neural Transm 33: 35–38

Weis S, Kimbacher M, Wenger E, Neuhold A (1993) Morphometric analysis of the corpus callosum using MR: correlation of measurements with aging in healthy individuals. AJNR 14: 637–645

Yamanouchi H, Sugiura S, Shimada H (1989) Decrease of nerve fibres in the anterior corpus callosum of senile dementia of Alzheimer's type. J Neurol 236: 491–492

Yamauchi H, Fukuyama H, Harada K, Nabatame H, Ogawa M, Ouchi Y, Kimura J, Konishi J (1993) Callosal atrophy paralles decreased cortical oxygen metabolism and neuropsychological impairment in Alzheimer's disease. Arch Neurol 50: 1070–1074

Yamauchi H, Funuyama H, Ogawa M, Ouchi Y, Kimura J (1994) Callosal atrophy in patients withlacunar infarctions and extensive leukoaraiosis. An indicator of cognitive impairment. Stroke 25: 1788–1793

Yamauchi H, Pagani M, Fukuyama H, Ouchi Y, Nagahama Y, Matsuzaki S, Kimura J, Yonekura Y, Konishi J (1995) Progression of atrophy of the corpus callosum with deterioration of cerebral cortical oxigen metabolism after carotid artery occlusion: a follow up study with MRI and PET. J Neurol Neurosurg Psychiatry 59: 420–426

Yoshii F, Duara R (1989) Size of corpus callosum in normal subjects and patients with Alzheimer's disease. Clin Neurol (Tokyo) 29: 1–7

Authors' address: Dr. med. J. Pantel, Section of Geriatric Psychiatry, University of Heidelberg, Voßstrasse 4, D-69115 Heidelberg, Federal Republic of Germany

What do we learn from a few familial Alzheimer's disease cases?

C. Haass[1] and R. Baumeister[2]

[1]Central Institute for Mental Health, Department of Molecular Biology, J5, Mannheim, and [2]Laboratory for Molecular Biology/Genzentrum, University of Munich, Munich, Federal Republic of Germany

Summary. Alzheimer's disease is the most common form of dementia. About 90% of the cases occur sporadically whereas in 10% of the cases mutations were found within three different genes. Mutations in the gene encoding the β-Amyloid precursor protein (βAPP) are located in the ultimate neighborhood of the three proteases (secretases) involved in proteolytic processing of βAPP. These mutations cause an increased production of the long form of Amyloid β-peptide (Aβ) the major component of Amyloid plaques. In contrast to the 40 amino acid form (Aβ40), the 42 amino acid form (Aβ42) aggregates more rapidly, kills cultured neurons more efficiently, and precipitates preferentially in amyloid plaques. Interestingly, mutations in the Presenilin genes which are responsible for more then 40% of all familial AD cases also cause enhanced production of the elongated form of Aβ. Therefore mutations in three different genes directly effect Aβ production in a pathological manner, which strongly supports the amyloid cascade hypothesis.

Mutations in three genes are involved in familial Alzheimer's disease

Alzheimer's disease (AD) is the most common form of dementia world wide. Pathologically, AD is characterized by the invariant accumulation of amyloid plaques in the brains of effected people (Selkoe, 1996). Amyloid plaques are predominately composed of the amyloid β-peptide (Aβ). Aβ itself is derived by proteolytic processing from a large precursor, the β-amyloid precursor protein (βAPP; Haass and Selkoe, 1993; see also Fig. 1a). Three proteases are involved in βAPP processing, called α-, β-, and γ-secretase. Cleavage by α-secretase occurs within the Aβ domain and therefore inhibits Aβ production (Fig. 1a). The cleavage results in the secretion of the soluble N'-terminal part of βAPP which is then found in biological fluids and conditioned media from cultured cells. In contrast, the combined action of β-secretase (at the N'-terminus of the Aβ domain) and γ-secretase (at the C'-terminus of the Aβ-domain) results in the secretion of Aβ (Shoji et al., 1992; Busciglio et al., 1993; Haass et al., 1992; Fig. 1a). Two types of peptides are frequently found in cultured media: the most abundant 40 amino acid Aβ40 (>90%) and the

A

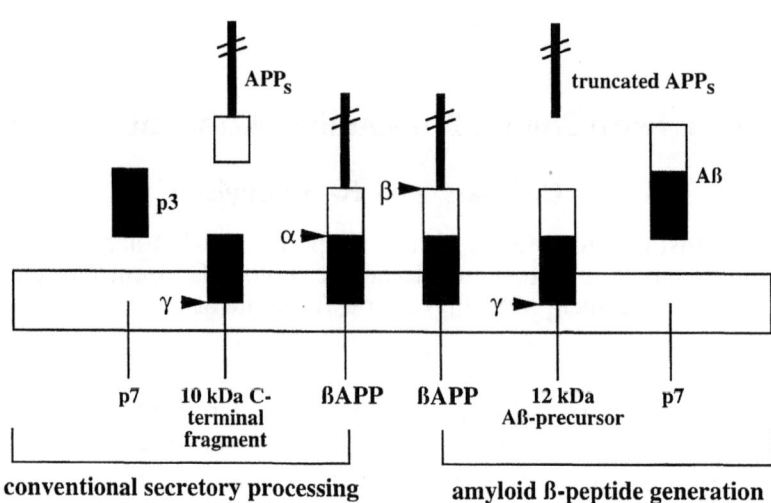

B

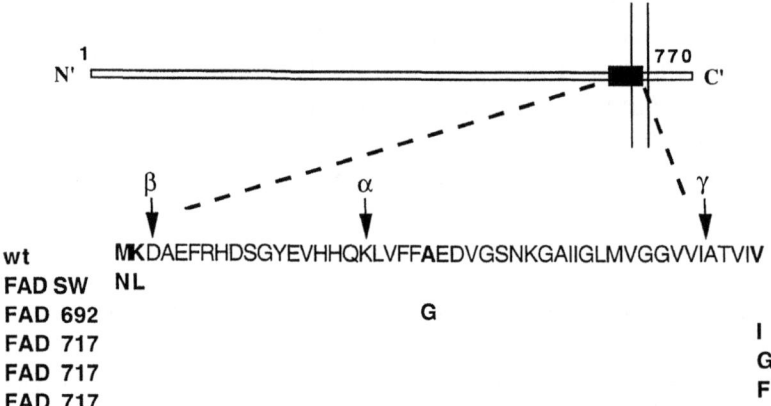

Fig. 1. A Proteolytic processing of βAPP by three secretases. Two general proteolytic processing pathways can be discriminated, an amyloidogenic pathway involved in the generation of Aβ as well as the conventional secretory pathway. In the secretory pathway Aβ generation is inhibited by α-secretase, which cleaves in the middle of the β-amyloid domain. This cleavage generates a 10 kDa C-terminal fragment which is either degraded in lysosomes or cleaved by γ-secretase leading to the secretion of p3. APPs is the secreted derivative of membrane bound βAPP generated by α-secretory processing. In the amyloidogenic pathway βAPP is cleaved by β- and γ-secretase which results in the secretion of Aβ. It is not yet clear if the cleavage at amino acid 42 and 40 is caused by one and the same secretase or two different enzymes. **B** Localization of FAD mutations within βAPP. The Aβ domain is shown as a black box. The cleavage sites of the three secretases are indicated by arrows. The five FAD mutations known to cause early onset FAD are shown. Note, that all mutations are located very close to cleavage sites of the secretases

much less abundant Aβ42 (elongated by two amino acids at its C'-terminus). Both are the result of a physiologically normal proteolytic process (Selkoe, 1996). The longer version of Aβ however is much more toxic for cultured neurons, it aggregates more rapidly, and it preferentially precipitates in amyloid plaques (Selkoe, 1996).

In most of the cases AD occurs as a sporadic disease, however, in about 10% of the cases, AD can also be inherited as an autosomal dominant trait (familial AD, FAD; Selkoe, 1996). In these cases mutations in three genes were linked to the early onset of the disease. The first mutations were not surprisingly found within the βAPP gene (Fig. 1b). βAPP mutations are close to the cleavage sites of each of the three types of secretases (Selkoe, 1996). These mutations have in common that they specifically enhance the production of Aβ40 and/or Aβ42 (Selkoe, 1996) by interfering with the corresponding secretase. In example, a double mutation at the N'-terminus of the Aβ domain (Fig. 1b) results in a ~ 6 fold increase of Aβ40 and Aβ42 production (Citron et al., 1992; Cai et al., 1993) by providing a better substrate for the β-secretase (Haass et al., 1995). Mutations close to the by γ-secretase site specifically enhance Aβ42 generation (Suzuki et al., 1994). However, these mutations are extremely rare and occur only in very few families.

Of the mutations causing early onset FAD most were mapped to a gene on chromosome 14 (Schellenberg et al., 1992). This gene was recently cloned and called Presenilin 1 (PS-1; Sherrington et al., 1995). Shortly after a second gene was cloned and named PS-2 (Rogaev et al., 1995; Levi-Lahad et al., 1995). Both genes are highly homologous and encode proteins which appear to contain 6–8 trans-membrane (TM) domains (Doan et al., 1997; DeStrooper et al., 1997; Fig. 2). Mutations cluster within the TM domains (specifically TM2)' or the large cytoplasmic loop (Haass, 1997). These mutations are responsible for the most aggressive forms of early onset FAD. Surprisingly, the Presenilins are proteolytically processed by a cleavage within the large loop (Thinakaran et al., 1996; Fig. 2). The biological role of the cleavage is unknown. Interestingly, work from many laboratories (Scheuner et al., 1996; Citron et al., 1997; Tomita et al., 1997; Xia et al., 1997; Borchelt et al., 1997; Duff et al., 1996) now showed that PS-1 and PS-2 mutations cause the enhance production of Aβ42. These data therefore provide the strongest possible support of the amyloid cascade hypothesis. Moreover, the identification of the novel genes involved in FAD now provide new tools to understand the molecular mechanisms of Alzheimer's disease, which might finally lead to the development of drugs which are able to slow AD pathology. In the following we will describe two examples from work out of our laboratories which demonstrates how knowledge derived from the analysis from FAD mutations can be used to understand the molecular events causing AD.

The biological and pathological function of the Presenilin genes

Although we know quite a bit about the role of mutant PS proteins in aberrant Aβ generation, very little is known about their biological and pathological

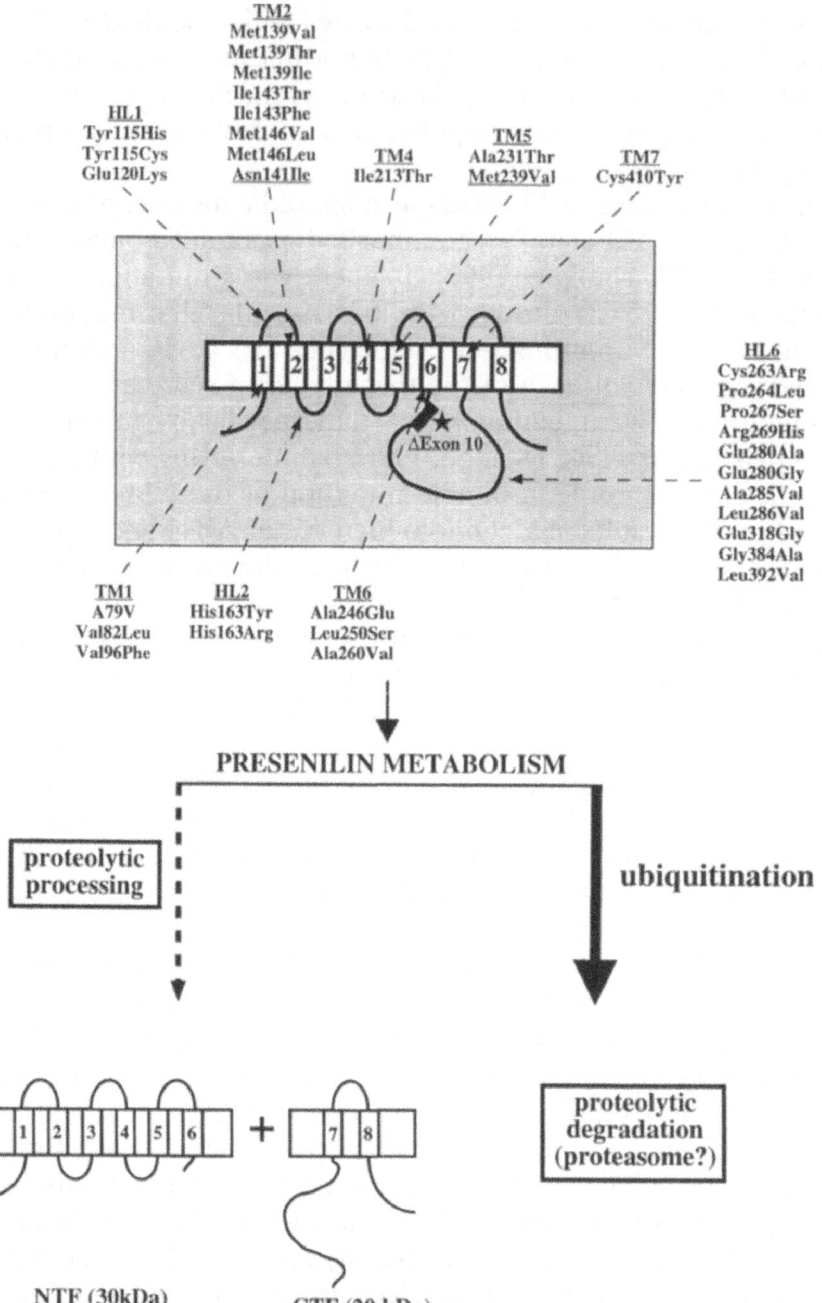

Fig. 2. Schematic representation of the Presenilin proteins. Point mutations as well as the exceptional splicing mutation which leads to the elimination of the domain encoded by exon 10 are indicated. PS proteins are proteolytically processed by cleavage within the exon 10 domain. The cleavage produces a N'-terminal fragment (NTF) of 30kDa and a C-terminal fragment (CTF) of 20kDa. A second pathway is involved in the ubiquitin dependent degradation of PS. The functional role of PS processing is unclear

function. Interestingly, a gene (sel-12) which is very homologous to the Presenilins was isolated in the nematode Caenorhabditis elegans (Levitan and Greenwald, 1996). Mutations in this gene cause a phenotype which is well known for defects in NOTCH signaling (Levitan and Greenwald, 1996). Genes encoding the components of the NOTCH signaling pathway mediate the specification of numerous cell fates during development (Artavanis-Tsakonas et al., 1995). We wanted to take advantage of this knowledge by trying to rescue the mutant phenotype simply by overexpressing the human PS-1 gene. Indeed, human PS-1 expressed in transgenic worms fully rescued the mutant phenotype of sel-12 thus strongly indicating that human PS-1 is involved in NOTCH signaling as well. Interestingly, mutations in the PS-1 gene which are responsible for early onset FAD lost their ability to rescue the mutant phenotype (Baumeister et al., 1997; Levitan et al., 1996). This might indicate that FAD causing mutations in the PS proteins occur at positions which are important for the their functional properties. This is supported by the fact that all point mutations identified so far occur at positions which are conserved in sel-12 (Levitan and Greenwald, 1996). We also used this biological test system to map domains which are essential for the functional role of PS-1 in NOTCH signaling. Using a deletion analysis, we found that the large cytoplasmic loop is essential for the biological function of PS-1 (Baumeister et al., 1997). This region of the protein is exposed in the cytoplasm and carries about 45% of PS-1 mutation identified so far. We also analyzed the functional role of proteolytic processing of PS-1 in C. elegans. By using a natural occurring deletion (Δexon 10, see Fig. 2), which is defective in proteolytic processing due to the lack of the cleavage site we found that processing is not a prerequisite for PS-1 function in NOTCH signaling (Baumeister et al., 1997; Levitan et al., 1996).

Further support for a role of PS-1 in NOTCH signaling was provided very recently by gene knock-out experiments in mice which showed that the lack of the PS-1 gene causes severe defects in somite segmentation and differentiation (Wong et al., 1997; Shen et al., 1997). Moreover, expression of NOTCH1 and its ligand is markedly reduced in PS-1$^{-/-}$ mice. Therefore these experiments provide strong support for a role of PS-1 in the spatiotemporal expression of NOTCH1 and its ligand, which are essential for somite segmentation and maintenance of somite borders. PS-1$^{-/-}$ mice do not survive beyond the first day of birth, making it difficult to understand the role of NOTCH in AD pathogenesis. However, the biological function of NOTCH in the adult organism is still unknown, and might be different from that during early development. A role of genes involved in NOTCH signaling in the pathology of dementia is also strongly supported by the recent cloning of the gene causing cerebral autosomal dominant arteriopathy with subcortical infarcts and leukoencephalopathy (CADASIL). CADASIL was found to be caused by mutations in the NOTCH3 gene (Joutel et al., 1996). Therefore, genes of the NOTCH signaling pathway play an important role in the pathology of the two abundant forms of dementias, AD and CADASIL.

142   C. Haass and R. Baumeister

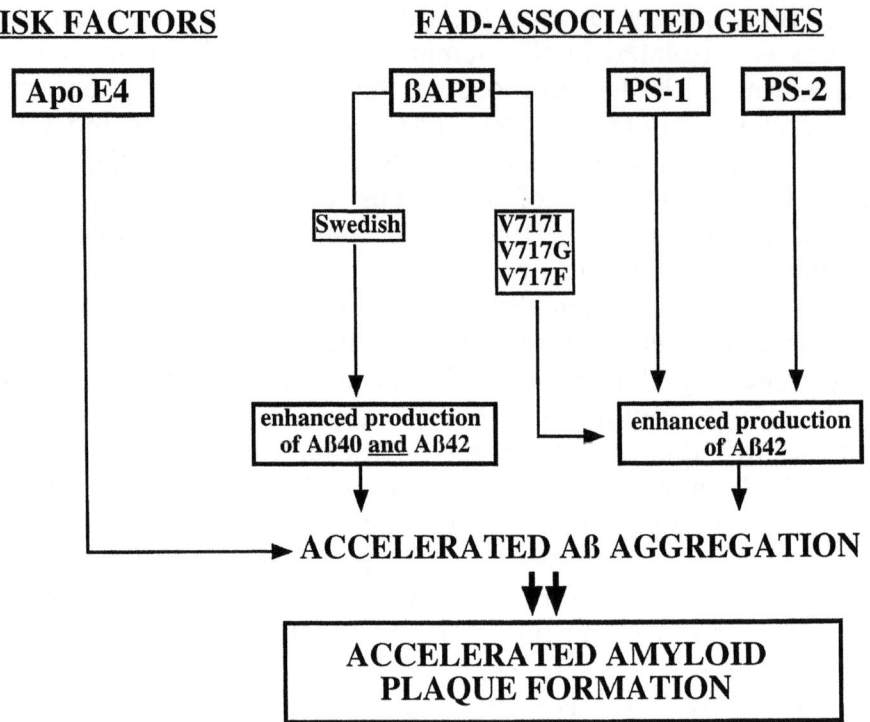

Fig. 3. The amyloid cascade. Mutations in three different genes have in common to produce enhanced levels of Aβ42, this leads to accelerated aggregation and amyloid plaque formation. Risk factors such as the apoE-4 allele and aging can also cause accelerated Aβ aggregation. Neurotoxicity based on Aβ aggregation and amyloid plaque formation might then induce other pathological phenomena such as inflammation, apoptosis, and tangle formation

The subcellular localization of PS proteins and Aβ42 generation

Using immunocytochemistry we identified the subcellular localization of PS proteins. Both PS proteins were found predominantly with the endoplasmic reticulum and early Golgi (Walter et al., 1996; Kovacs et al., 1996; DeStrooper et al., 1997; Cook et al., 1997). This is a surprising result, since Aβ generation is known to occur on the cell surface and during reinternalization within endosomes (Haass and Selkoe, 1993). However, as mentioned above most of the secreted forms of Aβ represent Aβ40. In all the work on the biological mechanism of Aβ generation, antibodies were used which could not discriminate Aβ40 from Aβ42. We therefore thought that it might be possible that the small amount of Aβ42 could be generated by a different cellular mechanism. This indeed turned out to be the case (Wilde-Bode et al., 1997). We found that Aβ42 can be generated within the ER and the early Golgi. Moreover, it appears that Aβ42 can accumulate in these compartments to much higher concentrations as in conditioned media (Wild-Bode et al., 1997). This might also explain the discrepancy that Aβ concentrations in biological fluids are to low to trigger aggregation. However, within intracellular compartments, local Aβ (specifically Aβ42) concentrations might very well reach concentrations which are sufficient for aggregation. Therefore, the knowledge about the localization of PS proteins helped to understand not only the biological mechanism of Aβ42 generation in cells which expressed the wild type βAPP and the wild type PS-1/PS-2 gene but might also contribute to our understanding of AD pathology in sporadic cases.

Taken together, the genetics of rare cases with early onset FAD allowed the identification of two novel genes involved in the pathology of AD. In addition, the biochemical analysis of these mutations in cultured cells or transgenic mice lead to fundamental knowledge about the pivotal role of Aβ42 in AD pathology. Moreover, since the mutations in all three genes lead to a common abnormality in the βAPP metabolism these findings strongly support the amyloid cascade hypothesis (Fig. 3).

References

Artavanis-Tsakonas A, Matsuno K, Fortini ME (1995) Notch signaling. Science 268: 225–232

Baumeister R, Leimer U, Zweckbronner I, Jakubek C, Grünberg J, Haass C (1997) Human presenilin-1, but not familial Alzheimer's disease FAD mutants, facilitate Caenorhabditis elegans Notch signaling independently of proteolytic processing. Genes & Function 1: 149–159

Borchelt DR, Thinakaran G, Eckman CB, Lee MK, Davenport F, Ratovitsky T, Prada C-M, Kim G, Eekins S, Yager D, Slunt HH, Wang R, Seeger M, Levey AI, Gandy SE, Copeland NG, Jenkins NA, Price DL, Younkin SG, Sisodia SS (1996) Familial Alzheimer's disease-linked presenilin 1 variants elevate Aβ 1–42/1–40 ratio in vitro and in vivo. Neuron 17: 1005–1013

Busciglio J, Gabuzda DH, Matsudaira P, Yankner B (1993) Generation of β-amyloid in the secretory pathway in neuronal and nonneuronal cells. Proc Natl Acad Sci USA 90: 2092–2096

Cai X, Golde TE, Younkin SG (1993) Release of excess amyloid β protein from mutant amyloid β protein precursor. Science 259: 514–516

Citron M, Oltersdorf T, Haass C, McConlogue L, Hung AY, Seubert P, Vigo-Pelfrey C, Lieberburg I, Selkoe DJ (1992) Mutation of the β-amyloid precursor protein in familial Alzheimer's disease increases β-protein production. Nature 360: 672–674

Citron M, Westaway D, Xia W, Carlson G, Diehl T, Levesque G, Johnson-Wood K, Lee M, Seubert P, Davis A, Kholodenko D, Motte R, Sherrington R, Perry B, Yao H, Strome R, Lieberburg I, Rommens J, Kim S, Schenk D, Fraser P, St. George Hyslop P, Selkoe DJ (1997) Mutant presenilins of Alzheimer's disease increase production of 42-residue amyloid β-protein in both transfected cells and transgenic mice. Nature Med 3: 67–72

Cook DG, Sung JC, Golde TE, Felsenstein KM, Wojczyk BS, Tanzi RE, Trojanowski JQ, Lee V M-Y, Doms RW (1996) Expression and analysis of presenilin 1 in a human neuronal system: localization in cell bodies and dendrites. Proc Natl Acad Sci USA 93: 9223–9228

De Strooper B, Beullens M, Contreras B, Levesque L, Craessaerts K, Cordell B, Moechars D, Bollen M, Fraser P, St. George-Hyslop P, van Leuven F (1997) Phosphorylation, subcellular localization and membrane orientation of the Alzheimer's disease-associated presenilins. J Biol Chem 272: 3590–3598

Doan A, Thinakaran G, Borchelt DR, Slunt HH, Ratovitsky T, Podlisny M, Selkoe DJ, Seeger M, Gandy SE, Price DL, Sisodia SS (1996) Protein topology of presenilin 1. Neuron 17: 1023–1030

Duff K, Eckman C, Zehr C, Yu X, Prada CM, Perez-Tur J, Hutton M, Buee L, Harigaya
    Y, Yager D, Morgan D, Gordon MN, Holcomb L, Refolo L, Zenk B, Hardy J,
    Younkin S (1996) Increased amyloid-β42 (43) in brains of mice expressing mutant
    presenilin 1. Nature 383: 710–713
Haass C (1997) Presenilins: genes for life an death. Neuron 18: 687–690
Haass C, Selkoe DJ (1993) Cellular processing of β-amyloid precursor protein and the
    genesis of amyloid β-peptide. Cell 75: 1039–1042
Haass C, Schlossmacher MG, Hung AY, Vigo-Pelfrey C, Mellon A, Ostaszewski BL,
    Lieberburg I, Koo EH, Schenk D, Teplow DB, Selkoe DJ (1992) Amyloid β-peptide
    is produced by cultured cells during normal metabolism. Nature 359: 322–325
Haass C, Lemere C, Capell A, Citron M, Seubert P, Schenk D, Lannfelt L, Selkoe DJ
    (1995) The Swedish mutation causes early onset Alzheimer's disease by β-secretase
    cleavage within the secretory pathway. Nature Med 1: 1291–1296
Joutel A, Corpechot C, Ducros A, Vahedi K, Chabriat H, Mouton P, Alamowitch S,
    Domenga V, Cécillion M, Maréchal E, Maciazek J, Vayssière C, Cruaud C, Cabanis
    E-A, Ruchoux MM, Weissenbach J, Bach JF, Bousser MG, Lasserve-Tournier E
    (1996) Notch3 mutations in CADASIL, a hereditary adult-onset condition causing
    stroke and dementia. Nature 383: 707–710
Kovacs DM, Faussett HJ, Page KJ, Kim T-W, Moir R, Merriam DE, Hollister RD,
    Hallmark OG, Mancini R, Felsenstein KM, Hyman BT, Tanzi RE, Wasco W (1995)
    Alzheimer-associated presenilin 1 and 2: neuronal expression in brain and localiza-
    tion to intracellular membranes in mamalian cells. Nature Med 2: 224–229
Levitan D, Greenwald I (1995) Facilitation of lin-12-mediated signalling by sel-12, a
    Caenorhabditis elegans S182 Alzheimer's disease gene. Nature 377: 351–354
Levitan D, Doyle TG, Brousseau D, Lee MK, Thinakaran G, Slunt HH, Sisodia SS,
    Greenwald I (1996) Assessment of normal and mutant human pesenilin function in
    Caenorhabditis elegans. Proc Natl Acad Sci USA 93: 14940–14944
Levy-Lahad E, Wasco W, Poorkaj P, Romano DM, Oshima J, Pettingell WH, Yu C,
    Jondro PD, Schmidt SD, Wang K, Crowley AC, Fu Y-H, Guenette SY, Galas D,
    Nemens E, Wijsman EM, Bird TD, Schellenberg GD, Tanzi RE (1995) Candidate
    gene for the chromosome 1 familial Alzheimer's disease locus. Science 269: 973–
    977
Rogaev EI, Sherrington R, Rogaeva EA, Levesque G, Ikeda M, Liang Y, Chi H, Lin C,
    Holamn K, Tsuda T, Mar L, Sorbi S, Nacmias B, Piacentini S, Amaducci L,
    Chumakkov I, Cohen D, Lannfelt L, Fraser PE, Rommens JM, St. George-Hyslop
    PH (1995) Familial Alzheimer's disease in kindreds with missense mutations in a
    gene on chromosome 1 related to the Alzheimer's disease type 3 gene. Nature 376:
    775–778
Schellenberg GD, Bird TD, Wijsman EM, Orr HT, Anderson L, Nemens E, White JA,
    Bonnycastle L, Weber JL, Alonso E, Potter H, Heston LL, Martin GM (1992)
    Genetic linkage evidence for a familial Alzheimer disease locus on chromosome 14.
    Science 3: 1–4
Scheuner D, Eckman C, Jensen M, Song X, Citron M, Suzuki N, Bird TD, Hardy J,
    Hutton M, Kukull W, Larson E, Levy-Lahad E, Viitanen M, Peskind E, Poorkaj P,
    Schellenberg G, Tanzi R, Wasco W, Lannfelt L, Selkoe D, Younkin S (1996) Secreted
    amyloid β-protein similar to that in the senile plaques of Alzheimer's disease is
    increased in vivo by the presenilin 1 and 2 and APP mutations linked to familial
    Alzheimer's disease. Nature Med 2: 864–870
Selkoe DJ (1996) Amyloid β-protein and the genetics of Alzheimer's disease. J Biol
    Chem 271: 18295–18298
Shen J, Bronson RT, Chen DF, Xia W, Selkoe DJ, Tonegawa S (1997) Skeletal and CNS
    defects in Presenilin-1-deficient mice. Cell 89: 629–639
Sherrington R, Rogaev EI, Liang Y, Rogaeva EA, Levesque G, Ikeda M, Chi H, Lin C,
    Li G, Holman K, Tsuda T, Mar L, Foncin J-F, Brni AC, Montesi P, Sorbi S, Rainero
    I, Pinessi L, Nee L, Chumakov I, Pollen D, Brookes A, Sanseau P, Polinsky RJ,

Wasco W, da Silva HAR, Haines JL, Pericak-Vance MA, Tanzi RE, Roses AD, Fraser PE, Rommens JM, St. George-Hyslop PH (1995) Cloning of a gene bearing missense mutations in early-onset familial Alzheimer's disease. Nature 375: 754–760

Shoji M, Golde TE, Ghiso J, Cheung TT, Estus S, Shaffer LM, Cai XD, McKay DM, Tintner R, Frangione B, Younkin SG (1992) Production of the Alzheimer anyloid β protein by normal proteolytic processing. Science 258: 126–129

Suzuki N, Cheung TT, Cai X-D, Odaka A, Otvos L, Eckman C, Golde TE, Younkin SG (1994) An increased percentage of long amyloid β protein secreted by familial amyloid β protein precursor (βAPP717) mutants. Science 264: 1336–1340

Thinakaran G, Borchelt DR, Lee MK, Slunt HH, Spitzer L, Kim G, Ratovitsky T, Davenport F, Nordstedt C, Seeger M, Hardy J, Levey AI, Gandy SE, Jenkins NA, Copeland NG, Pric DL, Sisodia SS (1996) Endoproteolysis of presenilin 1 and accumulation of processed derivatives in vivo. Neuron 17: 181–190

Tomita T, Maryuama K, Saido TC, Kume H, Shinozaki K, Tokuhiro S, Capell A, Walter J, Grünberg J, Haass C, Iwatsubo T, Obata K (1997) The presenilin 2 mutation (N141I) linked to familial Alzheimer disease (Volga German families) increases the secretion of amyloid β protein ending at the 42nd (or 43rd) residue. Proc Natl Acad Sci USA 94: 2025–2030

Walter J, Capell A, Grünberg J, Pesold B, Schindzielorz A, Prior R, Podlisny MB, Fraser P, St. George-Hyslop P, Selkoe DJ, Haass C (1996) The Alzheimer's disease — associated presenilins are differentially phosphorylated proteins located predominantly within the endoplasmic reticulum. Mol Med 2: 673–691

Wild-Bode C, Yamazaki T, Capell A, Leimer U, Steiner H, Ihara Y, Haass C (1997) Intracellular generation and accumulation of amyloid β-peptide terminating at amino acid 42. J Biol Chem 272: 16085–16088

Wong PC, Zheng H, Chen H, Becher MW, Sirinathsinghji DJS, Trumbauer ME, Chen HY, Price DL, van der Ploeg LHT, Sisodia SS (1997) Presenilin 1 is required for Notch 1 and D//1 expression in the paraxial mesoderm. Nature 387: 288–292

Xia W, Zhang J, Kholodenko D, Citron M, Teplow D, Haass C, Seubert P, Koo EH, Selkoe DJ (1997) Enhanced production and oligomeraization of the 42-residue amyloid β-protein by CHO cells stably expressing mutant presenilins. J Biol Chem 272: 7977–7982

Authors' address: Dr. C. Haass, Central Institute for Mental Health, Department of Molecular Biology, J5, D-68159 Mannheim, Federal Republic of Germany

Aberrancies in signal transduction and cell cycle related events in Alzheimer's disease

T. Arendt, M. Holzer, U. Gärtner, and **M. K. Brückner**

Department of Neuroanatomy, Paul Flechsig Institute of Brain Research, University of Leipzig, Federal Republic of Germany

Summary. Neurodegeneration in Alzheimer's disease (AD) is associated with the appearance of dystrophic neuronal growth profiles that most likely reflects an aberrant attempt of neuronal repair. This process of neuronal reorganisation, which eventually goes awry and becomes a disease itself, might be intitiated physiologically as a response to neuronal injuries. Minor neuronal damage due to a variety of life events or genetic pertubations that are usually compensated in the normal adult brain by adaptation and repair might thus be amplified and accumulated, thereby resulting in a progressive neurodegeneration. The present paper summarizes recent evidence supporting the hypothesis that a primary impairment of intracellular signal transduction that is mediated by a hierarchy of phosphorylation signals and associated with a aborted attempt of neurons to re-enter the cell-cycle is a key element in the pathomechanism of AD. These changes might result in malfunction of neuronal adaptation and repair and eventually lead to neuronal death.

During the process of aging as well as in chronic neurodegenerative disorders such as Alzheimer's disease (AD), the continuous but rather slow action of pathogenetic factors might give room for the activation of compensatory mechanisms, serving to regain a neuronal population much of its synaptic connectivity in the presence of cell loss. An upregulation in the capacity to synthesize and store neurotransmitters (Lapchak et al., 1991), an increased expression of trophic factors (Hellweg et al., 1990; Arendt et al., 1995a,b), as well as regenerative sprouting (Fritschy and Grzanna, 1992), synaptic enlargement (Scheff et al., 1990; Lippa et al., 1992), and neosynaptogenesis (Ramirez and Ulfhake, 1992) have been described among other processes.

Aberrant growth of neurites in AD

During normal aging, a compensatory dendritic growth has been observed in rodent (Hinds and McNelly, 1977; Connor et al., 1980, 1982), non-human primate (Cupp and Uemura, 1980; Uemura, 1985) and human (Buell and Coleman, 1979, 1980, 1981) brain. As opposed to the continuous growth during aging (Buell and Coleman, 1979; Flood et al., 1987), however, dendritic proliferation in AD is restricted to certain cell types and stages of the disease (Arendt et al., 1997). Growth processes in AD, furthermore, are aberrant with respect to their localization, morphological appearance (Arendt et al., 1986; Arendt and Brückner, 1992; Ferrer et al., 1990), and composition of cytoskeletal elements (McKee et al., 1989).

This aberrant growth in AD is accompanied by the re-expression of a number of developmentally regulated proteins, in particular those that are part of the cytoskeleton (Wolozin et al., 1988; Geddes et al., 1990; Morishima-Kawashima et al., 1991; Arendt et al., 1992a,b; Kanemaru et al., 1992; Bramblett et al., 1983; Goedert et al., 1993). More recent evidence that the formation of abnormal growth profiles might be associated with an aberrant and elevated expression of nerve growth factor receptor (Ernfors et al., 1990; Mufson and Kordower, 1992), which precedes the formation of neurofibrillary tangles (Arendt and Brückner, 1992), prompted us to suggest a sequence of events leading to neuronal degeneration and cell death in AD (Arendt, 1993a). This hypothesis is based on the assumption that as a result of a compensatory process of reorganization that becomes defective, a mitogenic overstimulation of terminally differentiated neurones leads to a developmentally immature condition, i.e., to a condition of dedifferentiation that is characterized by an expression of developmentally regulated genes, posttranslational modifications, and an accumulation of gene products to an extent that goes beyond those observed during regeneration. This process of dedifferentiation, which involves molecular events leading to neoplastic transformation in dividing cells, is not compatible with the state of a neurone being irreversibly blocked from the re-entry in the cell cycle and might, therefore, lead to neuronal death. From this hypothesis it can be predicted that those molecular events that are involved in neoplastic transformation might also play a key role in the pathomechanism of AD (Heintz, 1993). Here we provide evidence that has recently been obtained in our lab to support this hypothesis.

The elevation of mitogenic activity in AD

It has been shown in a number of experimental paradigms that prolonged cell death in the central nervous system may give rise to an enhanced proliferative force thereby stimulating the process of reparative sprouting (Arendt, 1993b; Standler and Bernstein, 1982; Sumner and Watson, 1971). This increased trophic activity induced by chronic brain injury might be triggered by a reduced competition of neighbouring neurones for afferent supply (Perry and Linden, 1982) as well as an elevated synthesis of trophic factors by locally activated glial cells (Arendt et al., 1995a,b). An increased expression of a variety of mitogenic factors as well as their binding sites has similarly been reported for AD (Table 1).

The intracellular transmission of growth-factor signals critically depends on a cycle of protein phosphorylation and dephosphorylation. This signal transduction from the neurotrophin receptors to the expression and posttranslational modifications of cytoskeletal proteins as one of the major molecular targets involved in neurite outgrowth is mediated by the tuned

Table 1. Increase in mitogenic activity in AD

NGF	Allen et al. (1991) Crutcher et al. (1993)
NGF-receptor p75	Ernfors et al. (1990) Mufson and Kordower (1992)
bFGF	Gomez-Pinilla et al. (1990) Stopa et al. (1990)
bFGF-receptor	Kato et al. (1991)
EGF	Biricree et al. (1988) Styren et al. (1990)
$APP_{751/770}$	Schubert et al. (1989) Alvarez et al. (1992) Milward et al. (1992)

activation of both protein phosphatases and protein kinases (tyrosine kinase, trk; mitogen-activated protein [MAP] kinase) with a number of proto-oncogenes (trk, p21ras, raf-1) being part of this cascade (for rev. see Meakin and Shooter, 1992; Nishida and Gotoh, 1993) (Fig. 1).

Molecular events that are sensitive to a disturbance of the balance between protein phosphorylation and dephosphorylation are involved in NGF-directed neurite outgrowth (Chiou and Westhead, 1992), in the reorganization of the neuronal cytoskeleton leading to axonal regeneration (Hall and Kosik, 1993), in the hyperphosphorylation of the microtubule associated protein tau present in PHF (Harris et al., 1993; Vandermeeren et al., 1993), as well as in the processing and secretion of the amyloid precursor protein (Buxbaum et al., 1993; Caporaso et al., 1992). More recent evidence suggests that the NGF effector pathway is not only involved in neurite outgrowth both under normal and pathological conditions but is probably also part of a cascade mediating the pathological effects of Aβ on the brain (Milward et al., 1992) as well as the formation of neurofibrillary tangles (Drewes et al., 1992).

The small G-protein p21ras

Stimulation of neurotrophin receptors is relayed to the downstream cascade of serine/threonine kinases by the small G-protein p21ras that is localized on the inner aspect of the plasma membrane (Heumann, 1994). In mammalian cells, the p21ras gene product is encoded by a family of ras proto-oncogenes that include at least three functional loci, H-ras, K-ras and N-ras (Shimizu et al., 1993). Binding of the neurotrophins to tyrosine kinase receptors converts p21ras from its inactive, GDP-bound, to active, GTP-bound, state. GTP-bound p21ras recruits raf-1 from the cytoplasm to the plasma membrane, where it is activated (Stokoe et al., 1994). Raf-1 phosphorylates and

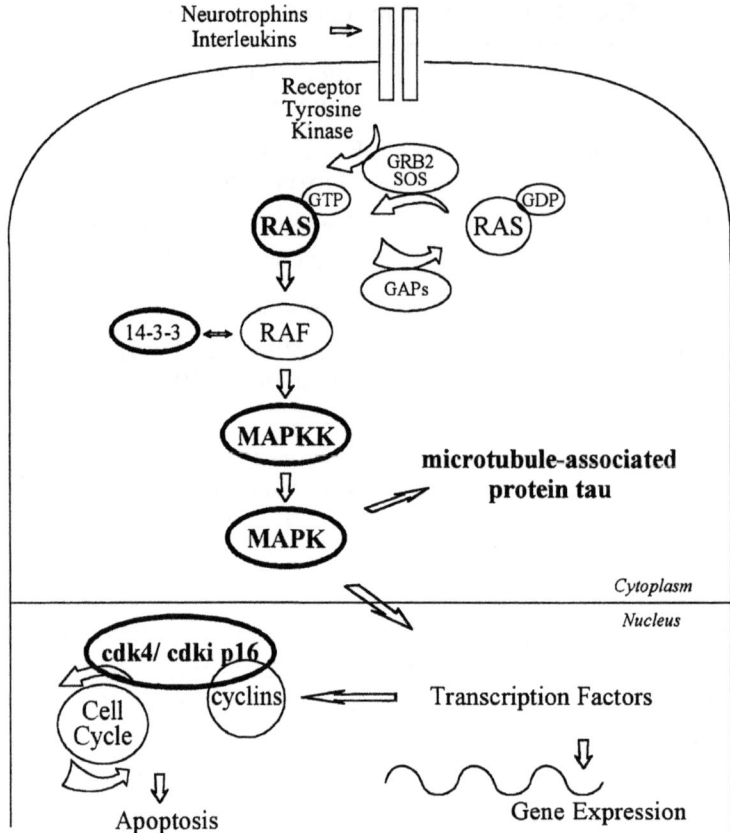

Fig. 1. Schematic link of p21ras dependent intracellular signalling, MAP kinase cascade, hyperphosphorylation of tau and cell cycle-related events. The expression of p21ras, 14-3-3, MAPKK, MAPK and cdki p16, key components of intracellular signal transduction, is closely associated with the formation of neurofibrillary tangles and neuritic plaques

activates the mitogen activated protein kinase kinase (MAPKK) leading to the activation of the mitogen activated protein kinase (MAPK) (see below). During certain stages of brain development, p21ras might be a critical regulator for cellular proliferation and differentiation. In the adult nervous system, expression of p21ras is involved in reactive dendritic proliferation and compensatory neosynaptogenesis (Phillips and Belardo, 1994) that occurs in response to injury, a process that might be disturbed in AD.

In both normal brain and in AD, the H-ras, K-ras and N-ras gene products can equally be detected in almost all neurones and occasionally also in glial cells. In AD, p21ras is highly expressed within neuritic plaques as well as in neurones and glial cells closely associated with plaques (Gärtner et al., 1995). Neurones containing tangle-bearing material also show a high expression (Fig. 2A,B). Since p21ras acts as a molecular switch that mediates the effects of mitogens on proliferation and structural reorganization it might be involved in the process of neurodegeneration and/or aberrant repair in AD.

The mitogen-activated protein kinase cascade

The activation of cell surface receptors of a number of mitogenic factors is linked to intracellular changes in enzyme activity and gene expression by the mitogen-activated protein (MAP) kinase cascade (Ahn, 1993). Running this cascade involves among others the sequential activation of mitogen-activated protein kinase kinase (MAPKK) and its substrate, the mitogen-activated protein kinases (MAPK). The MAPKs or intracellular signal regulated kinases (ERKs) and MAPKK or MAP/ERK kinase (MEK) belong to a group of protein kinases which is highly conserved from yeast to vertebrates (Boulton et al., 1990). They are key molecules in signal processing that become activated in response to a wide variety of reagents. Among these are tumour promotors, interleukins, growth factors whose receptors are tyrosine kinases, mitogens whose receptors couple to heterotrimeric guanine nucleotide binding proteins (G proteins), and agents that induce N-methyl-D-aspartate receptor activation (Boulton et al., 1991; Pelech and Sanghera, 1992). Regulation by MAPKs has been implicated in a wide array of physiological processes (Davis, 1993). When activated, ERKs rapidly phosphorylate targets that lead to changes in kinase cascades, protein function, or gene expression. Effectors include Ser/Thr kinases (pp^{90rsk}, MAPK-activated protein kinase-2 and 3p-kinase), transcription factors (Elk-1, c-Myc, c-Jun, NF-116 and ATF-2) and structural proteins (talin, microtubule-associated proteins and lamins (Pulverer et al., 1991; Lin et al., 1993; Chung et al., 1991).

The MAP kinase, referred to p42 or ERK2 (Drewes et al., 1992; Goedert et al., 1992) and perhaps other members of the ERK family have recently been shown in vitro to phosphorylate recombinant tau and convert it to a form which is similar to PHF tau.

In AD, the levels of MAPKK and MAPK are both increased in AD by about 35% to 40% compared with age matched controls (Arendt et al., 1995c). Elevation of both kinases is most pronounced during early stages of the disease and is inversely related to the tissue content of abnormally phosphorylated PHF-tau (Arendt et al., 1995c). Pronounced immunoreactivity of MAPKK and MAPK is present in unaffected neurones of the cerebral cortex as well as in tangle-bearing neurones that are likely to be metabolically highly compromized (Fig. 2C). Immunoreactive neurones are most often localized in the direct vicinity of neuritic plaques. The subcellular distribution of both MAPKK and MAK shows a translocation from the cytoplasmic to the nuclear compartment. These results suggest that the activation of the MAPK cascade that plays an essential role in transmitting proliferative responses is involved in early steps of the pathomechanism of AD.

A protein that has recently been suggested to participate in cell transformation and mitogenic signalling pathways is the 14-3-3 protein (Morrison et al., 1994). The 14-3-3 protein interacts with the Raf-kinase, a component of the MAPK cascade as well as with other proto-oncogenes and oncogene products, thereby modulating these signalling proteins. The 14-3-3 proteins represent a highly conserved family of dimeric proteins that are widely

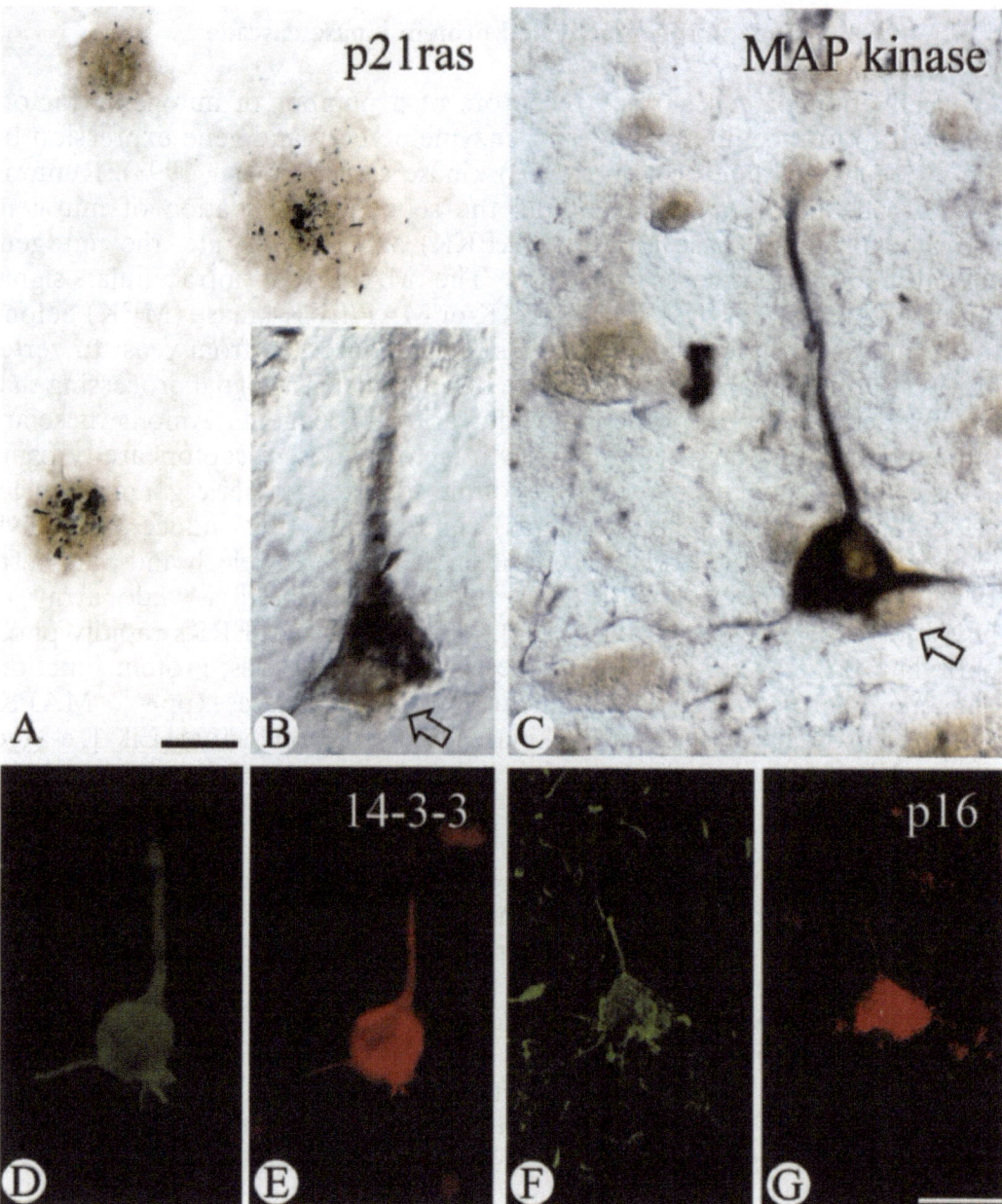

Fig. 2. Association of molecular components of intracellular signalling and cell cycle-related events with plaques and tangles in AD. **A** and **B** Immunohistochemical localization of p21ras (brown reaction product, mab Y13-259), counter-reacted for the immunocytochemical detection of PHF-tau (black reaction product; mab Alz50). **A** Localization of p21ras within neuritic plaques; **B** Expression of p21ras (arrow) in a tangle-bearing pyramidal neurone. **C** Localization of MAP kinase in both tangle-free neurones and in a tangle bearing neurone (arrow). **D** and **E** Colocalization of 14-3-3 protein (E, anti-14-3-3, K-19, Santa Cruz, Cy-3 conjugated secondary antibody) and highly phosphorylated PHF-tau (D, mab AT8, Cy-2 conjugated secondary antibody) simultaneously visualized by double immunofluorescence. **F** and **G** Colocalization of the cdki p16 (G, polyclonal antibody Santa Cruz Biotechnology, Cy-3 conjugated secondary antibody) and highly phosphorylated PHF-tau (F, mab AT8, Cy-2 conjugated secondary antibody) simultaneously visualized by double immunofluorescence; confocal laser image. Scale bars: **A** 50 mµ; **B–G** 20 µm

distributed among eucaryotic cells. At least seven isoforms have been identified in mammalian tissue. They are remarkably abundant in the brain where they constitute about 1% of the cytosolic protein.

In AD, expression of 14-3-3 protein is closely associated with neurofibrillary tangles (Fig. 2D/E) and dystrophic neurites within neuritic plaques (Gärtner et al., 1996).

The cell cycle marker p16

Expression of p21ras in AD is closely associated with the formation of the pathological hallmarks of the disease (see above). The small G-protein p21 ras is a proto-oncogene that in transforming cells is involved in the regulation of the G0/G1 transition of the cell cycle mediated through co-operation with cyclin D1. Cyclin-dependent kinases are likely to play a role in the pathomechanism of AD. The cdc2 kinase, for example, that appears to be increased in AD (Ledesma et al., 1992), is able to phosphorylate tau protein at sites shown to be phosphorylated in AD (Kobayashi et al., 1993; Ledesma et al., 1992). APP, furthermore, is phosphorylated both in vitro and in intact cells by a cdc2-like kinase in a cell cycle dependent manner which is associated with altered production of potentially amyloidogenic fragments containing the entire β/A4-domain (Suzuki et al., 1994). Activation of cyclin-dependent kinases (cdks) is negatively regulated by interaction with proteins of the cyclin-dependent kinase inhibitor (cdki) family (Cordon-Cardo, 1995). Deregulation of these cdki-proteins results in either uncontrolled proliferation and neoplastic transformation or activation of apoptosis. One notable candidate for this role is p16 (Serrano et al., 1993). Recent evidence implicates the p16 protein in pathways for control of cell growth and proliferation and demonstrates that p16 can function as a tumour suppressor protein to G1-arrest cells (Kamb et al., 1994; Caldas et al., 1994). p16 apparently inhibits cdk4 by binding in competition with cyclin D (Serrano et al., 1993). Malignant cellular transformation has been shown to produce major changes in the modulation of the cyclin-cdk complexes by associated cdki-proteins such as p16. A recent study (Kranenburg et al., 1996) provides evidence that the overexpression of the cyclin-dependent kinase-inhibitor p16 protects neurones from apoptotic cell death. In AD, we observed an increased expression of the cdki p16 that was closely related to neurofibrillary tangles (Fig. 2F/G) and neuritic components of plaques in AD (Arendt et al., 1996). These findings support the hypothesis that an aborted attempt to activate the cell cycle in terminally differentiated neurones might be a critical event of the pathomechanism of AD.

Conclusion — AD as a defective process of neuronal repair

Recent evidence indicates that a primary impairment of intracellular signal transduction that is mediated by a hierarchy of phosphorylation signals is a key element in the pathomechanism of AD. These changes might result in malfunction of neuronal adaptation and repair and eventually lead to neuronal death. Aberrancies in the neuronal response to degenerative stimuli might directly affect neuronal viability by triggering a self-perpetuating cascade of events leading to the formation of paired helical filaments (PHFs) and β/A4-amyloid. The process of neuronal reorganization, which eventually goes awry and becomes a disease itself, might be intitiated physiologically as a response to neuronal injuries. Minor neuronal damage due to a variety of life events or genetic pertubations that are usually compensated in the normal adult brain by adaptation and repair might thus be amplified and accumulated, thereby resulting in a progressive neurodegeneration. Through liberation of growth factors and cytokines mechanisms of repair are induced in the central nervous system that might lead to a mitogenic overstimulation of neurones. As a result, the activation of those molecular events might be triggered that in dividing cell populations would lead to a cellular transformation. Within terminally differentiated cells, that are irreversibly blocked from the re-entry into the cell cycle, however, activation of the same molecular events might lead to programmed cell death as an alternative effector pathway (Heintz, 1993). The disturbance of processes involved in signal transduction mechanisms might, therefore, represent an unifying framework that begins to emerge for the pathology of AD, linking it to such basic aspects as the understanding of mechanisms preventing neurones from re-entering the cell cycle.

Acknowledgements

This work was supported by the Bundesministerium für Bildung, Forschung und Technologie (BMBF), Interdisciplinary Centre for Clinical Research at the University of Leipzig (IZKF/01KS9504-C1).

References

Ahn NG (1993) The MAP kinase cascade. Discovery of a new signal transduction pathway. Mol Cell Biochem 127/128: 210–209

Allen SJ, MacGowan SH, Treanor JJS, Feeney R, Wilcock GK, Dawbarn D (1991) Normal β-NGF content in Alzheimer's disease cerebral cortex and hippocampus. Neurosci Lett 131: 135–139

Alvarez J, Moreno RD, Llanos O, Inestrosa NC, Brandan E, Colby C, Esch FS (1992) Axonal sprouting induced in the sciatic nerve by the amyloid precursor protein (APP) and other antiproteases. Neurosci Lett 144: 130–134

Arendt Th (1993a) Neuronal dedifferentiation and degeneration in Alzheimer's disease. Biol Chem Hoppe Seyler 374: 911–912

Arendt Th (1993b) The cholinergic deafferentation of the cerebral cortex induced by chronic consumption of alcohol — post-mortem and experimental studies. In: Hunt WA, Nixen SJ (eds) Alcohol-induced brain damage. National Institute on Alcohol Abuse and Alcoholism Research Monographs, NIH Publication No. 93-3549, Washington New York, pp 431–460

Arendt Th, Brückner MK (1992) Perisomatic sprouts immunoreactive for nerve growth factor receptor and neurofibrillary degeneration affect different neuronal populations in the basal nucleus in patients with Alzheimer's disease. Neurosci Lett 148: 63–66

Arendt Th, Zvegintseva HG, Leontovich TA (1986) Dendritic changes in the basal nucleus of Meynert and in the diagonal band nucleus in Alzheimer's disease — a quantitative Golgi investigation. Neuroscience 19: 1265–1278

Arendt Th, Brückner MK, Lange M, Bigl V (1992a) Changes in acetylcholinesterase and butyrylcholinesterase in Alzheimer's disease resemble embryonic development — a study of molecular forms. Neurochem Int 21: 381–396

Arendt Th, Brückner MK, Pagliusi S (1992b) Reexpression of developmentally regulated proteins in Alzheimer's disease. Eur J Neurosci [Suppl] 5: 18

Arendt Th, Brückner MK, Pagliusi S, Krell T (1995) Degeneration of rat cholinergic basal forebrain neurons and reactive changes in NGF expression after chronic neurotoxic injury. I. Degeneration and plastic response of basal forebrain neurons. Neuroscience 65: 633–645

Arendt Th, Brückner MK, Krell T, Pagliusi S, Kruska L, Heumann L (1995) Degeneration of rat cholinergic basal forebrain neurons and reactive changes in NGF expression after chronic neurotoxic injury. II. Reactive expression of the NGF gene in astocytes. Neuroscience 65: 647–659

Arendt Th, Holzer M, Großmann A, Zedlick D, Brückner MK (1995c) Increased expression and subcellular translocation of the mitogen activated protein kinase kinase and mitogen-activated protein kinase in Alzheimer's disease. Neuroscience 68: 5–18

Arendt Th, Rödel L, Gärtner U, Holzer M (1996) Expression of the cyclin-dependent kinase inhibitor p16 in Alzheimer's disease. NeuroReport 7: 3047–3049

Arendt Th, Schindler C, Brückner MK, Eschrich K, Bigl V, Zedlick D, Marcova L (1997) Plastic neuronal remodeling is impaired in patients with Alzheimer's disease carrying apolipoprotein epsilon 4 allele. J Neurosci 17: 516–529

Birecree E, Whetsell WO, Stoscheck C, King LE, Nanney LL (1988) Immunoreactive epidermal growth factors in neuritic plaques from patients with Alzheimer's disease. J Neuropathol Exp Neurol 47: 549–560

Boulton TG, Yancopoulos GD, Gregory JS, Slaughter C, Moomaw C, Hsu J, Cobb MN (1990) An insulin-stimulated protein kinase similar to yeast kinases involved in cell cycle control. Science 249: 64–66

Boulton TG, Nye SH, Robbins DJ, Ip NY, Radziejewska E, Morgenbesser SD, DePinho RA, Panayotatos N, Cobb MH, Yancopoulos GD (1991) ERKs: a family of protein-serin/threonine kinases that are activated and tyrosine phosphorylated in response to insulin and NGF. Cell 65: 663–675

Bramblett GT, Goedert M, Jakes R, Merrick SE, Trojanowski JQ, Lee VM-Y (1993) Abnormal tau phosphorylation at Ser396 in Alzheimer's disease recapitulates development and contributes to reduced microtubule binding. Neuron 10: 1089–1099

Buell SJ, Coleman PD (1979) Dendritic growth in the aged human brain and failure of growth in senile dementia. Science 206: 854–856

Buell SJ, Coleman PD (1980) Individual differences in dendritic growth in human aging and senile dementia. In: Stein D (ed) The psychobiology of aging: problems and pespectives. Elsevier, Amsterdam, pp 283–296

Buell SJ, Coleman PD (1981) Quantitative evidence for selective dendritic growth in normal human aging but not in senile dementia. Brain Res 214: 23–41

Buxbaum JD, Koo EH, Greengard P (1993) Protein phosphorylation inhibits production of Alzheimer amyloid β/A4 peptide. Proc Natl Acad Sci USA 90: 9195–9198

Caldas C, Hahn SA, da Costa LT, Redston MS, Schutte M, Seymour AB, Weinstein CL, Hruban RH, Yeo CJ, Kern SE (1994) Frequent somatic mutations and homozygous deletions of the p16 (MTS1) gene in pancreatic adenocarcinoma. Nature Genet 8: 27–32

Caporaso GL, Gandy SE, Buxbaum JD, Ramabhadran TV, Greengard P (1992) Protein phosphorylation regulates secretion of Alzheimer β/A4 amyloid precursor protein. Proc Natl Acad Sci USA 89: 3055–3059

Chiou J-Y, Westhead EW (1992) Okadaic acid, a protein phosphorylation inhibitor, inhibits nerve growth factor-directed neurite outgrowth in PC12 cells. J Neurochem 59: 1963–1966

Chung J, Pelech SL, Blenis J (1991) Mitogen-activated swiss mouse 3T3 RSK kinases I and II are related to p44mpk from sea star oocytes and participate in the regulation of pp90rsk activity. Proc Natl Acad Sci USA 88: 4981–4985

Connor JR, Diamond MC, Johnson RE (1980) Occipital cortical morphology of the rat: alterations with age and environment. Exp Neurol 68: 158–170

Connor JR, Beban SE, Hopper PA, Hansen B, Diamond MC (1982) A Golgi study of the superficial pyramidal cells of the somatosensory cortex of socially reared old adult rats. Exp Neurol 76: 35–45

Cordon-Cardo C (1995) Mutations of cell cycle regulators. Biological and clinical implications for human neoplasia. Am J Pathol 147: 545–560

Crutcher KA, Scott SA, Liang S, Everson WV, Weingartner J (1993) Detection of NGF-like activity in human brain tissue: increased levels in Alzheimer's disease. J Neurosci 13: 2540–2550

Cupp CJ, Uemura E (1980) Age-related changes in prefrontal cortex of Macaca mulatta: quantitative analysis of dendritic branching patterns. Exp Neurol 69: 143–163

Davis RJ (1993) The mitogen-activated protein kinase signal transduction pathway. J Biol Chem 268: 14553–14556

Drewes G, Lichtenberg-Kraag B, Döring F, Mandelkow E-M, Biernat J, Goris J, Dorée M, Mandelkow E (1992) Mitogen activated protein (MAP) kinase transforms tau protein into an Alzheimer-like state. EMBO J 11: 2131–2138

Ernfors P, Lindefors N, Chan-Palay V, Persson H (1990) Cholinergic neurons of the nucleus basalis express elevated levels of nerve growth factor receptor mRNA in senile dementia of the Alzheimer type. Dementia 1: 138–145

Ferrer I, Guionnet N, Cruz-Sanchez F, Tunon T (1990) Neuronal alterations in patients with dementia: a Golgi study on biopsy samples. Neurosci Lett 114: 11–16

Flood DG, Buell SJ, Horwitz GJ, Coleman PD (1987a) Dendritic extent in human dentate gyrus granule cells in normal aging and senile dementia. Brain Res 402: 205–216

Fritschy JM, Grzanna R (1992) Restoration of ascending noradrenergic projections by residual locus coeruleus neurons — compensatory response to neurotoxin induced cell death in the adult rat brain. J Comp Neurol 321: 421–441

Gärtner U, Holzer M, Heumann R, Arendt Th (1995) Induction of p21ras in Alzheimer pathology. NeuroReport 6: 1313–1316

Gärtner U, Holzer M, Arendt Th (1996) Neurofibrillary lesions in Alzheimer's disease are associated with 14-3-3 protein. Biol Chem 377 [Spec Suppl]: S180

Geddes JW, Wong J, Choi BH, Kim RC, Cotman CW, Miller FD (1990) Increased expression of the embryonic form of a developmentally-regulated mRNA in Alzheimer's disease. Neurosci Lett 109: 54–61

Goedert M, Cohen ES, Jakes R, Cohen Ph (1992) p42 map kinase phosphorylation sites in microtubule-associated protein tau are dephosphorylated by protein phosphatase 2A1. Implications for Alzheimers disease. FEBS Lett 312: 95–99

Goedert M, Jakes R, Crowther RA, Six J, Lübke U, Vandermeeren M, Cras P, Trojanowski JQ, Lee VM-Y (1993) The abnormal phosphorylation of tau protein at Ser-202 in Alzheimer disease recapitulates phosphorylation during development. Proc Natl Acad Sci USA 90: 5066–5070

Gomez-Pinilla F, Cummings BJ, Cotman CW (1990) Induction of basic fibroblast growth factor in Alzheimer's disease pathology. NeuroReport 1: 211–214

Hall GF, Kosik KS (193) Axotomy-induced neurofilament phosphorylation is inhibited in situ by microinjection of PKA and PKC inhibitors into identified lamprey neurons. Neuron 10: 613–625

Harris KA, Oyler GA, Doolittle GM, Vincent I, Lehman RAW, Kincaid RL, Billingsley ML (1993) Okadaic acid induces hyperphosphorylated forms of tau protein in human brain slices. Ann Neurol 33: 77–87

Heintz N (1993) Cell-death and the cell-cycle — a relationship between transformation and neurodegeneration. Trends Biochem Sci 18: 157–159

Hellweg R, Fischer W, Hock C, Gage FH, Björklund A, Thoenen H (1990) Nerve growth factor levels and choline acetyltransferase activity in the brain of aged rats with spatial memory impairments. Brain Res 537: 123–130

Heumann R (1994) Neurotrophin signalling. Curr Opin Neurobiol 4: 668–679

Kamb A, Gruis NA, Weaver-Feldhaus J, Liu Q, Harshman K, Tavtigian SV, Stockert E, Day RS-3rd, Johnson BE, Skolnick MH (1994) A cell cycle regulator potentially involved in genesis of many tumor types. Science 264: 436–440

Kanemaru K, Takio K, Miura R, Titani K, Ihara Y (1992) Fetal-type phosphorylation of the tau in paired helical filaments. J Neurochem 58: 1667–1675

Kato T, Sasaki H, Katagiri T, Sasaki H, Koiwai K, Youki H, Totsuka S, Ishii T (1991) The binding of fibroblast growth factor to Alzheimer's neurofibrillary tangles and senile plaques. Neurosci Lett 122: 33–36

Kobayashi S, Ishiguro K, Omori A, Takamatsu M, Arioka M, Imahori K, Uchida T (1993) A cdc2-related kinase PSSALRE/cdk5 is homologous with the 30 kDa subunit of tau protein kinase II, a proline-directed protein kinase associated with microtubule. FEBS Lett 335: 171–175

Kranenburg O, Vandereb A, Zantema A (1996) Cyclin D1 is an essential mediator of apoptotic neuronal cell death. EMBO J 15: 46–54

Lapchak PA, Jenden DJ, Hefti F (1991) Compensatory elevation of acetylcholine synthesis in vivo by cholinergic neurons surviving partial lesions of the septohippocampal pathway. J Neurosci 11: 2821–2828

Ledesma MD, Correas I, Avila J, Diaznido J (1992) Implication of brain Cdc2 and Map2 kinases in the phosphorylation of tau protein in Alzheimers disease. FEBS Lett 308: 218–224

Lin L-L, Wartmann M, Lin A, Knopf JL, Seth A, Davis RJ (1993) cPLA2 is phosphorylated and activated by MAP kinase. Cell 72: 269–278

Lippa CF, Hamos JE, Pulaskisalo D, Degennaro LJ, Drachmann DA (1992) Alzheimer's disease and aging — effects of perforant pathway perikarya and synapse. Neurobiol Aging 13: 405–411

McKee AC, Kowall NW, Kosik KS (1989) Microtubular reorganization and dendritic growth response in Alzheimer's disease. Ann Neurol 26: 652–659

Meakin SO, Shooter EM (1992) The nerve growth factor family of receptors. Trends Neurosci 15: 323–331

Milward EA, Papadopoulos R, Fuller SJ, Moir RD, Small D, Beyreuther K, Masters CL (1992) The amyloid protein precursor of Alzheimer's disease is a mediator of the effects of nerve growth factor on neurite outgrowth. Neuron 9: 129–137

Morishima-Kawashima M, Arai T, Ogawara M, Takio K, Titani K, Saitoh T, Kosik KS, Ihara Y (1991) A possible fetal antigen of MR-70,000 in neurofibrillary tangles. Brain Res 554: 316–320

Morrison D (1994) 14-3-3: modulators of signaling proteins? Science 266: 56–57

Mufson EJ, Kordower JH (1992) Cortical neurons express nerve growth factor receptors in advanced age and Alzheimer's disease. Proc Natl Acad Sci USA 89: 569–573

Nishida E, Gotoh Y (1993) The MAP kinase cascade is essential for diverse signal transduction pathways. Trends Biochem Sci 18: 128–131

Pelech SL, Sanghera JS (1992) MAP kinases: charting the regulatory pathways. Science 257: 1355–1356

Perry VH, Linden R (1982) Evidence for dendritic competition in the developing retina. Nature 297: 683–685

Phillips LL, Belardo ET (1994) Increase of c-fos and ras oncoproteins in the denervated neuropil of the rat dentate gyrus. Neuroscience 58: 503–514

Pulverer B, Kyriakis J, Avruch J, Nikolakaki E, Woodgett J (1991) Phosphorylation of c-jun mediated by MAP kinases. Nature 353: 670–674

Ramirez V, Ulfhake B (1992) Anatomy of dendrites in motoneurons supplying the intrinsic muscles of the foot sole in the aged cat — evidence for dendritic growth and neo-synaptogenesis. J Comp Neurol 316: 1–16

Scheff SW, DeKosky ST, Price DA (1990) Quantitative assessment of cortical synaptic density in Alzheimer's disease. Neurobiol Aging 11: 29–37

Schubert D, Cole G, Saitoh T, Oltersdorf T (1989a) Amyloid beta protein precursor is a mitogen. Biochem Biophys Res Commun 162: 83–88

Serrano M, Hannon GJ, Beach-D (1993) A new regulatory motif in cell-cycle control causing specific inhibition of cyclin D/CDK4. Nature 366: 704–707

Shimizu K, Birnbaum D, Ruley MA, Fasano O, Suard Y, Edlund L, Taparowsky E, Goldfarb M, Wigler M (1983) Structure of the Ki-ras gene of the human lung carcinoma cell line Calu-1. Nature 304: 497–500

Standler NA, Bernstein JJ (1982) Degeneration and regeneration of motoneuron dendrites after ventral root crush: computer reconstruction of dendritic fields. Exp Neurol 75: 600–615

Stokoe D, MacDonald SG, Cadwallader K, Symons M, Hancock JF (1994) Activation of Raf as a result of recruitment to the plasma membrane. Science 264: 1463–1467

Stopa EG, Gonzalez AM, Chorsky R, Corona RJ, Alvarez J, Bird ED, Baird A (1990) Basic fibroblast growth factor in Alzheimer's disease. Biochem Biophys Res Commun 171: 690–696

Styren SD, Mufson EJ, Styren GC, Civin WH, Rogers J (1990) Epidermal growth factor receptor expression in demented and aged human brain. Brain Res 512: 347–352

Sumner BEH, Watson, WE (1971) Retraction and expansion of the dendritic tree of motor neurones of adult rats induced in vivo. Nature 233: 273–275

Suzuki T, Oishi M, Marshak DR, Czernik AJ, Nairn AC, Greengard P (1994) Cell cycle-dependent regulation of the phosphorylation and metabolism of the Alzheimer amyloid precursor protein. EMBO J 13: 1114–1122

Uemura E (1985) Age-related changes in the subiculum of Macaca mulatta: dendritic branching pattern. Exp Neurol 87: 412–427

Vandermeeren M, Lübke U, Six J, Cras P (1993) The phosphatase inhibitor okadaic acid induces a phosphorylated paired helical filament tau epitope in human LA-N-5 neuroblastoma cells. Neurosci Lett 153: 57–60

Wolozin B, Scicutella A, Davies P (1988) Reexpression of a developmentally regulated antigen in Down syndrom and Alzheimer disease. Proc Natl Acad Sci 85: 6202–6206

Authors' address: Prof. Dr. T. Arendt, Department of Neuroanatomy, Paul Flechsig Institute of Brain Research, University of Leipzig, Jahnallee 59, D-04109 Leipzig, Federal Republic of Germany

Mechanisms of cell death in Alzheimer disease — immunopathology

P. L. McGeer and **E. G. McGeer**

Kinsmen Laboratory of Neurological Research, University of British Columbia,
Vancouver, Canada

Summary. Lesions in such chronic neurodegenerative disorders as Alzheimer disease, Parkinson disease, the parkinsonism dementia complex of Guam and amyotrophic lateral sclerosis have associated with them a variety of proteins known to be involved in inflammatory processes. This is particularly true of Alzheimer disease where inflammatory reactions are thought to be important contributors to the neuronal loss. They include complement proteins, complement inhibitors, acute phase reactants, inflammatory cytokines, proteases and protease inhibitors. Studies of cultured human astrocytes and microglia, obtained from postmortem brain, have established that nearly all of these proteins are produced by one or another of these cell types. Human neurons also produce many inflammatory proteins and their inhibitors, creating complex interactions. Accumulations of amyloid and extracellular tangles apparently act as irritants, causing the activation of complement, the initiation of reactive changes in microglia, and the release of potentially neurotoxic products. Such products include the membrane attack complex, oxygen free radicals and excess glutamate. Twenty epidemiological studies that have been published to data indicate that populations taking antiinflammatory drugs have a significantly reduced prevalence of Alzheimer disease or a slower mental decline. One small clinical trial with indomethacin showed arrest of the disease over a 6 month period. Thera peutic intervention in key inflammatory processes holds great promise for the amelioration of Alzheimer disease and possibly other neurodegenerative disorders.

The brain has traditionally been regarded as immunologically privileged. The existence of the blood/brain barrier, the absence of conventional lymphatic drainage, and the unusual tolerance of the brain to transplanted tissue have all reinforced this concept. Moreover, it does not show the pain and swelling typical of peripheral inflammatory reactions. However, immunohistochemical and molecular biological evidence accumulating over the past decade indicates that the brain has an active endogenous immune system and that chronic inflammation of the brain may play an important role in the progressive neuronal death in many neurodegenerative diseases. The evidence is strongest in Alzheimer's disease (AD) (McGeer and McGeer, 1995, 1997), possibly because it has been the focus of the majority of the work in this field. The importance of these findings is that they suggest that antiinflammatory medication may substantially slow the progress of these diseases and delay their clinical appearance.

Presumably the innate immune system of brain, like that of other tissues, is designed as a defense mechanism — to get rid of foreign invaders and clean up debris. But any chronic inflammatory process may damage healthy tissue, and the brain, instead of being immunologically privileged, may be particularly vulnerable in this regard since neurons are post-mitotic and, once lost, cannot be replaced.

The initial immunohistochemical finding that spurred work in this field was the identification of large numbers of reactive microglia in association with the lesions of AD and other neurodegenerative diseases. Microglia are the brain's representatives of the macrophage phagocytic system. They are quiescent in normal adult brain and do not then show the morphology or the high levels of various proteins characteristic of activated microglia (McGeer and McGeer, 1995). Like all macrophages, microglia produce, when activated, such potentially neurotoxic products as complement proteins (Walker et al., 1995), excess glutamate (Klegeris and McGeer, 1997) and a flood of oxygen free radicals (Klegeris and McGeer, 1994).

Subsequent immunohistochemical and other studies have revealed that the amyloid deposits in AD are also associated with many other extracellular molecules, including complement proteins, complement inhibitors, acute phase reactants, growth factors, heat shock proteins, proteoglycans, lipoproteins, cathepsins, cystatins, coagulation factors, proteases, protease inhibitors, integrin adhesion molecules and other miscellaneous proteins (Table 1). Many have also been shown to be associated with tangles. The accumulation is probably representative of what occurs around any chronic inflammatory lesion where attempts to resolve the irritant are unsuccessful. A situation occurs in which inflammatory forces compete with healing, or antiinflammatory forces. A stalemate results. In the case of brain, neurons and their processes may be the victims of toxic inflammatory products generated to overcome the adverse effects of protease inhibitors and other antiinflammatory products.

Of particular importance may be the membrane attack complex formed by the terminal components of the classical complement cascade. The membrane attack complex (MAC), or C5b-9, inserts into the membranes of intact cells causing lysis and death of the cell. The MAC is intended to destroy foreign cells and viruses, but host cells are at significant risk of bystander lysis. In AD, the MAC is seen in association with abnormal neurites in and around senile plaques, and in some tangled neurons (McGeer and McGeer, 1995).

Further evidence of a chronic inflammatory reaction in AD, as well as in some other neurodegenerative diseases, is provided by reports of increased levels of inflammatory cytokines and their receptors, such as interleukin-1β

Table 1. Some extracellular molecules reported associated with amyloid deposits and possible cellular sources

	Reported secreted by:		
	Microglia	Astrocytes	Neurons
Complement proteins			
C1 through C9	+	+	+
Complement Inhibitors			
C1 inhibitor	+		
C4-binding protein			+
Vitronectin		+	+
Clusterin		+	+
Protectin			+
Acute Phase Reactants			
Amyloid P component			
C-reactive protein		+	+
α1-Antichymotrypsin		+	+
α1-Antitrypsin			+
α2-Macroglobulin			+
Neuronal pentraxin			+
Growth Factors			
bFGF	+	+	
TGFβ-1	+	+	+
Midkine			+
Heat Shock Proteins			
HSP-72			+
HSP-27			+
Proteoglycans			
HSPG		+	+
CSPG	+	+	
DSPG			
Substrates for Lipoprotein Receptors			
Apolipoprotein E	+	+	+
LRP[1]			+
Lipoprotein lipase	+		+
Lactoferrin			+
Cathepsins & Cystatins			
Cathepsins B, D, E, H, L & S		+	+
Cystatins A & C			+
Tissue inhibitor of metalloproteinase			
Thrombin & Plasmin Systems			
Thrombin			
Tissue factor	+	+	+
Hageman factor			
Tissue plasminogen activator		+	+
Urokinase plasminogen activator	+		+
Other			
ICAM-1		+	+
Chromogranin A[2]			+

[1] *LPR* low density lipoprotein receptor-related protein. [2] Chromogranin A activates microglia (Taupenot et al., 1996)

(IL-1β), IL-6, the type B IL-8 receptor and the receptor for CSF-1 in brain tissue and/or CSF (for review see McGeer and McGeer, 1997). A number of in vitro interactions between cytokines and components that have been identified in AD senile plaques have been reported, suggesting a further way in which a vicious cycle might be generated (also reviewed in McGeer and McGeer, 1997). For example, beta-amyloid protein has been found to potentiate the secretion of IL-6 and IL-8 by IL-1β activated astrocytoma cells, and of IL-8 by monocytes. In turn, IL-1, IL-2, IL-6 and GM-CSF have all been reported to stimulate APP695 gene expression in neuronal cultures. IL-1 has also been found to increase the secretion of proteoglycans such as heparan sulfate by neuroblastoma cells and to induce expression of α1-antichymotrypsin, thromboplastin, complement protein C3 and apolipo-protein E by appropriate cell lines. Thus, secreted cytokines may stimulate neurons or glial cells to secrete a number of the proteins found in senile plaques.

The enhanced expression of nuclear factor-kappa B (NK-kB) in neurons in AD brain (Terai et al., 1996) is also consistent with an inflammatory reaction, since NF-kB is presently regarded as a central regulator of inflammatory, immune and acute phase reactions.

Studies of cultured human astrocytes and microglia, obtained from post-mortem brain, have established that nearly all of the inflammatory proteins seen in AD tissue can be produced by microglia, astrocytes or both (Table 1) (McGeer and McGeer, 1995). Human neurons also produce many inflammatory proteins and their inhibitors, indicating the possibility of complex interactions in vivo. In situ hybridization studies have shown that the mRNAs for all the complement proteins are prominently localized in neurons, as well as appearing to a lesser extent in glial cells (Shen et al., 1997). Thus, the brain clearly has the ability to initiate and sustain chronic inflammatory reactions.

But what initiates and promotes such a state? Our hypothesis (Fig. 1) is that some insult, perhaps complicated by a genetic weakness, causes initial neuronal damage with the deposition of debris that the microglia find hard to digest. They become activated, with initiation of the classical complement cascade. The toxic products thus produced lead to further neuronal death which, in turn, spurs the inflammatory reaction. This reaction is hypothesized to be more than just an epiphenomenon directed at detritus accumulating in the lesions. It may be a self-sustaining autodestructive force in which phagocytic attack injures bystander neurons in such a way that further lesions are produced. A vicious cycle of damage may be generated and sustained, all by localized glial cells. This autotoxic loop hypothesis may not be limited to AD or even to neurodegenerative brain disorders. It might apply to a diverse spectrum of chronic inflammatory diseases where evidence of systemic involvement is minimal or absent (Laskin and Pendino, 1995). Markers of peripheral immune system participation, such as specific antibodies or cloned T-cell subsets, need not be present. All that is required is that the inflammatory response reach a threshold necessary to produce autodestruction of viable host cells. Then the reaction can be sustained by

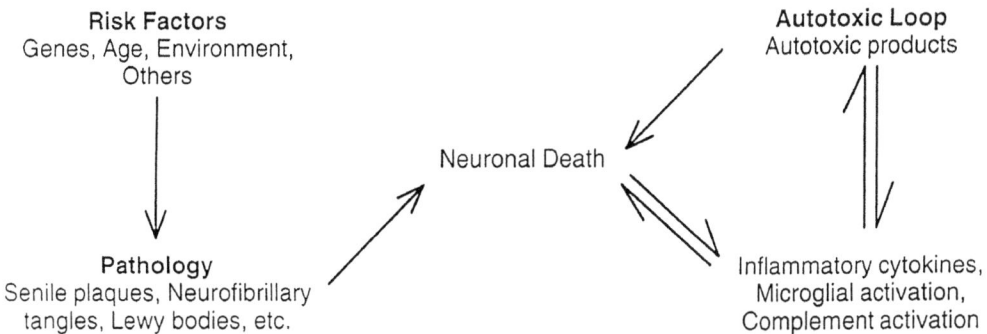

Fig. 1. Autotoxic loop hypothesized to be responsible for much of the neuronal damage in Alzheimer disease and possibly other neurodegenerative disorders

further production of inflammatory stimulants. Complement may be a key factor in this process.

This is not an autoimmune disease in the classical sense of the development of antibodies to host tissue. No reliable evidence exists for such antibodies in AD or many chronic neurodegenerative diseases (McGeer and McGeer, 1995). In experimental models of brain injury, activation of the complement pathway and appearance of reactive microglia occur much too rapidly to allow for the production of autoantibodies (e.g. Akiyama et al., 1994; Pasinetti et al., 1992). And it is now clear that the complement cascade can be activated in the absence of antibodies. Several of the proteins occurring in association with the lesions in AD have been found to activate the complement cascade in vitro. These include serum amyloid P, the Hageman factor, C-reactive protein and beta-amyloid itself (McGeer and McGeer, 1995). Thus, the brain seems capable of initiating and maintaining a chronic inflammatory reaction.

The accumulating evidence of a chronic innate immune reaction in AD brain led to the suggestion that treatment with antiinflammatory agents might slow the progress of AD or retard its onset (McGeer and Rogers, 1992). It is important to realize that this therapeutic approach to AD is very different from attempts to replace the lost cholinergic activity or stimulate the cortical glucose metabolism. Such pharmacological approaches do not attempt to slow the very rapid destruction of cortical neurons which is almost certainly the main cause of the mental deterioration. The suggestion is that antiinflammatory treatment may inhibit such neuronal death. There are now twenty published epidemiological studies and one reported clinical trial which generally support this possibility. Many of these studies are relevant because they considered arthritis, a major indication for the use of antiinflammatory drugs, or antiinflammatory drugs themselves, as risk factors for AD. In some of the studies, other diseases or drugs were considered as possible risk factors, but only arthritis and antiinflammatory drug use have generally shown negative associations with AD.

The outcome of a risk factor analysis is often expressed as an odds ratio. This is a commonly used statistic for estimation of the relative risk of developing the disorder if there is exposure to a particular factor. It measures the odds that a person in an exposed group will develop AD, relative to the corresponding odds for a person in a control, or non-exposed group. A negative risk, corresponding to a protective factor, yields an odds ratio less than one, while a positive risk factor is associated with an odds ratio greater than one. Estimating overall odds ratios using data from multiple reports requires that the studies be similar in design. We therefore grouped the seventeen studies published at the time of our analysis according to the risk factor employed and into case control or population based. For groups which passed a test of homogeneity (similarity in design), we did a meta-analysis to determine the overall risk factor and its significance (McGeer et al., 1996). Such an analysis on the relevant epidemiological studies, taken together, indicates that the use of NSAIDs will decrease the risk of AD by about 50%. Epidemiological studies are always plagued by problems such as ascertainment bias or differing genetic predispositions to various diseases. For this reason, the studies of Breitner et al. (1994, 1995) are of particular interest. They used twins and individuals genotyped for apolipoprotein E4, an established risk factor for AD (Roses, 1996). Breitner et al. came to the conclusion that use of an NSAID could delay the onset of AD by 5 to 7 years. Such a delay in onset, if generally applicable, would again mean that the prevalence of AD would be cut by about 50% since the prevalence doubles every 5 years after the age of 65.

A subsequent prospective study of a large aging Baltimore population also supports the hypothesis that people taking NSAIDs are relatively spared from AD (Stewart et al., 1997). And two additional papers (Rich et al., 1995; Doraiswamy et al., 1996) have reported retrospective studies of clinical charts which indicate that AD patients taking NSAIDs for other purposes have a slower progression of the disease. The only controlled clinical trial of the effects of an NSAID for the treatment of AD was a small, double blind, placebo controlled study in which AD cases given 75 mg/kg-day of indomethacin maintained their Mini Mental Status for the 6 month period of the trial while those on placebo showed the expected 10–12 percent loss (Rogers et al., 1993).

Taken together, these data suggest that the disciplined use of an effective NSAID should be able to cut the prevalence of Alzheimer disease at least in half. Reluctance to treat geriatric cases with NSAIDs exists in the medical community. This is based upon the known side effects of these drugs, the most dangerous of which is inducing gastrointestinal ulceration and bleeding. Although misoprostol offers some protection against this major side effect (Graham et al., 1988), it remains a concern. What needs to be balanced against such risks are the rewards that epidemiological studies suggest might result from NSAID use. These are economic as well as humanitarian. For example, the annual cost of caring for demented patients in Canada with its population of about 25 million has been estimated at $3.9 billion (after deducting costs associated with the medical care of age matched non-demented controls) (Ostbye and Crosse, 1994). One can readily calculate the pharmacoeconomic benefits of reducing the prevalence even by as little as half. And the benefit in alleviation of human suffering is obvious but incalculable. Thus any treatment which may inhibit the onset and slow the progress of AD seems worth thorough investigation.

Acknowledgments

Our research on Alzheimer disease is supported by grants from the Alzheimer Society of B.C., the Jack Brown and Family A.D. Research Fund and donations from individual British Columbians.

References

Akiyama H, Tooyama I, Kondo H, Ikeda K, Kimura H, McGeer EG, McGeer PL (1994) Early response of brain resident microglia to kainic acid-induced hippocampal lesions. Brain Res 635: 257–268

Breitner JCS, Gau BA, Welsh KA, Plassman BL, McDonald WM, Helmas MJ, Anthony JC (1994) Inverse association of anti-inflammatory treatments and Alzheimer's disease. Neurology 44: 227–232

Breitner JCS, Welsh KA, Helms MJ, Gaskell PC, Gau BA, Roses AD, Pericak-Vance MA, Saunders AM (1995) Delayed onset of Alzheimer's disease with nonsteroidal anti-inflammatory and histamine H2 blocking drugs. Neurobiol Aging 16: 523–530

Doraiswamy PM, Krishen A, Stallone F, Martin WL, Potts NLS, Metz A, DeVeaugh-Geiss J (1996) NSAIDs and cognition in Alzheimer's disease. Neurology 46: 1994

Graham DY, Agrawal NM, Roth SH (1988) Prevention of NSAID-induced gastric ulcer with misoprostol: multicentre, double-blind, placebo-controlled trial. Lancet ii: 1277–1280

Klegeris A, McGeer PL (1994) Rat brain microglia and peritoneal macrophages show similar responses to respiratory burst stimulants. J Neuroimmunol 53: 83–90

Klegeris A, McGeer PL (1997) β-Amyloid protein and glutamine enhance macrophage production of oxygen free radicals and glutamate. J Neurosci Res 49: 229–235

Laskin DL, Pendino KJ (1995) Macrophages and inflammatory mediators in tissue injury. Ann Rev Pharmacol Toxicol 35: 655–677

McGeer PL, Rogers J (1992) Anti-inflammatory agents as a therapeutic approach to Alzheimer's disease. Neurology 42: 447–449

McGeer PL, McGeer EG (1995) The inflammatory system of brain: implications for therapy of Alzheimer and other neurodegenerative disorders. Brain Res Rev 21: 195–218

McGeer EG, McGeer PL (1997) Inflammatory cytokines in the CNS. CNS Drugs 7: 214–228

McGeer PL, Schulzer M, McGeer EG (1996) Arthritis and antiinflammatory agents as negative risk factors for Alzheimer disease: a review of seventeen epidemiological studies. Neurology 47: 425–432

Ostbye T, Crosse E (1994) Net economic costs of dementia in Canada. Can Med Assoc J 151: 1457–1464

Pasinetti GM, Johnson SA, Rozovsky I, Lampert-Etchells M, Morgan DG, Gordon MN, Morgan TE, Willoughby D, Finch CE (1992) Complement C1qB and C4 mRNAs responses to lesioning in rat brain. Exp Neurol 118: 117–125

Rich JB, Rasmusson DX, Folstein MF, Carson KA, Kawas C, Brandt J (1995) Nonsteroidal anti-inflammatory drugs in Alzheimer's disease. Neurology 45: 51–55

Rogers J, Kirby LC, Hempelman SR, Berry DL, McGeer PL, Kaszniak AW, Zalinski J, Cofield M, Mansukhani L, Willson P, Kogan F (1993) Clinical trial of indomethacin in Alzheimer's disease. Neurology 43: 1609–1611

Roses AD (1996) Apolipoprotein E alleles as risk factors in Alzheimer's disease. Ann Rev Med 47: 387–400

Shen Y, Li R, McGeer EG, McGeer PL (1997) Neuronal expression of mRNAs for complement proteins of the classical pathway in Alzheimer brain. Brain Res 769: 391–395

Stewart WF, Kawas C, Corrada M, Metter EJ (1997) Risk of Alzheimer's disease and duration of NSAID use. Neurology 48: 626–632

Taupenot L, Ciesielski-Traska J, Ulrich G, Chasserot-Golaz S, Aunis D, Bader MF (1996) Chromogranin A triggers a phenotypic transformation and the generation of nitric oxide in brain microglial cells. Neuroscience 72: 377–389

Terai K, Matsuo A, McGeer PL (1996) Enhancement of immunoreactivity for NF-κB in the hippocampal formation and cerebral cortex of Alzheimer's disease. Brain Res 735: 159–168

Walker DG, Kim SU, McGeer PL (1995) Complement and cytokine gene expression in cultured microglia derived from postmortem human brains. J Neurosci Res 40: 478–493

Authors' address: Dr. P. L. McGeer, Kinsmen Laboratory of Neurological Research, University of British Columbia, 2255 Wesbrook Mall, Vancouver, B.C., V6T 1Z3, Canada

Pathological immuno-reactions of glial cells in Alzheimer's disease and possible sites of interference

P. Schubert[1], T. Ogata[1], H. Miyazaki[1], C. Marchini[1,2], S. Ferroni[2], and K. Rudolphi[3]

[1] Department of Neuromorphology, Max Planck Institute for Neurobiology, Martinsried, and [3] Hoechst Marion Roussel, Frankfurt, Federal Republic of Germany
[2] Department of Physiology, University of Bologna, Italy

Summary. A significant role of a pathological glial cell activation in the pathogenesis of Alzheimer's disease is supported by the growing evidence that inflammatory proteins, which are produced by reactive astrocytes, promote the transformation of diffuse β-amyloid deposits into the filamentous, neurotoxic form. A number of vicious circles, driven by the release of TNF-a and free oxygen radicals from microglial cells, may cause an upregulated microglial activation and their production of interleukin-1 which triggers, secondarily, the crucial activation of astrocytes. Reactive functional changes of glial cells seem to be controlled by an altered balance of the second messengers Ca^{2+} and cAMP and can be counterregulated by the endogenous cell modulator adenosine which strenghtens the cAMP-dependent signalling chain. A further reinforcement of the homeostatic adenosine effects on glial cells by pharmaca, such as propentofylline, may add to neuroprotection in Alzheimer's disease.

Evolving role of reactive glial cell changes in the pathomechanism of neuronal death

The activation of glial cells is a common event which occurs in a rather similar manner under different pathological conditions, such as brain ischemia, trauma, infection, and also during the course of neurodegenerative diseases. The observed reactive glial cell changes reflect a response of the brain-immanent cellular defense system in which the microglia represent the local immune-competent cells (for a review see Kreutzberg, 1996). Their ability of antigene presentation allows them to cooperate with the general blood cell linked immune system and they acquire a number of immunological weapons designed for cell attack. Thus, activated microglial cells produce extraordinary high amounts of free oxygen radicals, NO, and also aggressive cytokines like the tumor necrosis factor α (TNF-a). The activation of microglial cells is a graded response and may cause by the additional release of the cytokine interleukine-1 (Il-1) a secondary activation of astrocytes (Giulian, 1987). If so, the astrocytes undergo hyperplasia and/or start to proliferate which forces them to give up the differentiated state and to retract their cell processes e.g. from synaptic complexes. One of the consequences is that their capacity of taking up synaptically released K^+ and glutamate, the major physiological function of astrocytes, will be reduced. Paying such a price is presumably worth, if the newly adopted functions, such as an increased production of growth factors and of various cytokines, are required in conjunction with the microglial immune properties for defense or repair. But if such reactive glial cell changes escape from their rigorous endogenous control and may even cooperate with other pathological alterations, the potentially toxic microglial functions and an impaired maintenance of the extracellular ion homeostasis by reactive astrocytes may add to neuronal death (Fig. 1).

Such glia-related pathomechanisms are discussed to enhance secondary nerve cell damage occuring e.g. in the penumbra of an ischemic brain infarct. They may contribute to neuronal loss during the development of Alzheimer-type dementia for which brain ischemia is thought to be an aggravating factor. The appearance of a marked glial cell reaction in conjunction with Alzheimer's disease has been already demonstrated by Alzheimer himself. Later histological examination revealed that microglia together with large numbers of reactive astrocytes often form a halo surrounding the core of an

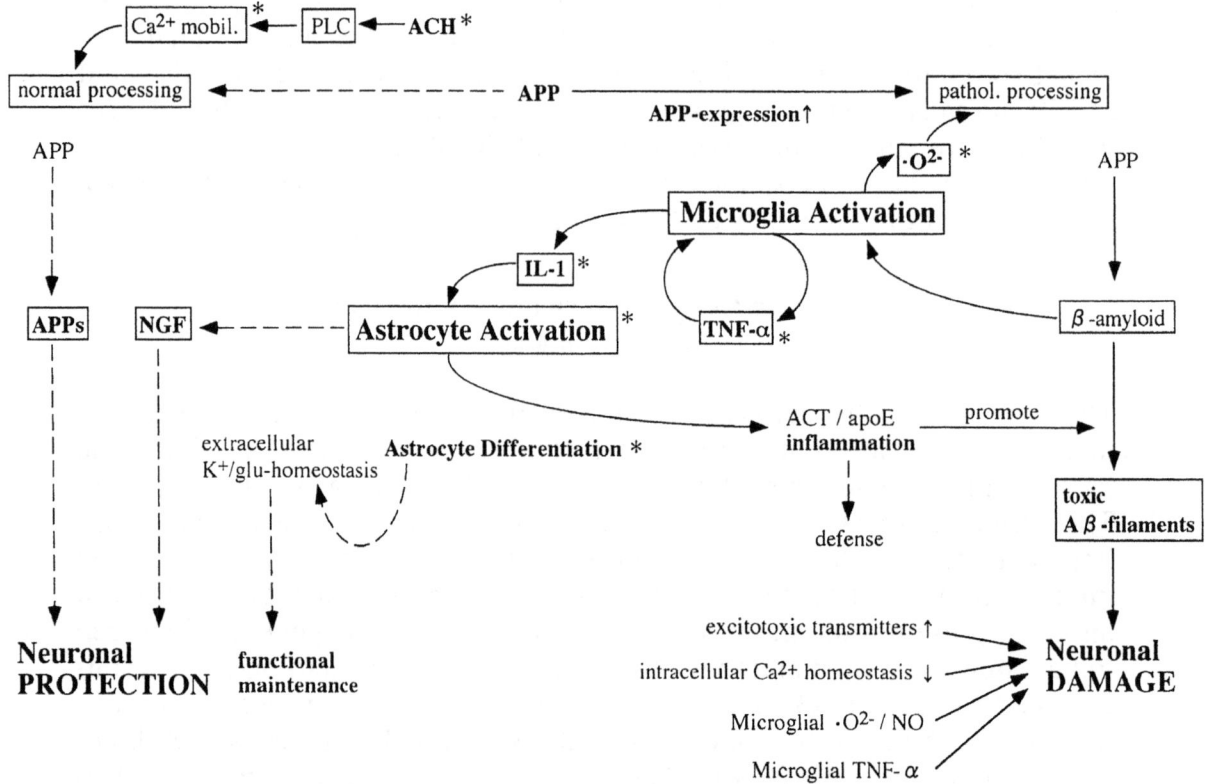

Fig. 1. Cascade of pathological glial reactions, suggested to contribute to local inflammation, toxic β-amyloid formation, and neuronal damage in Alzheimer's disease. Possible sites of interference are marked by asterics. Physiological paths are indicated by broken arrows

amyloid plaque (McGeer et al., 1993). The phenomenologically obvious association with the hallmark of this disease suggested that a pathological glial cell activation represents a causal factor in the complex process leading to progredient nerve cell death and to the development of dementia. This possibility was being strongly supported by the growing evidence that brain inflammation plays an essential role in the pathogenesis of Alzheimer's disease.

In conjunction with the observation that patients treated with anti-inflammatory drugs have a reduced incidence of Alzheimer's disease, inflammatory proteins, i.e. antichymotrypsin (ACT) or apolipoprotein-E (apoE), were found to be associated with Alzheimer plaques (Abraham et al., 1989; Wisniewsky and Frangione, 1992). Consecutive in vitro experiments by H. Potter's group showed that ACT and apoE4, the apolipoprotein-E isoform known to be linked to late-onset Alzheimer's disease, transformed amorphous β-amyloid into the filamentous form which is neurotoxic (Ma et al., 1994). If ACT or apoE4 were applied in conjunction with the β-amyloid peptide, they caused almost complete nerve cell death in vitro. A recent analysis of different plaque types in the brain of Alzheimer's disease patients revealed that more than 85% of the neuron-associated dense core plaques were aopE-positive, whereas more than 90% of the diffuse non-neuritic amyloid deposits and also the "burned out" dense core plaques were apoE-negative (Sheng et al., 1996). Taken together, these findings support that the neurotoxicity of amyloid plaques is largely dependent on the presence of such inflammatory proteins. Interestingly, they are apparently produced by reactive astrocytes. Thus, those cells which contained human apoE protein in the brains of transgenic mice were identified as astrocytes (Bowman et al., 1996) and human astrocytes produced ACT upon stimulation with the microglial cytokine Il-1 (Das and Potter, 1995).

It follows that the deleterious formation of neurotoxic β-amyloid filaments from amorphous β-amyloid by the promoting action of inflammatory proteins is apparently closely linked to reactive functional changes of astrocytes which were triggered by a pathological microglial activation (Fig. 1). A number of vicious circles are presumably involved leading to a gradual reinforcement of the glial reaction over time. The primary trigger causing the initial activation of microglial cells in Alzheimer's disease is not defined. Brain ischemia may play a role. More specific candidates are the β-amyloid peptides, formed as the result of an altered β-amyloid precursor protein (β-APP) processing. They were reported to have an activating effect on rat microglial cells in vitro (Araujo and Cotman, 1992). Activated microglial cells may, in turn, reinforce a pathological β-APP processing by the massive release of reactive oxygen intermediates which induced the oxidation of the β-APP C-terminal residues in vitro, causing the formation of aggregating β-amyloid (Dyrcks et al., 1993). A pathological APP processing can be expected to be particularly pronounced in reactive astrocytes which had been activated by the release of Il-1 from neighbouring microglial cells. The reason is that Il-1 has been shown in vitro to enhance markedly the expression of β-APP in astrocytes (Forloni et al., 1992) inducing an accelerated cycle of β-APP processing which increases its sensitivity to pathological influences. The resulting augmented formation of β-amyloid proteins may stimulate the release of TNF-a and NO, as shown in rat microglial cultures. This caused neuronal death in vitro (Meda et al., 1995). On the other hand, TNF-a also seems to exert an aggravating feed-back effect on still resting microglial cells favoring their recruitment to activated cells. The latter is indicated by the observation that intracerebral injection of TNF-a and interferon-γ induced a wide-spread upregulation of MHC-classII antigens in resident microglial cells (Wekerle et al., 1986), indicating their transformation into immuno-effective cells. This may provide another vicious circle by which a primarily mild microglial reaction could be further exaggerated. As a consequence, an upgraded level of microglial activation may be reached which is sufficient to cause the release of Il-1 and a secondary activation of astrocytes (Fig. 1). The final outcome would be a "mature" Alzheimer plaque which became neurotoxic because of the β-amyloid promoting effect of the specific inflammatory proteins produced by Il-1 activated astrocytes.

The presumed significance of a microglia coupled astrocyte reaction for the pathomechanism of Alzheimer's disease prompted H. Potter to propose a blockade of the microglial Il-1 production or a blockade of the astrocytic Il-1 receptor as new therapeutic approach. We propose a more general inhibition of activated microglial cell functions and a recovery of astrocyte differentiation by reinforcement of endogenous counterregulatory mechanisms.

Pathologically altered Ca^{2+}/cAMP signalling in glial cells and its endogenous counterregulation by adenosine

The list of specific molecular signals which participate in the complex intra- and intercellular information processing underlying reactive changes of astrocytes and microglial cells is steadily growing, but the logistics of their integrated interactions are just at the beginning of being understood. We therefore think, that it is a promising strategy to use the know-how of an endogenous cell modulator which has learned during evolution how to influence the interwoven networks of the different signal-evoked metabolic cascades underlying glial cell activation. The cell metabolite adenosine is such an ancient molecular signal which acts via different receptor subtypes and influences the cell metabolism and functions of neurons and also of glial cells (Schubert et al., 1994). The major target of the adenosine action is a homeostatic regulation of the intracellular signals Ca^{2+} and cAMP. The cross-talk of these second messengers represents a bottle neck of the molecular signalling network that controls a multitude of different receptor-mediated cell functions and also their reactive changes in response to pathological glial activation. There is evidence that a strengthening of the Ca^{2+}-dependent signalling favors cell activation, whereas the cAMP-dependent signalling serves as negative control. Under physiological conditions, the functional balance between the Ca^{2+}/cAMP signalling is under strict control in which adenosine participates by a "yin/yang" regulation of the cAMP synthesis. Under pathological conditions, going along with an increased extracellular concentration of the excitotoxic transmitter glutamate, a sustained activation of ionotropic receptors causes an excessive membrane depolarization and hence, an increased Ca^{2+} influx through voltage-dependent membrane channels. The cellular calcium load is augmented by the additional activation of metabotropic glutamate receptors (mGluR) which trigger a pronounced Ca^{2+} release from intracellular stores via a phospholipase-C (PLC)-linked pathway. The concomitant activation of those mGluR subtypes, which are negatively coupled to the adenylcyclase, causes an inhibition of the cAMP synthesis. The latter may be further enhanced by a pathological upregulation of the mRNA levels for these mGluR subtypes, as shown e.g. in response to transient brain ischemia (Diemer et al., 1994). There is evidence that the cyclic nucleotide dependent signalling is reduced in Alzheimer's disease brains by a downregulation of the Gs-protein coupled stimulatory regulation of the cyclases (O'Neill et al., 1994). As a consequence of the pathologically increased intracellular Ca^{2+} load and decreased cAMP synthesis, one can expect a dramatic change of the Ca^{2+}/cAMP balance in favor of a prevalent Ca^{2+} dependent signalling.

Effects on astrocytes

The generation of an increased Ca^{2+} signal associated with a reduced intracellular cAMP concentration can be observed under experimentally mimicked pathological mGluR activation in cultured rat astrocytes. They resemble in several aspects (high proliferation rate, dedifferentiated phenotype) reactive astrocytes. Using this experimental model, we tested the effect of adenosine agonists on the evoked Ca^{2+} and cAMP signals during continued mGluR activation by means of the Ca^{2+} fluorescence imaging technique and a biochemicdal cAMP assay (Ogata et al., 1996). Surprisingly, adenosine A1-receptor activation further increased the PLC-mediated intracellular Ca^{2+} mobilization by even subthreshold concentrations of mGluR agonists. In view of the fact that a deficiency of acetylcholine (ACH), another PLC-stimulating transmitter, is a cardinal symptom of Alzheimer's disease, we are testing in current experiments whether a deficient Ca^{2+} mobilization at reduced ACH concentrations can also be reinforced in astrocytes by bringing the action of adenosine into play. This may have therapeutic consequences since a maintained Ca^{2+} mobilization is known to support the regular β-APP processing by favoring the release of the soluble form of β-APP and diminishing the formation of aggregating β-amyloid protein (Buxbaum et al., 1994).

The observed facilitation of the intracellular Ca^{2+} mobilization by adenosine in metabotropically stimulated astrocytes did, however, not further increase the pathological Ca^{2+}/AMP dys-balance. In contrast, we found a Ca^{2+} dependent dramatic increase of the intracellular cAMP content which more than counterbalanced the mGluR -evoked depression of the cAMP synthesis (Ogata et al., 1996). The seemingly paradoxical cAMP increase under these conditions by adenosine apparently results from a reduced enzymatic cAMP break down by a Ca^{2+} dependent selective inhibition of phosphodiesterases (unpublished observation). We conclude from these studies that adenosine maintains its action as a homeostatic signal also under pathological conditions by counterbalancing an increased Ca^{2+} signalling via a parallel increase of the cAMP signalling.

In order to test the effect of such a strengthened cAMP signalling on the astrocyte differentiation state, we treated cultures of non-differentiated, immature astrocytes for several days with the membrane-permeable dibutyryl-cAMP. This initiated the outgrowth of extended cell processes suggesting cell differentiation. The latter was supported by patch clamp experiments revealing that cAMP-treated astrocytes had acquired newly expressed specific K^+ and Cl^- membrane channels which were not present in non-treated astrocytes (Ferroni et al., 1995). These ion channels support the voltage-sensitive uptake of neuronally released K^+ and glutamate and are required for the physiological maintenance of the extracellular ion homeostasis by differentiated astrocytes. The findings suggest that a strengthening of the cAMP signalling which promotes the differentiation and functional maturation of astrocytes in vitro, could also help reactive and dedifferentiating astrocytes to regain their physiological mature state.

The described homeostatic actions of adenosine which tend to maintain a balanced Ca^{2+}/cAMP signalling may be reinforced pharmacologically. In this respect, pharmaca which raise the effective endogenous adenosine concentration in the extracellular space and/or strengthen the cAMP signalling by mimicking the adenosine induced Ca^{2+} dependent blockade of phosphodiesterases, are indicated. Such a pharmacon is propentofylline (Hoechst AG). It elevates the extracellular adenosine concentration by blocking the cellular reuptake (Parkinson and Fredholm, 1991) and exerts a selective blockade of various phosphodiesterase subtypes (Meskini et al., 1994). In vivo studies on gerbils revealed that pretreatment with propentofylline prevented the ischemia-induced astrocyte reaction and protected neurons against delayed neuronal death (DeLeo et al., 1987).

Effects on microglial cells

Whether the production of the astrocyte-stimulating cytokine Il-1 by pathologically activated microglial cells is also under the homeostatic control of adenosine, has not been examined so far. But we have experimental evidence that the pathologically stimulated release of the cytokine TNF-a, elicited in cultured rat microglial cells by stimulation with lipopolysaccharides (LPS) was markedly depressed by even submicromolar adenosine concentration which may easily be reached under pathological conditions (Schubert et al., 1997). The TNF-a depression is apparently a cyclic nucleotide-mediated effect which could also be obtained by selective adenosine A2 receptor agonists known to stimulate the adenylcyclase. Via an A1 receptor-mediated action, low nanomolar concentrations of selective adenosine agonists inhibited the proliferation (^{3}H-thymidine uptake) of cultivated microglial cells when their proliferation rate was pathologically stimulated by protein kinase C activating phorbol esters (Si et al., 1996). Similar depressive effects were obtained with propentofylline. This neuroprotective pharmacon has further been shown to depress significantly the release of reactive oxygen compounds from microglia-derived macrophages (Banati et al., 1994). Prolonged treatment with propentofylline prevented the in vitro spontaneously occuring transformation of microglial cells into macrophages. Prolonged posttreatment in vivo counteracted the ischemia-induced microglial antigen expression (McRae et al., 1994, 1997).

Taken together: the in vitro studies indicate several sites (marked with asterics in Fig. 1) at which the cascade of pathological microglia and astrocyte activation can apparently be interrupted by a counterbalancing effect of adenosine on the pathologically altered Ca^{2+}/cAMP signalling (see also Schubert et al., 1997). Further in vivo studies on adequate experimental models are certainly required to support a pharmacological reinforcement of such homeostatic adenosine actions on reactive glial changes as a useful strategy for the treatment of Alzheimer's disease.

Acknowledgements

The studies have been supported by a grant from the German Minister of Research and Technology (BMBF "Neurotrauma, project A3). We appreciate the valuable technical help by R. Gleich and W. Kofler.

References

Abraham CA, Potter H (1989) Alzheimer's disease: recent advances in understanding the brain amyloid deposits. Biotechnology 7: 147–153

Araujo DM, Cotman CW (1992) β-amyloid stimulates glial cells in vitro to produce growth factors that accumulate in senile plaques in Alzheimer's disease. Brain Res 569: 141–145

Banati R, Schubert P, Rothe G, Gehrmann J, Rudolphi K, Valet G, Kreutzberg GW (1994) Modulation of intracellular reactive oxygen intermediates in peritoneal macrophages and microglia/brain macrophages by propentofylline. J Cereb Blood Flow Metab 14: 145–149

Bowman BH, Yang F, Buchanan JM, Adrian GS, Martinez AO (1996) Human APOE protein localized in brains of transgenic mice. Neurosci Lett 219: 57–59

Buxbaum JD, Ruefli AA, Parker CA, Cypess AM, Greengard P (1994) Calcium regulates processing of the Alzheimer amyloid protein precursor in a protein kinase C-independent manner. Proc Natl Acad Sci USA 91: 4489–4493

Das S, Potter H (1995) Expression of the Alzheimer amyloid-promoting factor antichymotrypsin is induced in human astrocytes by Il-1. Neuron 14: 447–456

DeLeo J, Tóth L, Schubert P, Rudolphi K, Kreutzberg GW (1987) Ischemia-induced neuronal cell death, calcium accumulation and glial response in the hippocampus of the gerbil and protection by the xanthine derivative HWA 285. J Cereb Blood Flow Metab 7: 745–752

Diemer NH, Seitzberg D, Rosdahl D, Nielsen M, Christensen T, Balchen T, Johansen FF (1994) AMPA receptor and metabotropic glutamate receptor mRNA expression after transient global ischemia in the rat. Pathophysiology 1: 107

Dyrcks T, Dyrcks E, Masters CL, Beyreuther K (1993) Amyloidogenicity of rodent and human β A4 sequences. FEBS Lett 324: 231–236

Ferroni S, Marchini C, Schubert P, Rapisarda C (1995) Two distinct inward rectifying conductances are expressed in cultured rat cortical astrocytes after long term dibutyryl-cyclic-AMP treatment. FEBS Lett 267: 319–325

Forloni G, Demicheli F, Giorgi S, Bendotti C, Angeretti N (1992) Expression of amyloid precursor protein mRNAs in endothelial, neuronal and glial cells: modulation by interleukin-1. Mol Brain Res 16: 128–134

Giulian D (1987) Amoeboid microglia as effector of inflammation in the central nervous system. J Neurosci Res 18: 155–171

Kreutzberg GW (1996) Microglia: a sensor for pathological events in the CNS. TINS 19: 312–318

Ma J, Yee A, Brewer HB, Das S, Potter H (1994) Amyloid-associated proteins alpha 1-antichymotrypsin and apolipoprotein E promote assembly of beta-protein into filaments. Nature 372: 92–94

McGeer PL, Kawamata T, Walker D, Abyama H, Toyama I, McGeer EG (1993) Microglia in degenerative neurological disease. Glia 7: 84–92

McRae A, Rudolphi K, Schubert P (1994) Propentofylline depresses amyloid and Alzheimer's CSF microglial antigens after ischemia. NeuroReport 5: 1193–1196

McRae A, Schubert P, Ogata T, Nakamura Y, Ling EA, Kaur C, Rudolphi K (1997) Postischemic glial responses and amyloid accumulation are modified by propentofylline: a neuroprotective pharmacon for Alzheimer's disease? In: Iqbal K, Winblad B, Nishimura T, Takeda M, Wisniewski HM (eds) Biology, diagnosis and therapeutics. Wiley, New Jersey, pp 759–767

Meda L, Cassatella MA, Szendrei I (1995) Activation of microglial cells by β-amyloid protein and interferon-γ. Nature 374: 647–650

Meskini N, Némoz G, Okyayuz-Baklouti I, Lagard M, Prigent AF (1994) Phosphodiesterase inhibitory profile of some related xanthine derivatives pharmacologically active on the peripheral microcirculation. Biochem Pharmacol 47: 781–788

O'Neill C, Fowler CJ, Winblad B, Cowburn RF (1994) G-protein coupled signal transduction systems in the Alzheimer's disease brain. Biochem Soc Transact 22: 167–171

Ogata T, Nakamura Y, Schubert P (1996) Potentiated cAMP rise in metabotropically stimulated rat cultured astrocytes by a Ca^{2+}-related A_1/A_2 adenosine receptor cooperation. Eur J Neurosci 8: 1124–1131

Parkinson FE, Fredholm BB (1991) Effects of propentofylline on adenosine A_1 and A_2 receptors and nitrobenzylthioinosine-sensitive neucleoside transporters: quantitative autoradiographic analysis. Eur J Pharmacol 202: 361–366

Schubert P, Rudolphi K, Fredholm F, Nakamura Y (1994) Modulation of nerve and glial cell function by adenosine — role in the development of ischemic brain damage. Int J Biochem 26: 1227–1236

Schubert P, Ogata T, Rudolphi K (1997) Depression of TNF-a release from microglial cells by adenosine and propentofylline. J Cereb Blood Flow Cell Metab 17 [Suppl 1]: S718

Schubert P, Ogata T, Rudolphi K, Marchini C, McRae A, Ferroni S (1997) Support of homeostatic glial cell signalling: a novel therapeutic approach by propentofylline. In: de la Torre JC, Hachinski V (eds) Cerebrovascular pathology in Alzheimer's disease. Ann NY Acad Sci 826: 337–347

Sheng JG, Mrak RE, Griffin WS (1996) Apolipoprotein E distribution among different plaque types in Alzheimer's disease: implications for its role in plaque progression. Neuropathol Appl Neurobiol 22: 334–341

Si Q, Nakamura Y, Schubert P, Rudolphi K, Kataoka K (1996) Adenosine and propentofylline inhibit phorbol ester-induced proliferation of cultured microglia. Exp Neurol 137: 345–349

Wekerle H, Linington C, Lassmann H, Meyermann R (1986) Cellular immune reactivity within the CNS. TINS 9: 271–277

Wisniewsky T, Frangione B (1992) Apolipoprotein E: a pathological chaperone in patients with cerebral amd systemic amyloid. Neurosci Lett 135: 235–238

Authors' address: P. Schubert, MD, Department of Neuromorphology, Max Planck Institute for Neurobiology, am Klopferspitz 18a, D-82152 Martinsried, Federal Republic of Germany

Therapeutic strategies based on immunological hypotheses of Alzheimer's disease

H.-J. Möller

Psychiatric Hospital, Ludwig-Maximilians-University, Munich,
Federal Republic of Germany

Summary. There are several findings demonstrating the importance of inflammatory or immunological processes in the etiopathogenesis of Alzheimer's disease (AD).

Several studies on nonsteroidal anti-inflammatory drugs (NSAID) give evidence for a therapeutic effect of these drugs in AD, among other the prospective double-blind placebo-controlled study on indomethacin, strongly support the therapeutic effect of these agents. Possibly also the therapeutic effects of propentofylline might be interpreted in the light of this theory.

Introduction

Inflammatory processes contribute to the etiopathology of AD (Rogers und O'Barr, 1997). Neuropathologic studies of brain tissue from AD patients have identified reactive microglia densely embedded around the core of senile plaques. Post mortem analyses of brains from Alzheimer's patients also revealed the presence of several immunoprotective proteins that are normaly absent or expressed at very low levels in brain (McGeer und Rogers, 1992). Among other Interleukin-6 (IL-6), a proinflammatory cytokine, was demonstrated as indicator of this process in post mortem brain (Bauer et al., 1991; Huell et al., 1995).

Given the fact that at this moment a very powerful drug therapy for AD is not available — not only the nootropics, but also the recently introduced cholinergic drugs demonstrated only a more or less small effect size — it seems reasonable that therapy strategies which focus on the different aspects of the complex etiopathogenesis of the disease should be developed. Possibly one of these drug strategies will reach a higher effect size or the theoretically meaningful combination of drugs targeted for different etiopathogenetical aspects will increase efficacy. Under this aspect it seems reasonable to look for a drug therapy based on the immunological hypothesis of AD.

The research in this field started with the epidemiological and clinical observations and case control studies of Jenkinson et al. (1989). They demonstrated a lower frequency of rheumatoid arthritis among geriatric hospital patients with senile dementia than among other residents in the same facility. McGeer et al. (1990) have also shown an inverse association between AD and rheumatoid arthritis (a condition commmonly treated with anti-inflammatory drugs (AIs)) in autopsy, clinic and hospital discharge data. French et al. (1985) noted an odds ratio (OR) for arthritis (type unspecified) of 0,62 (confidence interval (CI), 0,29 to 1,29) when comparing hospitalized AD cases with hospital controls. The EURODEM collaborative meta-analysis of 11 case-control studies of AD (Breteler et al., 1991) reported an OR for osteoarthritis of 0,7 (CI, 0,5 to 1,0). Broe et al. (1990) found an OR for arthritis of 0,56 (CI, 0,36 to 0,87) in a matched pair analysis from Australia that included older subjects. Henderson et al. (1992) found a significant inverse association between AD and extended analgesic use (nature of treatments not specified) in older subjects from the same sample (OR, 0,52; p = 0,03) and a significant interaction with age (Breitner et al., 1994).

High risk studies demonstrated a delayed onset of Alzheimer disease under NSAIDs

Breitner et al. (1994) conducted a co-twin control study among 50 elderly twin pairs with onsets of Alzheimer's disease separated by 3 or more years. Twenty-three male pairs (46%) were screened from the (U.S.) National Academy of Sciences — National Research Council Registry (NAS-NRC Registry) of World War II veteran twins; others (mostly women) had responded to advertisements or were referred from AD clinics. Twenty-six pairs (52%) were monozygous. The onset of AD was inversely associated with prior use of corticosteroids or ACTH (OR, 0,25; 95% CI, 0,06 to 0,95; p = 0,04). Similar but weaker trends were present among pairs discordant for history of arthritis or for prior daily use of nonsteroidal anti-inflammatory drugs or aspirin. The association was strongest when use of steroids/ACTH or NSAIDs was combined post hoc into a single variable of anti-inflammatory drugs (OR, 0,24; CI, 0,07 to 0,74; p = 0,01). The inverse relation was strong in female (volunteer) twin pairs but was not present in the younger men from the NAS-NRC Registry. AIs had typically been taken for arthritis or related conditions, but a similar result was apparent after controlling statistically for the arthritis variable (OR, 0,08; CI, 0,01 to 0,69; p = 0,02). AIs have been proposed as a means of retarding the progression of AD symptoms, and these data suggest that AIs may also prevent or delay the initial onset of AD symptoms (Breitner et al., 1994). Breitner et al. (1995) gave further evidence for the hypotheses that non-steroidal antiinflammatory drugs might be relevant for the incidence of AD by their study on siblings at high risk of AD. They identified sipships meeting either of two conditions that could yield information regarding environmental modification of onset: (a) Presence of two or more cases of AD with onsets that differed in age by 3 or more years; or (b) at least one affected individual and one or more unaffected sibs who had survived 3 or more years beyond the onset age of the index case. Altogether they approached 205 individuals whose diagnoses and ages at onset of AD, if any, had been previously established by consideration of all relevant data, including extensive longitudinal observations, laboratory testing and autopsy information when available (Table 1). They used survival analytical methods to assess alteration in risk of AD among sibs with particular illnesses or treatment. This approach categorizes subjects by their reported exposures before onset of AD (if any) and relies on subjects' censoring age (current age or age at death) or age at onset. The data were used to estimate and compare the age-specific hazard (incidence) of AD among groups with various reported exposures. Daily use of NSAIDs for one month or more was reported most commonly with various forms of ibuprofen (39% of those endorsing such use of any NSAID), naproxen (16%), sulindac or indomethacin (8% for each) and piroxicam (5%). Figure 1 shows survival curves for the subjects categorized by prior daily exposure to any nonaspirin NSAIDs for more than one month. To avoid the possible effects of disproportionate reporting of exposures in autobiographical data, the fig. shows the results with information from collateral informants only. Similar results were obtained however, when autobiographical data were included (Table 2). Presumably because of the nature of the sample (which includes several sibships in which all subjects eventually developed AD) the lifetime risk of AD in the unexposed group is extreme. By comparison the age-specific risk among subjects exposed to NSAIDs is substantially lower (p = 0.0005). The horizontal line at 20% cumulative incidence of AD (as an example) ist intersected 11 years later in exposed subjects. The hazard risks listed up in Table 2 is similar to the more familiar odds ratio but is preferable for conditions like AD, because it deals with onset of AD as a time-dependent process. A hazard risk (h.r.) of less than 1 implies reduced risk of AD with exposure. Thus, the h.r. of 0.228 with NSAIDs indicates that the 20 NSAID users experienced about $\frac{1}{4}$ of the age-adjusted risk of the 111 nonusers. The h.r. with use of NSAIDs for >1 year (n = 17, median duration of exposure 5 years), was 0.075, implying that long term users of these drugs showed less than 1/10 the risk of nonusers for developing AD (from: Breitner et al. 1995). These results corroborate the above mentioned prior observations of the same group suggesting that antiinflammatory treatments are associated with delayed onset of AD. All other antiinflammatory drugs like aspirin or acetaminophen (Paracetamol), taken alone, without comedication with NSAIDs, produced only a weak, but similar effect to NSAIDs. An unexpected result was that also histamin-H_2-receptor blocking drugs, commonly prescribed for acid-peptid disease was associated with a visibly late onset of disease. The effect of glucocorticoids could not be estimated adequately because of the low proportion of exposed patients. As with NSAIDs the effect with H_2-blockers showed an increase of strength with duration of treatment (Fig. 2).

The principal action of NSAIDs (Vane, 1994; Breitner et al., 1995) is the suppression of cyclooxygenase (COX). One isoform of COX promotes inflammation through the synthesis of prostaglandines after being induced by interleukin 1β (IL-1β) and related cytokines (Mitchell et al., 1993). IL-1β is elevated in Alzheimer brain (Griffin et al., 1989). Other markers of

Table 1. Characteristics of affected and unaffected sibs (Breitner et al., 1995)

Status	Number	No. deceased	Censoring age or onset*
Affected	107	63	69.1 (9.4 years)
Unaffected, with			
collat. informants only	16	13	} 74.0 (9.0 years)
collateral + self	43	0	
self-report only	20	0	74.1 (11.3 years)
Total unaffected	79	13	74.0 (9.5 years)
Grand total	186	76	71.2 (9.8 years)

* Mean (SD); Censoring age is age at death, or current age if living

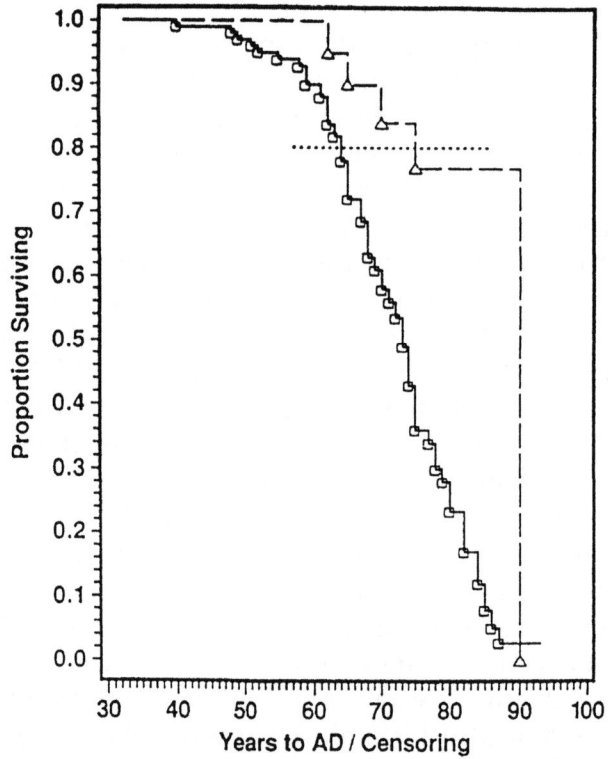

Fig. 1. Disease-free survival in subjects exposed to NSAIDs. Survival curve plots the estimated probability of remaining free of disease as a function of age. The squares and triangles at the bottom of each riser in the step-plot indicate appearance of one or more new cases among the unexposed and exposed groups, respectively. The method intrinsically adjusts for attrition in the numbers at risk as older ages are considered. The cumulative survival estimates are obtained by chain multiplying the individual survival fractions (number surviving free of disease divided by number at risk) at the appearance of each new case through the age in question. The cumulative incidence before age 90 in the exposed group is 1 minus the survival fraction of 0,75 or 0,25. The comparable figure for unexposed subjects is 0,97. The difference in lifetime risk between the two groups is highly significant (Breitner et al., 1995)

Table 2. Hazard ratios for risk of AD with exposure to anti-inflammatory or analgesic drugs (Breitner et al., 1995)

Exposure	Source of data*	Proportion exposed	Hazard ratio (95% e.i.)†	p value‡
Glucocorticoids	COL only	6/130	0.542 (0.114–2.570)	0.4405
	COL + AU	9/151	0.569 (0.123–2.633)	0.4703
NSAIDs	COL only	20/131	0.228 (0.068–0.722)	0.0175
	COL + AU	25/151	0.192 (0.058–0.639)	0.0071
(1–12 month)	COL + AU	4/129	0.188 (0.024–1.491)	0.1450
(>1 year)	COL + AU	17/142	0.075 (0.022–0.261)	0.0001
(affected only)	COL only	5/58	0.272 (0.031–2.367)	0.2381
(age ≤ 70)	COL + AU	7/56	0.583 (0.179–1.899)	0.3708
(age > 70)	COL + AU	18/76	0.215 (0.051–0.909)	0.0366
(no ε4 allele)	COL + AU	14/48	0.139 (0.018–1.057)	0.0566
(≥1 ε4 allele)	COL + AU	11/84	0.556 (0.200–1.547)	0.2611
(women)	COL + AU	17/96	0.181 (0.056–0.580)	0.0040
(men)	COL + AU	8/55	0.415 (0.098–1.757)	0.2320
(AD since 1980)	COL + AU	25/124	0.254 (0.074–0.872)	0.0295
(ignoring exposures for unaffected in last 5 years)	COL + AU	21/151	0.229 (0.068–0.771)	0.0174
Aspirin	COL only	31/136	0.349 (0.130–0.938)	0.0368
	COL + AU	40/157	0.343 (0.139–0.844)	0.0199
(1–12 month)	COL + AU	4/121	0.625 (0.086–4.558)	0.6410
(>1 year)	COL + AU	35/152	0.369 (0.171–0.796)	0.0123
Acetaminophen	COL only	10/131	0.157 (0.020–1.222)	0.0770
	COL + AU	17/152	0.104 (0.014–0.787)	0.0283

*AU autobiographical; COL collateral informant(s); †from Cox proportional hazards models; ‡probability of observed data under null hypothesis (h.r. = 1.0). Results with data from collateral informants (COL) and also, for comparison, with addition of autobiographical data from unaffected subjects lacking collaterals (AU). To improve statistical power, the latter method was used for stratified analyses of main effects or for analyses of interactions. Genotype at APOE was determined using the polymerase chain reaction and restriction fragmentation isotyping. The sample was stratified by sibship, except for male versus female, young versus old, and APOE genotype comparisons. Owing to small numbers available, simple odds ratios instead of hazard ratios are given for dose-response effects with NSAIDs and aspirin. The variable numbers in the denominators for proportion exposed reflect results of stratification or of variable numbers of subjects with missing data

inflammatory change, including glial synthesis of several components of the classical complement pathway, have been demonstrated immunohistochemically in and around the amyloid plaque of AD (Eikelenboom et al., 1989; Rogers et al., 1988). It is not clear, however, that inhibition of COX-mediated prostaglandin synthesis in classical inflammation explains the effect of NSAIDs in AD. The alternative explanation of the authors is based on the unexpected finding concerning the H_2-blockers. Those types of drug curtail NMDA glutamatergic excitotoxicity. COX-dependent events are part of the

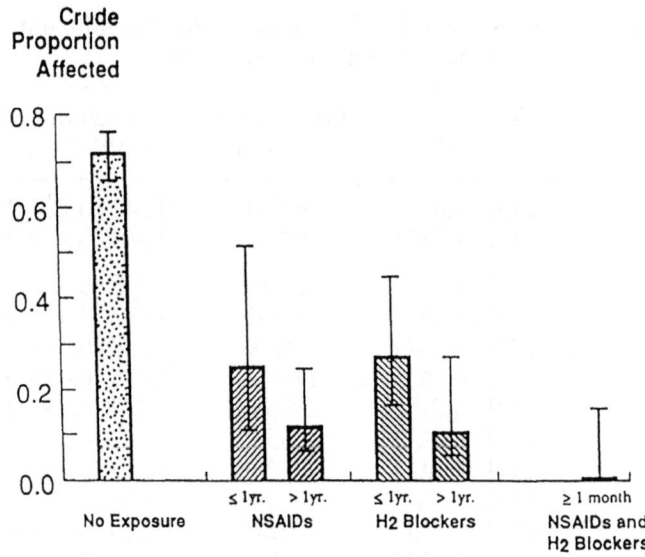

Fig. 2. Alteration in proportion affected by AD with exposure to NSAIDs, H_2 blockers, or both. Crude proportions of subjects who had developed AD (means with standard errors shown). Subjects exposed to NSAIDs were evaluated without consideration of exposure to H_2 blockers, and vice versa. Reduced proportions of subjects with 1 to 12 months exposure to NSAIDs or H_2 blockers were affected with AD. With >1 year of exposure, the proportions were reduced further. No subject exposed to both types of drugs (not necessarily concurrently) was affected (Breitner et al., 1995)

calcium-dependent postsynaptic cascade that follows stimulation of NMDA receptors (Lerea und McNamara, 1993) and result in induction of immediate early genes including c-fos that may effect either long-term potentiation or with excessive stimulation, excitotoxic cell death. Vulnerability to the latter is increased in presence of the β-amyloid peptide of AD (Koh et al., 1990). The NMDA response cascade is also potentiated by histamine action of H receptors. COX-mediated pro-staglandin synthesis has also been implicated in postsynaptic transduction of histamin signals. The disparate findings of NSAIDs and H_2 blockers thus may eventually be linked conceptually by several known aspects of the NMDA pathway.

Better cognitive function of NSAIDs patients in a cohort of Alzheimer patients

Rich et al. (1995) examined the records of 210 consecutive patients in the Johns Hopkins Alzheimer's Disease Research Center. This cohort consists of patients diagnosed with probable or possible AD who entered the ADRC in the period 1984 to 1987. The initial evalation for entry into the ADRC included a medical history review, neurologic, psychiatric and neuropsychologic examinations, brain CT, and appropriate laboratory studies. The medical history included a survey of current medications and those taken over the previous 12 months, regardless of duration. Medications were categorized as NSAIDs, beta blockers, diuretics, antidementia drugs (e.g. ergoloid mesylates, lecithin) etc. The coding of over-the-counter anti-inflammatory medications such as aspirin or ibuprofen, depended on the reported frequency of their use. When used on a daily basis, they were coded as "NSAIDs"; when used on an as-needed basis, they were coded as "miscellaneous over-the-counter medication". 32 patients were identified who were taking NSAIDs at the time of entry into the ADRC. The two most common NSAIDs were aspirin, used by 12 patients, and ibuprofen, used by seven patients. All subjects received a battery of neuropsychological tests to assess mental status, various language functions, spatial cognition, learning and memory, mood and the ability to carry out activities of daily living. To determine whether there was any influence of NSAIDs on the rate of progression of AD, the change scores from visit 1 to visit 3 (1 year later) for each neuropsychologic measure was calculated. Because the NSAIDs group had higher MMSE scores than did non-NSAID patients at visit 1, however, it was possible that the two groups would have different rates of cognitive change associated with the different starting points rather than with medication status per se. Specifically, one could argue on rational grounds that higher initial scores allow more "room" to decline over time and therefore may be associated with greater change scores; others (Morris et al., 1993) however, have found empirically that higher initial MMSE scores are associated with slower rates of decline. In the cohort investigated, the initial MMSE scores were positively correlated with 1-year change scores on the MMSE ($r = 0.15$) and the Category Fluency Test ($r = 0,26$). Those with greater initial MMSE scores also had increased behavior problems as measured by the Psychogeriatric Dependency Rating Scale (DGDRS, $r = 0.26$). The mean raw change scores on the clinical and cognitive measures for each group are provided in Table 3. Despite the fact that NSAID patients had higher MMSE scores than did non-NSAID patients at visit 1 and that those with higher initial MMSE scores showed greater decline after 1 year on the measures listed above in the cohort as a whole, the patients taking NSAIDs actually declined less than those who were not taking the drugs on the Category Fluency Test, Delayed Recognition Span Test and Orientation Subscale of the PGDRS. The other differences between the groups were not statistically significant.

Because patients may have been taking aspirin in low doses for cardiac or stroke prophylaxis rather than the larger doses used for antiinflammatory purposes, and because other studies involving antiinflammatories did not include aspirin as an NSAID, additional analyses excluded patients taking aspirin or aspirin containing medications. This reduced the NSAID group to 21 patients. The results of this additional analysis showed into the same directions (Rich et al., 1995).

Positive results of a prospective study on indomethacin

The study of Rogers et al. (1993) is a study to examine the effect of one NSAID, namely indomethacin (100–150 mg p.d.) on Alzheimer patients based on a prospective 6-month double blind placebo-controlled design.

Table 3. Clinical and cognitive 1-year change scores (visit 1 to visit 3) for probable/possible AD patients (Rich et al., 1995)

	NSAID	Non-NSAID	p
Mini-Mental State Examination	3.93	4.76	NS
Category Fluency Test	3.67	6.31	0.038
Boston Naming Test	3.74	4.29	NS
Block Design	1.94	3.39	NS
Responsive Naming Test	1.13	1.68	NS
Token Test	16.94	10.28	NS
Benton Visual Retention Test			
immediate	2.00	2.68	NS
delayed	0.50	0.44	NS
Gollin Incomplete Figures Test*	−0.12	−0.12	NS
Delayed Recognition Span Test	−0.13	1.25	0.0002
Psychogeriatric Dependency Rating Scale			
Orientation*	−0.29	−1.49	0.004
Behavior*	3.50	3.65	NS
Physical*	−3.14	−5.08	NS
Hamilton Depression Scale*	2.09	2.52	NS
Extrapyramidal Rating Scale*	−0.26	−0.4	NS

NSAID Nonsteroidal anti-inflammatory drug, *NS* Not significant. * Low scores indicate better performance on these measures; therefore, positive change scores indicate improvement

Sixty-six patients with a diagnosis of AD were recruited for this study. Of these, 44 patients met the entrance criteria for inclusion in the study. They had to fill among other the diagnosis of probable AD and a Mini-Mental State Examination (MMSE) score of 16 or more. 28 of the original 44 patients completed the trial. Gastrointestinal side effects of indomethacin were the most common cause of drop-out in the drug treatment group (5 patients). Other reasons for drop-out were stroke (1 patient), head-ache (1 patient), loss of care-giver (2 patients) and death of the patient (1 patient). Interestingly 4 placebo patients were droped out because they developed increasingly severe behavioral problems during the trial. No indomethacin patients were lost because of such changes.

The patients of the indomethacin and placebo-group were matched for age, sex and entry-level of cognitive measures. Across the battery of mental status tests (MMSE, ADAS, Boston Naming Test, Token Test), indomethacin patients exhibited in general improvement after six months of treatment, whereas placebo patients declined. With respect to the individual mental status tests, the most consistent differences between indomethacin and placebo patients were recorded on the MMSE and the ADAS. These differences were significant, although the sample size was small (Table 4).

In general these results seem positive. Comparing these efficacy results with the effects of other antidementia studies, for example the studies on cholinergic drugs, the extreme differences between verum and placebo are remarkable. However it has to be mentioned, that the total score of ADAS

Table 4. Patient demographics and response to treatment (Rogers et al., 1993)

Group	N	Age	Sex	Percent change from baseline ($\pm$ SEM)				
				ADAS	MMSE	BNT	TK	X all tests
Indomethacin	14	78 $\pm$ 2	9M/5F	+1.4 $\pm$ 4.9	−0.9 $\pm$ 4.8	+4.4 $\pm$ 3.7	+0.5 $\pm$ 1.0	+1.3 $\pm$ 1.8*
Placebo	14	77 $\pm$ 1	6M/8F	−13.3 $\pm$ 5.6	−13.4 $\pm$ 4.4	−6.6 $\pm$ 5.5	−0.4 $\pm$ 2.9	−8.4 $\pm$ 2.3

* $p < 0.003$ compared with placebo

was given here, while in most of the studies of recently developed anticholinergic drugs mostly the ADAScog score was the basis of evaluation. Nevertheless also the great differences between the change courses for the MMSE are indicating a remarkable cognitive effect. As to tolerability, it has to be considered that over 20% of indomethacin treated patients developed drug related adverse effects of such degree, primarily gastro-intestinal, as to warrant their removal from the study.

The authors conclude with the caveat that the choice of antiinflammatory drugs for the treatment of AD should be carefully considered. In an earlier pilot study, for example 10 mg p.d. of prednisone were administered to 4 Alzheimer patients for a period of 6 months. Over the course of study these patients developed increasingly severe behavioral problems including sleep impairments and increased wandering. These adverse effects may reflect interactions of the psychogenic effects of steroids (Lewis and Smith, 1983) with dementia, the possibility that steroids are neurotoxic to hyppocampal neurons (Landfield und Eldridge, 1989) or both. Under this aspect NSAIDs like indomethacin seem to be preferable.

The right candidate for further studies of NSAIDs in dementia

Of great interest for the further evaluation of NSAIDs in Alzheimer disease is the study of Fiebich et al. (1996). Under the hypothesis, that interleukin IL-6, a proinflammatory cytokine, is found in the brains of AD-patients but not in the brains of normal control persons, the authors investigated the effects of seven NSAIDs on Interleukin-1β (IL-1β) induced IL-6 mRNA expression and protein synthesis in a human astrocytoma cell line. Tenidap, naproxen and meloxicam inhibited the IL-1-β induced synthesis of IL-6, whereas ibupren, piroxicam, diclofenac and indomethacin showed no effect. While the effects of naproxen and meloxicam were small and restricted to protein synthesis, tenidap strongly inhibited IL-6 protein synthesis and also affected IL-6 mRNA levels. These results also suggested that particularly tenidap might be of special interest for the evaluation of NSAIDs in Alzheimer patients. However it should be considered that perhaps the focus of this investigation is to much restricted to IL-6-protein synthesis and that other inflammatory processes, which might also be of importance for AD are not considered. Under the assumption that the validity of the human astrocytoma cell model is not questionable, the results of the studies mentioned above, among other the positive study on indomethacine, suggest that apparently not only the effects on IL-6 is of clinical relevance.

Efficacy of propentofylline in Alzheimer disease

Propentofylline is a neuroprotective agent that readily crosses the blood-brain barrier. In view of recent evidence that excessive microglial and immunological markers are associated with the plaque pathology of AD, the inhibitory effect of propentofylline on the formation of oxygene free radicals by reactive microglia, and the propentofylline induced increase in immunostaining for reactive microglia, it seems that propentofylline might interfere with the disease process itself (Banati et al., 1994; McRae et al., 1994; Marcusson et al., 1997).

In the randomized double-blind 12 months-study of Marcusson et al. (in press) 129 patients received propentofylline (300 mg p.d.) and 131 patients placebo 3 times a day. This study only included outpatients with mild or moderate dementia (MMSE scores between 15 and 25) according to the DSM-III-R definition. The investigators classified patients as suffering from AD or vascular dementia. Patients who were diagnosed as suffering from both types of dementia were classified to the vascular dementia group.

The investigators evaluated the psychopathological state of the patient by means of the Gottfries-Brane-Steen-Scale (GBS) and the Clinical Global Impression (CGI). The positive effects in favor of propentofylline shown in the GBS were dominated by the improvement of the subscore for the intellectual function. All global measures showed a beneficial effect in favor of propentofylline. Additionally the psychological test (Syndrome Short Test, Minimental State Examination, Digit Symbol Substitution Test, Psychological Test of Cognitive Functions) showed positive results for propentofylline. An additional analysis considering the subgroup of Alzheimer Dementia and vascular dementia came to the result that propentofylline is effective in both AD and vascular patients.

Also further large sample size studies, the results of which are not yet published, demonstrate a positive effect on cognitive functions of Alzheimer patients. These positive results might be interpreted in the light of immunological hypotheses of AD, but also the metabolic actions of propentofylline should be taken into consideration.

References

Banati RB, Schubert P, Rothe G, Gehrmann J, Rudolphi K, Valet G, Kreutzberg GW (1994) Modulation of intracellular formation of reactive oxygen intermediates in peritoneal macrophages and microglia/brain macrophages by propentofylline. J Cereb Blood Flow Metab 14: 145–149

Bauer J, Strauss S, Schreiter Gasser U, Ganter U, Schlegel P, Witt I, Yolk B, Berger M (1991) Interleukin-6 and alpha-2-macroglobulin indicate an acute-phase state in Alzheimer's disease cortices. FEBS Lett 285: 111–114

Breitner JC, Gau BA, Welsh KA, Plassman BL, McDonald WM, Helms MJ, Anthony JC (1994) Inverse association of anti-inflammatory treatments and Alzheimer's disease: initial results of a co-twin control study. Neurology 44: 227–232

Breitner JC, Welsh KA, Helms MJ, Gaskell PC, Gau BA, Roses AD, Pericak Vance MA, Saunders AM (1995) Delayed onset of Alzheimer's disease with nonsteroidal anti-inflammatory and histamine H_2 blocking drugs. Neurobiol Aging 16: 523–530

Breteler MM, van Duijn CM, Chandra V, Fratiglioni L, Graves AB, Heyman A, Jorm AF, Kokmen E, Kondo K, Mortimer JA, et al (1991) Medical history and the risk of Alzheimer's disease: a collaborative re-analysis of case-control studies. EURODEM Risk Factors Research Group. Int J Epidemiol 20 [Suppl 2]: S36–42

Broe GA, Henderson AS, Creasey H, McCusker E, Korten AE, Jorm AF, Longley W, Anthony JC (1990) A case-control study of Alzheimer's disease in Australia. Neurology 40: 1698–1707

Eikelenboom P, Hack CE, Rozemuller JM, Stam FC (1989) Complement activation in amyloid plaques in Alzheimer's dementia. Virchows Arch B Cell Pathol Incl Mol Pathol 56: 259–262

Fiebich BL, Lieb K, Hull M, Berger M, Bauer J (1996) Effects of NSAIDs on IL-1 beta-induced IL-6 mRNA and protein synthesis in human astrocytoma cells. Neuroreport 7: 1209–1213

French LR, Schuman LM, Mortimer JA, Hutton JT, Boatman RA, Christians B (1985) A case-control study of dementia of the Alzheimer type. Am J Epidemiol 121: 414–421

Griffin WS, Stanley LC, Ling C, White L, MacLeod V, Perrot LJ, White CL, Araoz C (1989) Brain interleukin 1 and S-100 immunoreactivity are elevated in Down syndrome and Alzheimer disease. Proc Natl Acad Sci USA 86: 7611–7615

Henderson AS, Jorm AF, Korte AE, Creasey H, McCusker E, Broe GA, Longley W, Antony JC (1992) Environmental risk factors for Alzheimer's disease: their relationship to age of onset and to familial or sporadic types. Psychol Med 22: 429–436

Huell M, Strauss S, Volk B, Berger M, Bauer J (1995) Interleukin-6 is present in early stages of plaque formation and is restricted to the brains of Alzheimer's disease patients. Acta Neuropathol (Berl) 89: 544–551

Jenkinson ML, Bliss MR, Brain AT, Scott DL (1989) Rheumatoid arthritis and senile dementia of the Alzheimer's type. Br J Rheumatol 28: 86–88

Koh JY, Yang LL, Cotman CW (1990) Beta-amyloid protein increases the vulnerability of cultured cortical neurons to excitotoxic damage. Brain Res 533: 315–320

Landfield PW, Eldridge JC (1989) Increased affinity of type II corticosteroid binding in aged rat hippocampus. Exp Neurol 106: 110–113

Lerea LS, McNamara JO (1993) Ionotropic glutamate receptor subtypes activate c-fos transcription by distinct calcium-requiring intracellular signaling pathways. Neuron 10: 31–41

Lewis DA, Smith RE (1983) Steroid-induced psychiatric syndromes. A report of 14 cases and a review of the literature. J Affect Disord 5: 319–332

Marcusson J, Rother M, Kittner B, Rössner M, Smith J, Babic T, Folgenovic-Smalc V, Möller HJ, Labs KH (1997) A 12-month, randomized, plazebo-controlled trial of propentofylline (HWA 285) in patients with dementia according to DSM-III-R. Dement Geriatr Cogn Dis 8: 320–328

McGeer PL, Rogers J (1992) Anti-inflammatory agents as a therapeutic approach to Alzheimer's disease. Neurology 42: 447–449

McGeer PL, McGeer E, Rogers J, Sibley J (1990) Anti-inflammatory drugs and Alzheimer disease. Lancet 335: 1037

McRae A, Rudolphi KA, Schubert P (1994) Propentofylline depresses amyloid and Alzheimer's CSF microglial antigens after ischaemia. Neuroreport 5: 1193–1196

Mitchell JA, Akarasereenont P, Thiemermann C, Flower RJ, Vane JR (1993) Selectivity of nonsteroidal antiinflammatory drugs as inhibitors of constitutive and inducible cyclooxygenase. Proc Natl Acad Sci USA 90: 11693–11697

Morris JC, Edland S, Clark Ce (1993 43) The consortium to establish a registry for Alzheimer's Disease (CERAD), part IV. Rates of cognitive change in the longitudinal assessment of probable Alzheimer's disease. Neurology 43: 2457–2465

Rich JB, Rasmusson DX, Folstein MF, Carson KA, Kawas C, Brandt J (1995) Nonsteroidal anti-inflammatory drugs in Alzheimer's disease. Neurology 45: 51–55

Rogers J, O'Barr S (1997) Inflammatory mediators in Alzheimer's disease. In: Wasco W, Tanzi RE (eds) Molecular mechanisms of dementia. Humana Press, Totowa New Jersey, pp 177–98

Rogers J, Luber Narod J, Styren SD, Civin WH (1988) Expression of immune system-associated antigens by cells of the human central nervous system: relationship to the pathology of Alzheimer's disease. Neurobiol Aging 9: 339–349

Rogers J, Kirby LC, Hempelman SR, Berry DL, McGeer PL, Kaszniak AW, Zalinski J, Cofield M, Mansukhani L, Willson PL, et al (1993) Clinical trial of indomethacin in Alzheimer's disease. Neurology 43: 1609–1611

Vane J (1994) Towards a better aspirin. Nature 367: 215–216

Author's address: Prof. Dr. med. H.-J. Möller, Psychiatric Hospital, Ludwig-Maximilians-University Munich, Nußbaumstrasse 7, D-80336 Munich, Federal Republic of Germany

Risk factors for Azheimer's disease during aging. Impacts of glucose/energy metabolism

S. Hoyer

Department of Pathochemistry and General Neurochemistry, University of Heidelberg, Heidelberg, Federal Republic of Germany

Summary. The majority of Alzheimer patients is of late onset and with unknown etiology. However, several risk factors have been discussed among which age is a most important one with respect to sporadic Alzheimer type dementia (SDAT). Age includes changes in brain glucose/energy metabolism, in both insulin and acetylcholine signal transduction and in membrane function to name the functionally most important ones. Variations in these parameters can form the basis for ongoing changes in terms of the principle of self-organized criticality inducing catastrophic i.e. disease processes. Subsequent abnormalities at the cellular and molecular levels may develop including the formation of both amyloid plaques and neurofibrillary tangles.

Introduction

Alzheimer's disease is a heterogeneous neurodegenerative disorder. The majority of cases is sporadic and with late onset. Clear evidence has been provided that the prevalence of late-onset sporadic dementia of the Alzheimer type (SDAT) increases exponentially beyond the age of 65 years (Gottfries, 1985; Evans et al., 1989; Ott et al., 1995). Thus, age per se can be considered as a major risk factor for SDAT (Storandt et al., 1988). During the aging process, numerous morphologic and metabolic variations occur in the brain (Hoyer, 1995), but not all can be assumed to be risk factors for SDAT. Among the latter, abnormalities in cerebral glucose/energy metabolism and its control may be of pivotal significance. Two different disturbances may result from the latter: 1. the reduced availability of energy necessary to maintain cellular and molecular work, and 2. an increase in advanced glycation end products (AGE). Both abnormal processes may forward neuronal damage in a cascade-like way starting very early in the disease process. In this short review, it is demonstrated in which way functionally important cellular and molecular parameters shift from normality to increasing abnormality the latter being the basis for SDAT.

Glucose/energy metabolism in the normal adult mammalian brain

Normal cellular and molecular work depends on the availability of sufficient amounts of biological energy. In the healthy, mature, nonstarved mammalian brain, energy in the form of ATP is formed exclusively from the oxidation of glucose (Erecinska and Silver, 1989; Hoyer, 1992). There is clear evidence that the neuronal glucose metabolism is controlled by brain insulin via the neuronal insulin receptor (for review see Henneberg and Hoyer, 1995). Glucose breakdown yields the high-energy compound acetyl CoA, a constituent of acetylcholine synthesis which is accomplished at a rate in proportion to that of pyruvate oxidation (Sims et al., 1981). Any impairment in glucose oxidation altered the cellular redox state and led to a perturbed formation of acetylcholine without changing the ATP concentration or the energy charge potential (Gibson and Blass, 1976).

Numerous metabolic processes require ATP: synaptic transmission, the multiple steps of protein processing and maintenance of membrane stability to name some functionally most important ones (for review see Hoyer, 1997; Wu et al., 1996).

The normal pathway of glucose and related metabolism is schematically demonstrated in Fig. 1. Glucose is transported across the blood-brain barrier into the extracellular space by means of glucose transport protein 1. This process is controlled by circulating insulin. The transport from the extracellular space into the neuron is mediated by means of glucose transport protein 3 which is controlled by neuronal insulin receptor signal transduction. Acetlycholine acts on APP metabolism via acetylcholinergic muscarinic m1 and m3 receptors by favoring the formation of the secreted form of APP. Advance glycation end (AGE) products are formed in small concentrations and when localized extracellularly taken up into the cell via the AGE receptor (RAGE). Interestingly, βA4 formed from APP competes with AGE for RAGE.

From these results, it becomes obvious that numerous metabolites originating from normal glucose breakdown in neurons act in a widespread manner in the brain. It may, therefore, be deduced from these data that any impairment in the control of cerebral glucose metabolism in general, and in glucose oxidation/energy production in particular may change the functional state of the neuron. This will be discussed in the following related to the aging process.

Glucose/energy metabolism in the aging brain

Numerous studies had clearly demonstrated a decrease of blood flow, oxygen and glucose consumption of the human brain during normal aging beyond the 7th the 8th decade of life (Hoyer, 1986). The same holds true for glycolytic glucose breakdown, the concentration of creatine phosphate and the ATP turnover (Hoyer, 1985, 1992). Mental activity enhanced the size of the energy pool but did not prevent its decrease with aging (Dutschke et al., 1994). The

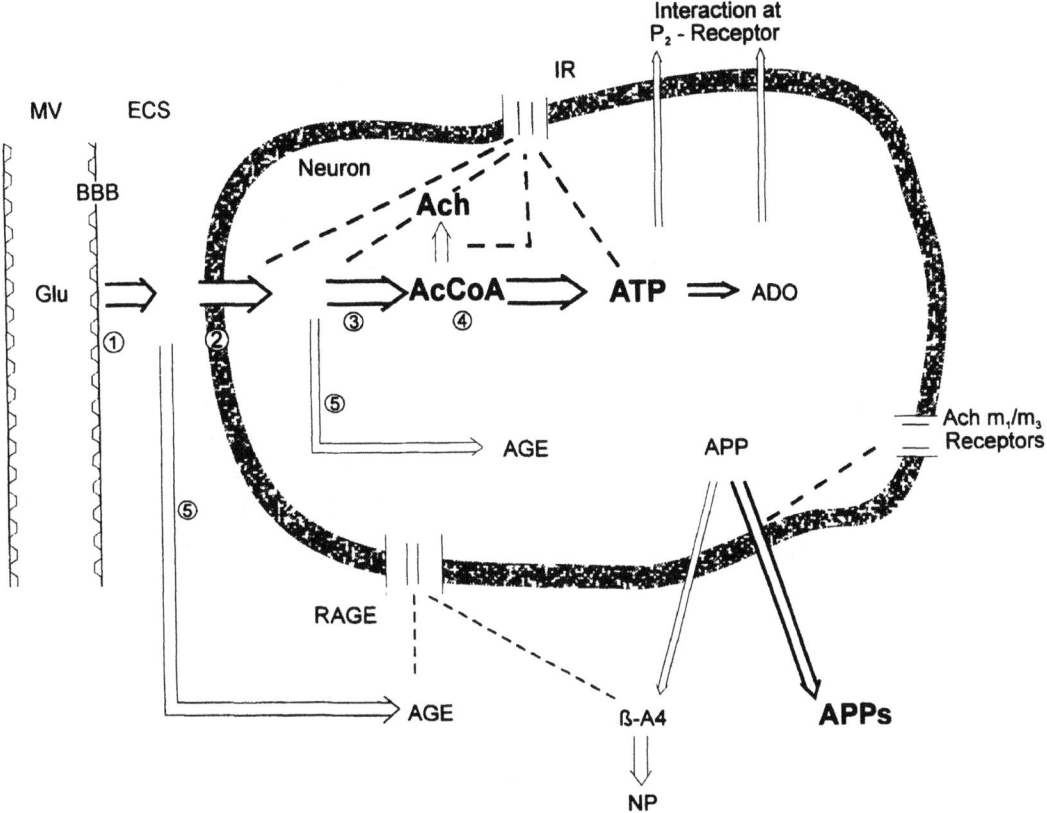

Fig. 1. Pathway of glucose (⟹) from arterial blood into the neuron, its control (-----),
metabolism and interactions of metabolites under normal conditions. Main normal pathways and metabolites are presented as accentuated. ①: glucose transport protein 1, ②:
glucose transport protein 3, ③: glycolytic chain, ④: tricarboxylic acid cycle, respiratory
chain, ⑤: nonenzymatic glycation, *Ach* acetylcholine, *ADO* adenosine, *AGE* advanced
glycation end product, *APP* amyloid precursor protein, *BBB* blood brain barrier, *ECS*
extracellular space, *Glu* glucose, *IR* insulin receptor, m_1/m_3 muscarinergic m_1/m_3 —
receptors, *MV* microvessel, *NP* neuritic plaque, *RAGE* advanced glycation end product
receptor

intracellular pH and the cytoplasmic redox potential shift to the acidic milieu
(Hoyer, 1985; Roberts and Sick, 1996). The concentration of insulin, the
density of the insulin receptors and the activity of tyrosine kinase decrease
beyond the age of 60 years (Frölich et al., 1997). The cerebral glucose metabolism is jeopardized, too, with cortisol (Plaschke et al., 1996) which was found
to increase with aging in both arterial blood and cerebral spinal fluid (Lupien
et al., 1994; Sapolsky et al., 1986; Swaab et al., 1994).

From all neurotransmitters, the most remarkable age-related changes
were found in acetylcholine and glutamate which both were reduced in synthesis and release (Bowen, 1984; Mullany et al., 1996) which may contribute to
the age-related deficits in learning and memory capacities (Drachman et al.,
1980). Another aspect is the functional imbalance of acetylcholine and noradrenaline with respect to cortical microvessels. In contrast to acetylcholine,
the presynaptic noradrenaline concentration increases with aging (Ida et al.,

1982; Harik and McCracken, 1986). Thus, the noradrenergic function predominates and causes a constriction of the microvasculature resulting in reduced blood flow (sympathetic tone of the aging brain).

Advanced glycation endproducts (AGE)

From glucose or other hexoses, AGE can be formed via several non-enzymatic reactions. AGE binds to high affinity receptors (RAGE) whereby the expression of growth factors or transcription factors, and changes in membrane permeability are induced (Vlassara et al., 1994). The amyloidogenic APP-derivative β-A4 was found to bind to RAGE (Yan et al., 1996). RAGE are present in the nervous tissue (Brett et al., 1993). During aging, AGE are found in the pericaria of larger neurons in the hippocampus and the dentate gyrus, and in pyramidal cells of the cortical cell layers (Li et al., 1995).

Age-related membrane changes

During aging, the fluidity of the exofacial membrane layer was found to be reduced as compared to the cytofacial membrane layer which was due to the increase of cholesterol in the exofacial layer (Igbavboa et al., 1996). Accordant with the reduction in fluidity is the increase in membrane viscosity causing an elevation of protein tyrosine phosphatase activity which impairs the activation of the insulin receptor tyrosine kinase (Nadiv et al., 1994). This disturbance in the control of the neuronal glucose metabolism may be one important reason for the age-related reduction in energy production (Hoyer, 1985). The latter changes the biophysical membrane properties whereby the cells are injured (Wu et al., 1996).

Normally, the amyloid precursor protein (APP) is cleaved in non-amyloidogenic derivatives by α-secretase. In the opposite, cholesterol favors the formation of amyloidogenic derivatives (Bodovits and Klein, 1996) obviously due to its increase in the exofacial membrane layer.

The principle of self-organized criticality

From the metabolic variations discussed above, it can be deduced that the cerebral glucose metabolism, its control and related metabolic pathways are involved during the normal aging process in that imbalances in homeostatic equilibria become obvious between

— acetylcholine and norarenaline,
— insulin and cortisol
— energy production and energy turnover, and

— cholesterol in cytofacial and exofacial membrane layer, to name only some functionally most important ones.

These age-related changes may be assumed to be of minor quantity only, but they are numerous in total number and exist for a longer period. This pattern may reflect a distinct metalabile steady state in aged neurons. Any small additional abnormality, even one that is ineffective in itself, may change the former steady state and may cause a catastrophic reaction representing another new but detrimental steady state. In this general context, age may be considered as a risk factor for neuronal damage, and, thus, for age-related brain disorders such as sporadic dementia of the Alzheimer type.

Age-related cellular changes, β-amyloid and tau-protein

With aging, the secretion of the amyloid precursor protein (APP) was found to be elevated (Wallace et al., 1995) which may contribute to the increase of β-amyloid formation (Cai et al., 1993). Reduction of the acetylcholine-mediated neurotransmission via the m3-receptor may inhibit the release of secreted APP (Petryniak et al., 1996). An increase in the cellular cholesterol content inhibited the secretory processing of APP (Racchi et al., 1997). The decrease in the pool of available energy may lower or even arrest the transport of newly synthesized membrane proteins (such as APP) in the endoplasmic reticulum, the intermediate compartment and the Golgi complex obviously due to a shift of pH from mildly acidic to neutral (Seksek et al., 1995; Verde et al., 1995).

   Recently, it was demonstrated that β-A4 can be generated by β-secretase cleavage in the trans-Golgi network (Stephens and Austen, 1996) what is obviously mediated by a reduced transport within the Golgi complex (Wild-Bode et al., 1997) due to an energy deficit (Gabuzda et al., 1994). With respect to the formation of hyperphosphorylated tau-protein, the activities of the tau-protein kinases PK40 and PK36 were highest when ATP was low (Roder and Ingram, 1991).

Conclusion

A great variety of cellular and molecular changes takes place in the brain during normal aging among which changes in glucose/energy metabolism are of pivotal significance: reduced acetylcholine synthesis, formation of advanced glycation end products, membrane instability and reduced energy availability are consequences of the abnormality in insulin receptor signal transduction. These changes can be assumed to be the basis for the formation of β-amyloid and hyperphosphorylated tau-protein which both contribute to sporadic dementia of the Alzheimer type.

References

Bodovitzs S, Kelin WL (1996) Cholesterol modulates α-secretase cleavage of amyloid precursor protein. J Biol Chem 271: 4436–4440

Bowen DM (1984) Cellular aging: selective vulnerability of cholinergic neurons in human brain. Monogr Dev Biol 17: 42–59

Brett J, Schmidt AM, Yan SD, Zou YS, Weidman E, Pinsky D, Nowygrod R, Neeper M, Przysiecki C, Shaw A, Migheli A, Stern D (1993) Survey of the distribution of a newly characterized receptor for advanced glycation end products in tissues. Am J Pathol 143: 1699–1712

Cai XD, Golde TE, Younkin SG (1993) Release of excess amyloid β protein from a mutant amyloid β protein precursor. Science 259: 514–519

Drachman DA, Noffsinger D, Sahakian BJ, Kurdziel S, Fleming P (1980) Aging, memory and the cholinergic system: a study of dichotic listening. Neurobiol Aging 1: 39–43

Dutschke K, Nitsch RM, Hoyer S (1994) Short-term mental activation accelerates the age-related decline of high-energy phosphates in rat cerebral cortex. Arch Gerontol Geriatr 19: 43–51

Erecinska M, Silver IA (1989) ATP and brain function. J Cereb Blood Flow Metab 9: 2–19

Evans DA, Funkenstein HH, Albert MS, Scherr PA, Cook NR, Chown MJ, Hebert LE, Hennekens CH, Taylor JO (1989) Prevalence of Alzheimer's disease in a community population of older persons: higher than previously reported. J Am Med Assoc 262: 2551–2556

Frölich L, Blum-Degen D, Hoyer S, Beckmann H, Riederer P (1997) Insulin, insulin receptors and IGF-I receptors in post-mortem human brain in ageing and in dementia of Alzheimer type. In: Iqbal K, Winblad B, Nishimura T, Takeda M, Wisniewski HM (eds) Alzheimer's disease: biology, diagnosis and therapeutics. Wiley, Chichester, pp 457–465

Gabuzda D, Buciglio J, Chen LB, Matsudaira P, Yankner BA (1994) Inhibition of energy metabolism alters the processing of amyloid precursor protein and induces a potentially amyloidogenic derivative. J Biol Chem 269: 13623–13628

Gibson GE, Blass JP (1976) Impaired synthesis of acetylcholine in brain accompanying mild hypoxia and hypoglycemia. J Neurochem 27: 37–42

Gottfries CG (1985) Alzheimer's disease and senile dementia: biochemical characteristics and aspects of treatment. Psychopharmacology 86: 245–252

Harik SI, McCracken KA (1986) Age-related increase in presynaptic noradrenergic markers of the rat cerebral cortex. Brain Res 381: 125–130

Henneberg N, Hoyer S (1995) Desensitization of the neuronal insulin receptor: a new approach in the etiopathogenesis of late-onset sporadic dementia of the Alzheimer type (SDAT)? Arch Gerontol Geriatr 21: 63–74

Hoyer S (1985) The effect of age on glucose and energy metabolism in brain cortex of rats. Arch Gerontol Geriatr 4: 193–203

Hoyer S (1986) Senile dementia and Alzheimer's disease: brain blood flow and metabolism. Progr Neuropsychopharmacol Biol Psychiatry 10: 447–478

Hoyer S (1992) Oxidative energy metabolism in Alzheimer brain. Studies in early-onset and late-onset cases. Mol Chem Neuropathol 16: 207–224

Hoyer S (1995) Age-related changes in cerebral oxidative metabolism. Implications for drug therapy. Drugs Aging 6: 210–218

Hoyer S (1997) Models of Alzheimer's disease: cellular and molecular aspects. J Neural Transm [Suppl] 49: 11–21

Ida Y, Tanaka M, Kohno Y, Nakagawa R, Iimori K, Tsuda A, Hoaki Y, Nagasaki N (1982) Effects of age and stress on regional noradrenaline metabolism in the rat brain. Neurobiol Aging 3: 233–236

Igbavboa U, Avdulov A, Schroeder F, Wood WG (1996) Increasing age alters transbilayer fluidity and cholesterol asymmetry in synaptic plasma membranes of mice. J Neurochem 66: 1717–1725

Li JJ, Surini M, Catsicas S, Kawashima E, Bouras C (1995) Age-dependent accumulation of advanced glycosylation end products in human neurons. Neurobiol Aging 16: 69–76

Lupien S, Lecours AR, Lussier I, Schwartz G, Nair NPV, Meaney MJ (1994) Basal cortisol levels and cognitive deficits in human aging. J Neurosci 14: 2893–2903

Mullaney P, Conolly S, Lynch MA (1996) Ageing is associated with changes in glutamate release, protein tyrosine kinase and Ca^{2+}/calmodulin-dependent protein kinase II in rat hippocampus. Eur J Pharmacol 309: 311–315

Nadiv O, Shinitzky M, Manu H, Hecht D, Robert CT, Le Roith D, Zick Y (1994) Elevated protein tyrosine phosphatase activity and increase membrane viscosity are associated with impaired activation of the insulin receptor kinase in old rats. Biochem J 298: 443–450

Ott A, Breteler MMB, van Harskamp F, Claus JJ, van der Cammen TJM, Grobbee DE, Hofman A (1995) Prevalence of Alzheimer's disease and vascular dementia: association with education. The Rotterdam study. Br J Med 310: 970–973

Petryniak MA, Wurtman RJ, Slack BE (1996) Elevated intracellular calcium concentration increases secretory processing of the amyloid precursor protein by a tyrosine-phosphorylation-dependent mechanism. Biochem J 320: 957–963

Plaschke K, Müller D, Hoyer S (1996) Effects of adrenalectomy and corticosterone substitution on glucose and energy metabolism in rat brain. J Neural Transm 103: 89–100

Racchi M, Baetta R, Salvietti N, Ianna P, Franceschini G, Paoletti R, Fumagalli R, Govoni S, Trabucchi M, Soma M (1997) Secretory processing of amyloid precursor protein is inhibited by increase in cellular cholesterol content. Biochem J 322: 893–898

Roberts EL jr, Sick TJ (1996) Aging impairs regulation of intracellular pH in rat hippocampal slices. Brain Res 735: 339–342

Roder HM, Ingram VM (1991) Two novel kinases phosphorylate tau and the KSP site of heavy neurofilament subunits in high stoichiometric ratios. J Neurosci 11: 3325–3343

Sapolsky RM, Krey LC, McEwen BS (1986) The neuroendocrinology of stress and aging: the glucocorticoid cascade hypothesis. Endocr Res 7: 284–301

Seksek O, Biwersi J, Verkman AS (1995) Direct measurement of trans-Golgi pH in living cells and regulation by second messengers. J Biol Chem 270: 4967–4970

Sims NR, Bowen DM, Davison AN (1981) (^{14}C) acetylcholine synthesis and (^{14}C) carbon dioxide production from (U-^{14}C) glucose by tissue prisms from human neocortex. Biochem J 196: 867–876

Stephens DJ, Austen BM (1986) Metabolites of the β-amyloid precursor protein generated by β-secretase localise to the trans-Golgi network and late endosome in 293 cells. J Neurosci Res 46: 211–225

Storandt M, Bäkman L, Baltes MM, Blass JP, Braak H, Gutzmann H, Hauw JJ, Hoyer S, Jorm AF, Kauss J, Kliegl R, Mountjoy CQ (1988) Relationships of normal aging and dementing disease in later life. In: Henderson AS, Henderson JH (eds) Etiology of dementia of Alzheimer's type. Wiley, Chichester, pp 231–239

Swaab DF, Raadsheer FC, Endert EF, Hofman MA, Kamphorst W, Ravid R (1994) Increases of cortisol levels in aging and Alzheimer's disease in postmortem cerebrospinal fluid. J Neuroendocrinol 6: 681–687

Verde C, Pascale MC, Martire G, Lotti LV, Torrisi MR, Helenius A, Bonatti S (1995) Effect of ATP depletion and DTT on the transport of membrane proteins from the endoplasmic reticulum and the intermediate compartment to the Golgi complex. Eur J Cell Biol 67: 267–274

Vlassara H, Bucala R, Striker L (1994) Biology of disease. Pathogenetic effects of advanced glycosylation: biochemical, biologic, and clinical implications for diabetes and aging. Lab Invest 70: 138–151

Wallace WC, Lieberburg I, Schenk D, Vigo-Pelfrey C, Davis KL, Haroutunian V (1995) Chronic elevation of secreted amyloid precursor protein in subcortically lesioned rats, and its exacerbation in aged rats. J Neurosci 15: 4896–4905

Wild-Bode C, Yamazaki T, Capell A, Leimert U, Steiner H, Ihara Y, Haass C (1997) Intracellular generation and accumulation of amyloid β-peptide terminating at amino acid 42. J Biol Chem 272

Wu Y, Sun FF, Tong DM, Taylor BM (1996) Changes in membrane-properties during energy depletion-induced cell injury studied with fluorescence microscopy. Biophys J 71: 91–100

Yan SD, Chen X, Fu J, Chen M, Zhu H, Roher A, Slattery T, Zhao L, Nagashima M, Morser J, Migheli A, Nawroth P, Stern D, Schmidt AM (1996) RAGE and amyloid-β peptide neurotoxicity in Alzheimer's disease. Nature 382: 685–691

Author's address: Prof. Dr. S. Hoyer, Department of Pathochemistry and General Neurochemistry, University of Heidelberg, Im Neuenheimer Feld 220/221, D-69120 Heidelberg, Federal Republic of Germany

Aging, dementia and calcium metabolism

S. Kanowski

Psychiatrische Klinik und Poliklinik, Universitätsklinikum Rudolf Virchow, Berlin,
Federal Republic of Germany

Summary. After a brief discussion of the theory of disturbed neuronal calcium metabolism an overview is given on the results of clinical studies with nimodipine in the treatment of vascular and Alzheimer's dementia.

Calcium seems to be the essential if not the only intracellular signal transmitter, on which all the signals transduced by the different transmitter systems converge, modulating the intracellular calcium concentration. Secondly disturbance to the intracellular calcium homeostasis is the common mechanism by which noxious interventions, like for instance hypoxia, deteriorate cell function, and finally even lead to cell death. There have been many experimental data showing that the ability of cells to sustaine calcium homeostasis might be impaired by the aging process itself. The hypothesis has been postulated, that this impairment might also be of central importance for brain aging, associated cognitive decline and development of dementia. In that sense the age dependent increasing incapacitation of the intraneuronal calcium regulating processes could be viewed as risk factors causing the increasing susceptibility of brain cells against any noxious agents including etiology of dementia in general and Alzheimer's dementia in particular. Khachaturian (1989) has argued that a longlasting continuous and rather small impairment of calcium homeostasis may have the same effect as an acute and massive calcium overloading of neuronal cells as for example induced by acute ischemic states.

This rather clear cut vision of a chronic calcium overload of neuronal cells as a central process of brain aging has been critically questioned by recent publications of Hartmann et al. (1996) and Müller et al. (1996). Based on experimental data of this research group and in agreement with those of other ones using dissociated preparations of neuronal cells of mice and rats it has been demonstrated that there is no elevation of calcium concentration in neuronal cells of the aged compared to young animals. In contrary a diminished calcium concentration appeared in the older ones. Acute depolarisation of the cells by calcium chloride surprisingly enough results in a lower increase of calcium concentration in the older animals compared to the younger ones. The lower level of stimulated calcium increase continued stable over a longer period of time. So in light of these experiments the calcium hypothesis of brain aging has to be modified: brain aging seems to be associated with a diminished intraneuronal calcium concentration accompanied by a greater sensitivity of regulating processes when intracellular calcium concentration is stimulated. However, although the underlying mechanisms are not clear as yet, the age dependent alteration of calcium homeostasis may nevertheless be the cause of impaired adaptation to external or internal cell toxic mechamisms. Concerning dementia of Alzheimer's type the situation is rather less clear because results of research are conflicting. Of course, that is due to the fact that direct experimentation with neuronal cells of patients is not possible, and animal models of Alzheimer's disease have not been accessible until recently. However, there is an interesting correlation between beta-amyloid deposition and calcium homeostasis. Beta-amyloid in higher concentrations seems to be neurotoxic itself, whereas in lower concentrations it has neuroprotective effects. Neurotoxicity of Beta-amyloid might be mediated by destabilisation of intraneuronal calcium homeostasis. Müller et al. (1996) found that low Beta-amyloid concentrations amplify stimulated increase of intracellular calcium concentration while higher concentration lead to a direct calcium influx. The same effects could be shown in human lymphocytes. In patients with Alzheimer dementia this calcuim amplifying effect of Beta-amyloid is considerably reduced. These results have been confirmed by other working groups. Müller et al. refer furthermore to experimental results of Etcheberrigary's working group (1994). They demonstrated that in normal human skin fibroblasts the stimulated increase of calcium concentration by tetraethylammoniumchlorid is blocked by low concentrations of beta-amyloid. This blocking effect cannot be seen in fibroblasts from patients with Alzheimer's dementia. Without going into details this still indicates that calcium regulation may play an important part in neuronal cell degeneration of Alzheimer's type.

Based on that general assumption central acting calcium antagonists have been introduced into antidementia drug treatment. Nimodipine represents this type of a nootropic drug and its clinical efficacy has been proven. The magnitude of ist effects are comparable to that of other wellknown nootropic drugs. The first study to be cited has been performed during the late 80th and has been published first in a German journal in 1988 (Kanowski et al., 1988), one year later in English (Kanowski et al., 1989). The trial was randomized and doubleblinded, for the controlled design using three parallel treatment groups (nimodipine, coerdocrinemesylate, placebo), involving inpatients in a psychiatric hospital in Vienna. The twelve week treatment phase was preceeded by a single blinded placebo run in phase; after six and twelve weeks treatment the target and associated variables were measured. The inclusion criteria were age between 60 and 85 years, and the clinical diagnosis of milde to moderate organic brain syndrome according to the Lausanne grading, and a total score between 41 and 90 on the Shader Clinical Assessment Geriatric Scale (SCAG). Cognitive status was measured by the Mental Status Questionnaire. The target outcome parameters on the basis of which confirmatory statistical analysis has been done were 1. SCAG, 2. Assessment Scale for the Behaviour of Geriatric Patients (BGP), 3. Syndrome Short Test (SKT), and 4. The Trail Making Test (ZVT-G). The Clinical Global Impression and subscales of SCAG, BGP and SKT were analyzed in a descriptive, respectively exploratory way. Nimodipine was given in a daily dose of 3 × 30 mg, Coerdocrinemesylate 4 mg per day, and as an active placebo Silecea-tablets (strenght D 6) were used. The overall clinical results can be seen from Table 1. After adjustment for multiple measurements nimodipine was shown to be effective on all four target parameters compared to placebo, and there was a superiority of nimodipine over coerdocrinemesylate on most parameters. The second drug was also superior to placebo. Figures 1–3 examplify the efficacy and a global view on the effects on the global psychopathology (SCAG) and two psychometric tests. Confirmation by replication has been achieved using a very similar design only omitting the coerdocrinemesylate treatment group (Fischhoff et al., 1989). Furthermore a careful à priori stratification of primary degenerative dementia and multi-infarct dementia has been performed. This study came out with identical results. In accordance with the ex post stratification between PDD and MID in the former study there were no differences seen in therapeutic efficacy between these two groups. Zirn et al. (1994) have published a well designed study on a total of

Table 1. Overall clinical results

Psychometrische Testverfahren	Nimodipin/ Placebo	Hydergin/ Placebo	Nimodipin/ Hydergin
SCAG	p < 0,01	p < 0,01	p < 0,01
GBP	p < 0,01	—	p < 0,05
SKT	p < 0,01	p < 0,01	p < 0,01
ZVT-G	P < 0,01	p < 0,01	p < 0,01

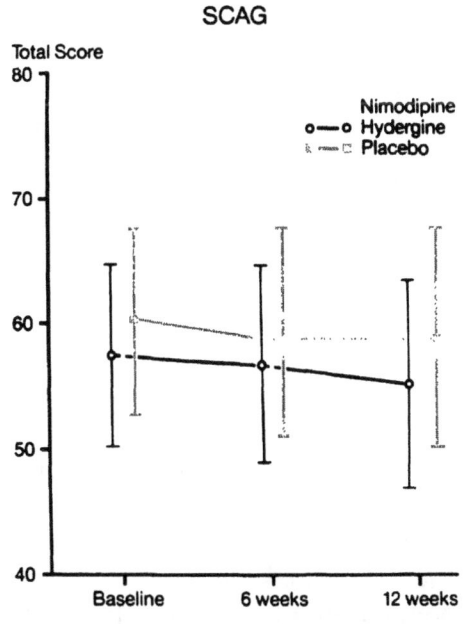

Fig. 1

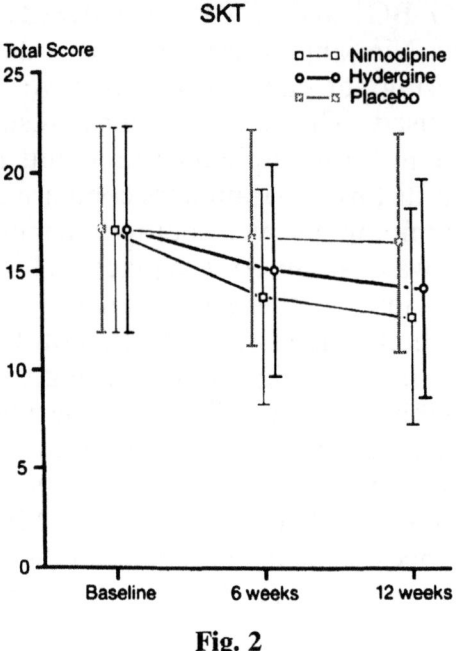

Fig. 2

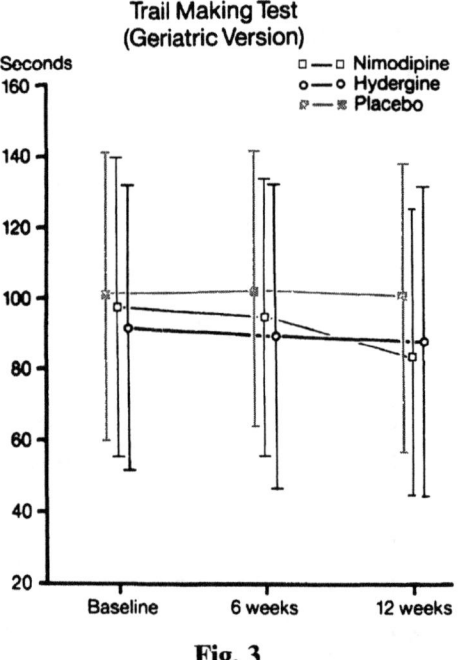

Fig. 3

60 patients suffering either from primary degenerative dementia or multi-infarct dementia comparing nimodipine and piracetam (30 patients in each treatment group). They found superiority of nimodipine against piracetam on the two target variables: Trailmaking Test, version G, and Clinical Clobal Improvement (therapeutic outcome). The difference between both treatment groups must be seen on a relative low dosage of piracetam (2.4 g/day),

whereas nimodipine was given in the usual dosage of 3×30 mg/day. The difference in therapeutic efficacy between nimodipine and piracetam is interesting because there was also a difference in favour of nimodipine compared to coerdocrinemesylate in the first study cited.

From US studies there is evidence that 1. nimodipine may slow down progression, 2. Patients with more severe cognitive disability show better improvement than those with milder disturbances, and 3. patients with higher dosage of nimodipine (3×60 mg per day) may benefit more than those on lower dosage (see Grobe-Einsler, 1993; Morich et al., 1996).

Finally Schmage et al. (1991; 1992) performed a meta-analysis of 12 doubleblind placebo controlled studies on patients with dementia related cognitive impairment. Treatment period varied between 8 and 16 weeks. In most studies dosage was 3×30 mg nimodipine per day. The data were based on 933 patients. 2 out of the 12 studies did not demonstrate any therapeutic difference between nimodipine and placebo. Of course, there were methodological differences between the studies concerning methods of assessment and definition of target variables. However, Sandoz Clinical Assessment Geriatric Scale, Clinical Global Improvement and Trail Making Test were most frequently used. Taking these methods into account there was considerable and statistically significant greater improvement on these three outcome measures under nimodipine compared to placebo.

Coming to conclusion: Important involvement of calcium metabolism in brain aging and development of Alzheimer's disease as well is still supported by experimental data and clinical evaluation of nimodipin's therapeutic efficacy. At present it seems that the first hypothesis by Khachaturian of chronic calcium overload of neuronal cells has to be substituted by greater sensitivity of calcium regulation and lower intraneuronal calclium concentration resulting in an impaired capability of neuronal cells to adapt to internal or environmental influences of noxious stress conditions.

References

Etcheberrigaray R, Ito E, Oka K, et al (1994) Soluble β-amyloid induction of Alzheimer's phenotype for human fibroblast K^+ channels. Science 264: 276–279

Fischhof P, Wagner G, Littschauer, et al (1989) Therapeutic results with nimodipine in primary degenerative dementia and multi-infarct dementia. In: Bergener M, Reisberg B (eds) Diagnosis and treatment of senile dementia. Springer, Berlin Heidelberg New York Tokyo, pp 350–359

Grobe-Einsler R (1993) Clinical aspects of nimodipine. Clin Neuropharmacol 16 [Suppl 1]: 39–45

Hartmann H, Eckert A, Velbinger K, et al (1996) Down-regulation of free intracellular calcium in dissociated brain cells of aged mice and rats. Life Sci 59: 435–449

Kanowski S, Fischhof P, Hiersemenzel R, et al (1988) Wirksamkeitsnachweis von Nootropika am Beispiel von Nimodipin — ein Beitrag zur Entwicklung geeigneter klinischer Prüfmodelle. Z Gerontopsychol psychiatr 1: 35–44

Kanowski S, Fischhof P, Hiersemenzel R, et al (1989) Therapeutic efficacy of nootropic drugs — A discussion of clinical phase III studies with nimodipine as a model. In:

Bergener M, Reisberg B (eds) Diagnosis and treatment of senile dementia. Springer, Berlin Heidelberg New York Tokyo, pp 339–349

Khachaturian ZS (1989) The role of calcium regulation in brain aging: reexamination of a hypothesis. Aging 1: 17–34

Morich FJ, Bieber F, Lewis JM, et al (1996) Nimodipine in the treatment of probable Alzheimer's disease. Results of two multicenter trials. Clin Drug Invest 11: 185–195

Müller WE, Eckert A, Hartmann H, et al (1996) Zur Kalziumhypothese der Hirnalterung. Nervenarzt 67: 15–24

Schmage N, Dycka J (1991) Auswertung von verschiedenen psychometrischen Verfahren aus klinischen Studien mit Nimodipin. In: Möller H-J (Hrsg) Hirnleistungsstörungen im Alter. Springer, Berlin Heidelberg New York Tokyo, pp 97–104

Schmage N, Bergener M (1992) Global rating, symptoms, behaviour and cognitive performance as indicators of efficacy in clinical studies with nimodipine in elderly patients with cognitive impairment syndromes. Int Psychogeratr 4: 89–99

Zirm B, Steinwachs KC, Pracher G, et al (1994) Effects of nimodipine and piracetam on speed of information processing (ZVT: G) and clinical dementia symptoms — results of an unicenter randomized clinical trial. Z Gerontopsychol psychiatr 7: 157–168

Author's address: Prof. Dr. S. Kanowski, Psychiatrische Klinik und Poliklinik, Universitätsklinikum Rudolf Virchow, Eschenallee 3, D-14050 Berlin, Federal Republic of Germany

Changes of intracellular calcium regulation in Alzheimer's disease and vascular dementia

A. Eckert[1,4]**, H. Förstl**[2,*]**, R. Zerfass**[2]**, M. Oster**[3]**, M. Hennerici**[3]**, and W. E. Müller**[1,4]

Departments of [1]Psychopharmacology and [2]Psychiatry, Central Institute of Mental Health, J5, [3]Neurological Clinic, Klinikum Mannheim of the University of Heidelberg, Mannheim, and [4]Department of Pharmacology, Biocenter, University of Frankfurt, Frankfurt, Federal Republic of Germany

Summary. Free intracellular calcium ($[Ca^{2+}]_i$) represents probably the most important intracellular messenger for many signal transduction pathways. Due to this crucial role of $[Ca^{2+}]_i$, it has been assumed that alterations of $[Ca^{2+}]_i$ are critically involved in brain aging and in the pathophysiology of Alzheimer's disease (AD). This hypothesis is corroborated by several studies demonstrating changes of $[Ca^{2+}]_i$ in peripheral cells from AD patients. However, the findings are still controversial. Using blood lymphocytes and neutrophils as two different peripheral model systems, we evaluated several parameters of intracellular Ca^{2+} regulation in a very large group of AD patients and non-demented controls. We found no major difference in Ca^{2+} homeostasis, since neither the basal $[Ca^{2+}]_i$, nor the activation-induced Ca^{2+} responses differed among neutrophils or lymphocytes from aged controls and AD patients. However, we observed a delayed Ca^{2+} response of AD lymphocytes after phytohemagglutinin (PHA) stimulation indicating an impaired function of Ca^{2+} influx-controlling mechanisms. Furthermore, we studied whether differences exist in Ca^{2+} regulation between lymphocytes from patients with vascular dementia and AD patients, to define AD-specific alterations and to distinguish between the two dementia groups and non-demented control subjects respectively. First evidences indicate that Ca^{2+} mobilization in lymphocytes is specifically impaired in lymphocytes from patients with vascular dementia.

Introduction

Alzheimer's disease (AD) is usually considered a neurodegenerative disorder of certain brain regions only. Increasing evidence, however, indicates addi-

---

* Present address: Department of Psychiatry, Technical University, Munich, Federal Republic of Germany

tional abnormalities in metabolic, biochemical, and signal transducting processes in tissues outside the central nervous system (deLustig et al., 1994). Because of its broad function as an intracellular messenger and its generation by several second messenger generating systems, free intracellular calcium ($[Ca^{2+}]_i$) has been the major focus of many studies. In contrast to many other biochemical mechanisms, determination of the cellular regulation of $[Ca^{2+}]_i$ requires functioning vital cells and cannot be carried out in postmortem brain tissue. Since a valid animal model of AD or direct access to vital human brain cells from AD patients do not exist, nonneuronal peripheral cells have attracted specific attention. Data performed on human lymphocytes and skin fibroblasts so far are contradictory, since usually small samples were investigated (Adunsky et al., 1991; Bondy et al., 1994; Borden et al., 1991; Eckert et al., 1994; Eckert et al., 1996; Grossmann et al., 1993; Hartmann et al., 1994).

The present study focuses on AD-related alterations in $[Ca^{2+}]_i$ in two different cell types, lymphocytes and neutrophils using a sufficiently large sample size. Since the composition of the Ca^{2+} signal after cell activation is different in both cell types (O'Flaherty et al., 1991; Zweifach and Lewis, 1993), we were able to investigate major mechanisms of cellular Ca^{2+} signalling regulation in AD. N-formyl-methionyl-leucyl-phenylalanin (fMLP)-induced Ca^{2+} response in neutrophils is mediated mostly by the release of Ca^{2+} from intracellular stores via an inositol phosphate-sensitive pathway, whereas the mitogen-induced Ca^{2+} signal in lymphocytes is strongly dependent on Ca^{2+} influx from the extracellular space.

Vascular dementia is the second common cause of dementia in the western world, after Alzheimer's disease. While many studies investigated Ca^{2+} regulation in AD, only very few data are presently available giving detailed information about specific changes of $[Ca^{2+}]_i$ in patients with cerebrovascular dementia. Therefore, it was of great interest to search for differences in Ca^{2+} regulation between SVE and AD patients, and non-demented controls respectively. Considering the difficulties of diagnosis to differentiate exactly between vascular disease and the coexistence of vascular and degenerative dementia, specific care was taken to avoid inclusion of patients with mixed forms of dementia by investigating only a specific group of patients with subcortical vascular encephalopathy (SVE). The SVE patients represent a well characterized group of patients with white matter lesions especially in frontal regions.

Methods

Subjects

The experiments were performed using blood cells from 50 patients (22 men and 28 women) with "probable" (n = 27) or "possible" (n = 23) AD according to the NINCDS-ADRDA criteria. The patients were recruited from an ongoing longitudinal study. The mean age was 68.4 ± 9.2 years (range 50 to 86 years, median 69 years). The majority of cases exhibited moderate dementia. The clinical dementia ratings (CDR) ranged from mild to severe (CDR = 0.5–3.0). Blood cells from 41 non-demented individuals of similar age (mean age 67.5 ± 8.0 years, median 68 years, range 42 to 88 years, 21 men and 20 women) were used as controls as described previously (Eckert et al., 1997a).

In addition, blood cells from 26 patients (14 men and 12 women) with subcortical vascular encephalopathy (SVE) following the diagnostic criteria for research studies (NINDS-AIREN) were investigated. Patients underwent a structured medical and neurological examination as well as neuropsychological interviews as previously described (Eckert et al., 1997b). The mean age was 72 ± 6.2 years (range 59 to 84 years, median 71 years). Findings in lymphocytes of SVE patients were compared with those of 26 age- and sex-matched AD patients and control subjects.

Approximately half of the AD patients, half of the aged controls, and most of the SVE patients were taking cardiovascular and antidiabetic drugs. 9 SVE patients were taking calcium antagonists. None of the drugs used are known to interfere with intracellular Ca^{2+} homeastasis in lymphocytes. This is also the case for calcium antagonists, since lymphocytes do not express functional L-type Ca^{2+} channels (Zweifach and Lewis, 1993).

Cell separation and $[Ca^{2+}]_i$ measurements

Peripheral blood lymphocytes were separated from heparinized blood by centrifugation on Ficoll-Hypaque for $400 \times g$ for 40 min as previously described (Eckert et al., 1993a). The neutrophils in the bottom fraction of the Ficoll-Hypaque density centrifugation were separated from erythrocytes by dextran sedimentation (Hartmann et al., 1994).

Fura-2AM loading and measurements of $[Ca^{2+}]_i$ were performed as described previously (Eckert et al., 1993a). Freshly prepared lymphocytes were stimulated with phytohemagglutinin (PHA; Sigma, Germany) at a final concentration of 15 µg/ml. Neutrophils were stimulated with N-formyl-methionyl-leucyl-pheylalanin (fMLP) at a final concentration of 1 µmol/l.

Statistics

Significance was tested using analysis of variance (ANOVA; SAS-Institute, Cary, NC, USA).

Results

Alterations of $[Ca^{2+}]_i$ were investigated in human lymphocytes and neutrophils of forty-one elderly non-demented controls and fifty AD patients. Figure 1 demonstrates the difference in Ca^{2+} mobilization between both cell types showing a typical time course of $[Ca^{2+}]_i$ after fMLP (1 µmol/l) stimulation in neutrophils and after cell activation with PHA (15 µg/mL) in lymphocytes of one representative aged control. In neutrophils, the fMLP-induced Ca^{2+} increase reaches its maximum (ΔCa^{2+}: 490 nmol/l) within few seconds due to the quick and extensive Ca^{2+} release from intracellular stores (20, 53) (Fig. 1. In addition, $[Ca^{2+}]_i$ declines to basal $[Ca^{2+}]_i$ levels within 2 min (Fig. 1). In lymphocytes, however, PHA-induced Ca^{2+} response shows a slow increase of $[Ca^{2+}]_i$ after addition of the mitogenic stimulus (Fig. 1). The maximum Ca^{2+} signal (ΔCa^{2+}: 92.4 nmol/l) was reached after 60 s (Fig. 1) leading into a sustained plateau phase which is stable during 20–30 min.

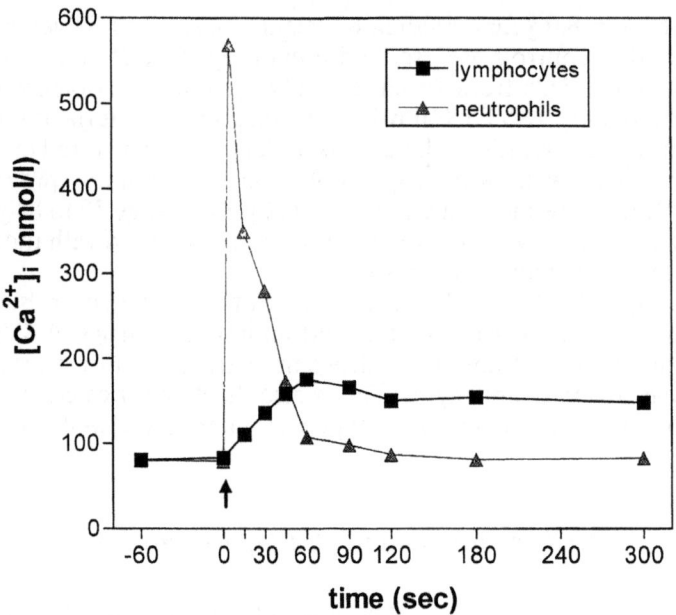

Fig. 1. Typical time course of the increase in $[Ca^{2+}]_i$ after cell activation in freshly isolated lymphocytes and neutrophils from one representative non-demented control (male, age: 58 years, no medication). As indicated by arrow, stimuli were added to cell suspension: PHA (15 µg/ml) to lymphocytes, fMLP (1 µmol/l) to neutrophils. The maximal Ca^{2+} response was reached in neutrophils within 7 s and within 60 s in lymphocytes respectively

Measurement of basal $[Ca^{2+}]_i$ in lymphocytes revealed no difference between the two groups (aged: 102.4 ± 17.8 nmol/l; AD: 100.5 ± 18.4 nmol/l) (Fig. 2, left panel). Moreover, the PHA-induced increase in $[Ca^{2+}]_i$ over baseline $[Ca^{2+}]_i$ (ΔCa^{2+}) was not different between aged controls and AD patients (aged: 91.4 ± 25.3 nmol/l, AD: 86.0 ± 23.4 nmol/l) (Fig. 2, right panel). In contrast to findings of Adunsky et al. (1), even after stimulation with a very high concentration of PHA (100 µg/ml) no AD-specific alterations were observed (aged: 116.8 ± 32.2 nmol/l, n = 34; AD: 128.7 ± 37.2 nmol/l, n = 32) (data not shown).

On the other hand, the time to reach maximum Ca^{2+} rise (t_{max}) was significantly increased in lymphocytes of AD patients (Fig. 2, right panel) (aged controls: range 45–120 s, mean $\pm$ SD 68 ± 24 s; AD: range 45–180 s, mean $\pm$ SD 93 ± 38 s, p < 0.001).

Basal Ca^{2+} levels were not different in neutrophils from the two groups (aged: 90.2 ± 18.7 nmol/l, AD: 91.6 ± 22.0 nmol/l) (Fig. 3, left panel) nor was fMLP-induced Ca^{2+} increase (aged: 471 ± 206 nmol/l, AD: 470 ± 116 nmol/l) (Fig. 3, left panel) confirming previous findings in a small group of patients (35). In addition, time course to reach the maximal Ca^{2+} increase was not altered among both groups (aged: 6.8 ± 1.5 s, AD: 7.0 ± 1.4 s) (Fig. 3, right panel).

Furthermore, alterations of $[Ca^{2+}]_i$ were investigated in freshly prepared peripheral lymphocytes of twenty-six SVE patients. Figure 4 shows the time

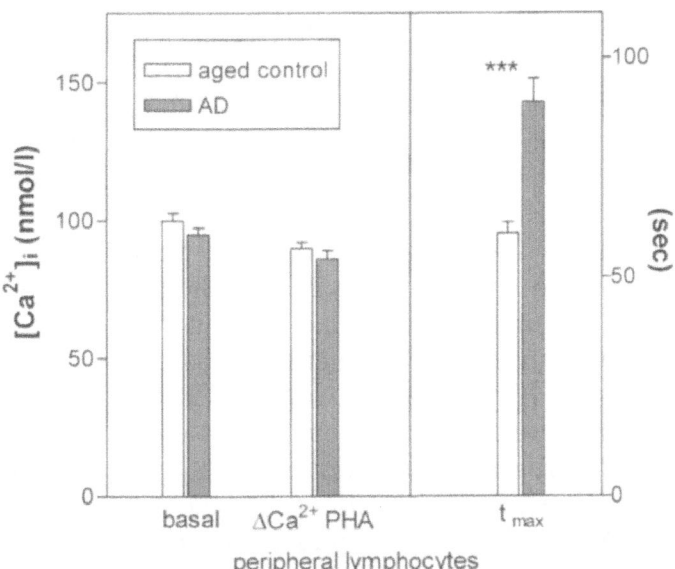

Fig. 2. *Left panel*: Basal $[Ca^{2+}]_i$ and the Ca^{2+} increase after stimulation with 15 µg/ml PHA over baseline (ΔCa^{2+}) were similar in lymphocytes from aged non-demented controls (n = 41) and AD patients (n = 50). Values represent the maximal response and are expressed as means ± SEM. *Right panel*: The time to reach the maximal Ca^{2+} response after PHA stimulation was significantly increased in lymphocytes of AD patients (n = 50) compared to aged controls (n = 41) (***p < 0.001, F = 14.04, ANOVA). Values represent the maximal response and are expressed as means ± SEM. (All data are taken from Eckert et al., 1997a)

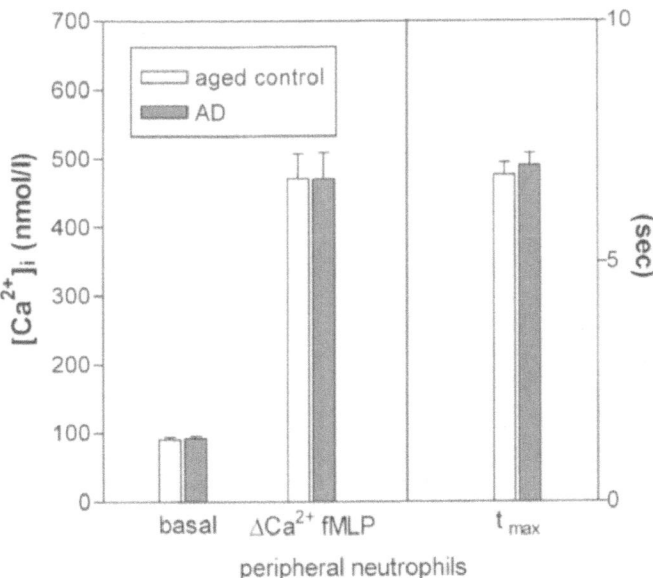

Fig. 3. *Left panel*: Basal $[Ca^{2+}]_i$ and the fMLP-induced Ca^{2+} increase over baseline (ΔCa^{2+}) were unaltered in neutrophils from aged non-demented controls (n = 32) and AD patients (n = 27). Values represent the maximal response and are expressed as means ± SEM. *Right panel*: There was no difference in the time to reach maximal Ca^{2+} release from intracellular stores. Values are expressed as means ± SEM. (All data are taken from Eckert et al., 1997a)

course of PHA-induced increase in $[Ca^{2+}]_i$ over baseline $[Ca^{2+}]_i$ (ΔCa^{2+}) after PHA stimulation in lymphocytes from aged controls and SVE patients. The maximum Ca^{2+} signal was reached after 1 min in both groups (Fig. 4). However, comparison of the time courses revealed a significantly impaired PHA-induced Ca^{2+} response in cells from SVE patients compared to controls (ANOVA, p = 0.002, F = 10.64; Fig. 4). The difference in intracellular Ca^{2+} mobilization between both groups was mainly pronounced in the inital phase of the Ca^{2+} response (ANOVA, p < 0.001 for the time points within the first 60 seconds), which is dominated by a Ca^{2+} release from intracellular stores.[24,25] In contrast, the PHA-induced Ca^{2+} increase was not different between AD patients and controls (Fig. 2) Moreover, measurement of basal $[Ca^{2+}]_i$ in lymphocytes revealed no difference between all groups.

The time rate to reach the maximum Ca^{2+} peak after stimulation with PHA was unaltered between SVE patients and aged controls (controls: 68.1 ± 26.6 seconds vs. SVE: 76.7 ± 29.8 seconds) (Fig. 4, inset). In contrast, time to reach maximum Ca^{2+} peak was significantly delayed (p < 0.01) in lymphocytes of AD patients compared to controls (AD: 96.4 ± 42.4 seconds vs. controls: 68.1 ± 26.6 seconds) by unaltered Ca^{2+} response height between both groups as mentioned earlier (Fig. 2).

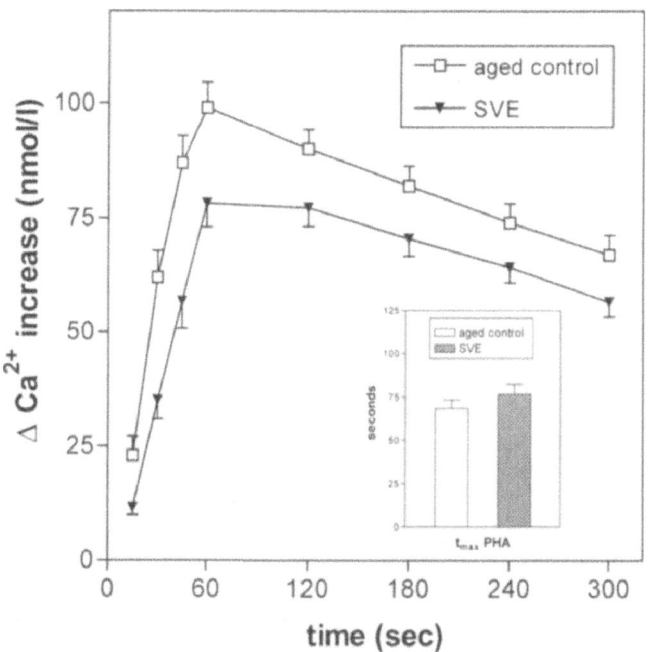

Fig. 4. Time course of the increase in $[Ca^{2+}]_i$ in freshly prepared lymphocytes from SVE patients (n = 26) and aged-matched non-demented controls (n = 26) after PHA (15 μg/ml) stimulation. Data are means ± SEM. ANOVA indicates that there is a significant reduction of the PHA-induced Ca^{2+} increase in lymphocytes from SVE patients (p = 0.002, F = 10.64). *Inset*: The time to reach the maximal Ca^{2+} response in lymphocytes revealed no differences between SVE patients and aged individuals. (All data are taken from Eckert et al., 1997b)

Discussion

Using lymphocytes as well as neutrophils, we were able to investigate two different mechanisms of Ca^{2+} signalling and their possible alterations in AD. Our findings demonstrate that neither basal $[Ca^{2+}]_i$, nor the PHA-induced Ca^{2+} influx in lymphocytes, nor the fMLP-mediated Ca^{2+} release in neutrophils are altered in AD confirming our previous data (Eckert et al., 1993b, 1994; Hartmann et al., 1994). Our observations that these aspects of $[Ca^{2+}]_i$ homeostasis are unaltered in AD are also consistent with findings from the most other groups using lymphocytes and PHA stimulation (Bondy et al., 1994; Gibson and Toral-Borza, 1992; Grossmann et al., 1993). Findings of Adunsky et al. (1991) about strongly increased Ca^{2+} responses after PHA stimulation using a supramitogen dose of PHA (100 µg/ml) could not be confirmed by our group and others (Bondy et al., 1994; Eckert et al., 1994). The same authors (Adunsky et al., 1991) additionally demonstrated a significant increase of Ca^{2+} signalling in lymphocytes of AD patients after crosslinked anti-CD3 stimulation. These findings have been disproved by Grossmann et al. (1993), demonstrating reduced Ca^{2+} levels after anti-CD3 stimulation in a specific T lymphocyte subpopulation ($CD4^+$ T cells) of AD patients. $CD8^+$ T cells did not differ between patients and aged controls. The reduced anti-CD3-induced Ca^{2+} response in $CD4^+$ cells of patients was not related to reduced CD3 receptor density, but to an impaired signal transduction pathway of tyrosine phosphorylation (Grossmann et al., 1993). After stimulation with the mitogen PHA, however, which also stimulates tyrosin kinase activity and Ca^{2+} mobilization through the CD3/T cell receptor complex (Weiss and Littmann, 1994), no AD-related differences have been observed by the same authors (Grossmann et al., 1993). An explanation for this inconsistency in signal transduction through the CD3/T cell receptor complex has not been given. Therefore, a rather general relevance of this observation is questionable. Although the number of lymphocytes is decreased with age, it is not further decreased with AD (Collins et al., 1991; Dysken et al., 1992). Moreover, there exist no evidence that lymphocyte subpopulations differ between AD patients and controls (Arage et al., 1990). Thus, alterations of Ca^{2+} signalling in one subset only should be reflected in the whole lymphocyte population. This assumption is further supported by findings about unaltered proliferative response in T cells of AD patients after PHA or anti-CD3 stimulation (Araga et al., 1990), a late event of the Ca^{2+}-initiated signal transduction cascade (Gelfand et al., 1984).

Our data on neutrophils indicate that the G protein-mediated fMLP receptor activation is also not altered in AD. These findings are in accordance with observations of an unchanged fMLP-induced Ca^{2+} mobilization in AD fibroblasts (Peterson et al., 1985) as well as unaltered bradykinin-induced Ca^{2+} activation, another G protein-coupled receptor, in fibroblasts (Borden et al., 1991). In addition, the number of neutrophils is similar in young, aged, and AD groups (Collins et al., 1991).

Confirming preliminary findings of Bondy et al. (1996), we observed a delayed Ca^{2+} peak after PHA stimulation in lymphocytes of AD patients compared to controls. Mainly Ca^{2+} influx-regulating events activated by intra-cellularly released Ca^{2+} seems to be impaired in AD, since Ca^{2+} release from intracellular stores appears to be unchanged (Eckert et al., 1997a). The importance of this observation is still under investigation.

In contrast to our findings in AD patients, Ca^{2+} increase after cell activation with the mitogen PHA was markedly reduced in lymphocytes from SVE patients compared to non-demented controls. Only very few data are presently available giving detailed information about specific changes of $[Ca^{2+}]_i$ in patients with cerebrovascular disease or dementia. Two investigators studied intracellular Ca^{2+} regulation in lymphocytes of patients with multi-infarct-dementia (MID) and compared them to aged controls and AD patients (Adunsky et al., 1991; Bondy et al., 1994). Consistent with our data, both authors did not observe any differences in basal $[Ca^{2+}]_i$ levels between all groups. However, they could not observe differences after PHA stimulation in lymphocytes from MID patients when compared to aged controls or AD patients respectively. One explanation for the inconsistency of the results could be the higher PHA concentrations used by Adunsky et al. (1991) and Bondy et al. (1994) (PHA 25 μg/ml and 100 μg/ml) superimposing the possibly impaired initial Ca^{2+} release from intracellular stores by intense Ca^{2+} influx through the plasma membrane into the cell during plateau phase of the Ca^{2+} response. Moreover, a different subgroup of patients has been investigated in our study. The SVE patients represent a well characterized group of patients with white matter lesions especially in frontal regions (Eckert et al., 1997b) whereas the diagnosis of MID may enclose a less prescisely defined group of patients (Gottfries et al., 1994). In respect to the heterogeneity of our findings in PHA-induced Ca^{2+} response in lymphocytes from SVE patients compared to those of others, the divergent subgroup type and the really small number of patients investigated by Adunsky et al. (1991) (MID patients, n = 6) and by Bondy et al. (1994) (MID patients, n = 6) have to be considered. The impaired PHA-induced Ca^{2+} response in lymphocytes of SVE patients over the whole time period of stimulation seems to be associated with a reduced Ca^{2+} mobilization from intracellular Ca^{2+} organelles, which mainly dominates the initial Ca^{2+} increase after cell activation (Zweifach and Lewis, 1993), whereas impaired Ca^{2+} influx mechanisms seem to be involved in the delayed time rate of the maximum Ca^{2+} response in lymphocytes of AD patients (Eckert et al., 1997a).

In lymphocytes, an increase in $[Ca^{2+}]_i$ represents an early event in the intracellular signal cascade of cell proliferation after PHA stimulation (Gelfand et al., 1984) Very importantly, Tarkowski et al. (1995) demonstrated that during stroke the proliferative responses of T lymphocytes to the mitogens PHA and concanavalin A were reduced compared to healthy controls. Therefore, we can assume that findings about an impaired Ca^{2+} activation in SVE lymphocytes are in accordance with these data and gain new insights in the pathogenesis of SVE in respect to a probably altered immunological function. Nervous system and immune system are known to interact at various levels. Moreover, cells of both systems share common membrane structures and communicate with hormones and cytokines. Some evidence of immune activation in AD brain suggest that enhanced CD8[+] T cell-derived suppressor activity initiates activation of brain microglia (Hartwig et al., 1995).

Therefore, lymphocytes may provide an easily accessible and powerful model to study cellular modulation in neurodegenerative disorders. In addition, our work offers a new approach to partially discriminate two different groups of patients with either cerebrovascular or Alzheimer's disease.

Acknowledgments

This study was supported by grants from the Deutsche Forschungsgemeinschaft, SFB 258, project K5, the Forschungsfond Fakultät Mannheim, and a H.G.F. Schilling professorship to H.F.

References

Adunsky A, Baram D, Hershkowitz M, Mekori YA (1991) Increased cytosolic calcium in lymphocytes of Alzheimer patients. J Neuroimmunol 33: 167–172

Araga S, Kagimoto H, Funamoto K, Takahashi K (1990) Lymphocyte proliferation and subpopulations in dementia of the Alzheimer's type. Jpn J Med 29: 572–575

Bondy B, Klages U, Müller-Spahn F, Hock C (1994) Cytosolic free [Ca^{2+}]$_i$ in mononuclear blood cells from demented patients and healthy controls. Eur Arch Psychiatry Clin Neurosci 243: 224–228

Bondy B, Hofmann M, Müller-Spahn F, Witzko M, Hock CH (1996) The PHA-induced calcium signal in lymphocytes is altered after blockade of K$^+$ channels in Alzheimer's disease. J Psychiat Res 30: 217–227

Borden LA, Maxfield FR, Goldman JE, Shelanski ML (1991) Resting [Ca^{2+}]$_i$ and [Ca^{2+}]$_i$ transients are similar in fibroblasts from normal and Alzheimer's donors. Neurobiol Aging 13: 33–38

Collins JM, Scott RB, McClish DK, Taylor JR, Grogan WM (1991) Altered membrane anisotropy gradients of plasma membranes of living peripheral blood leukocytes in aging and Alzheimer's disease. Mech Ageing Dev 59: 153–162

deLustig ES, Kohan S, Famulari AL, Dominguez RO, Serra JA (1994) Peripheral markers and diagnostic criteria in Alzheimer's disease: critical evaluations. Rev Neurosci 5: 213–225

Dysken MW, Minichielleo MD, Hill JL, Skare S, Little JT, Molchan SE, Sunderland T (1992) Distribution of peripheral lymphocytes in Alzheimer patients and controls. J Psychiat Res 26: 213–218

Eckert A, Hartmann H, Müller WE (1993a) β-Amyloid protein enhances the mitogen-induced calcium response in circulating human lymphocytes. FEBS Lett 330: 49–52

Eckert A, Förstl H, Hartmann H, Müller WE (1993b) Decreased β-amyloid sensitivity in Alzheimer's disease. Lancet 342: 805–806

Eckert A, Hartmann H, Förstl H, Müller WE (1994) Alterations of intracellular calcium regulation during aging and Alzheimer's disease in nonneuronal cells. Life Sci 55: 2019–2029

Eckert A, Förstl H, Zerfass R, Hartmann H, Müller WE (1996) Lymphocytes and neutrophils as peripheral models to study the effect of β-amyloid on cellular calcium signalling in Alzheimer's disease. Life Sci 59: 499–510

Eckert A, Förstl H, Zerfass R, Hennerici M, Müller WE (1997a) Free intracellular calcium in peripheral cells in Alzheimer's disease. Neurobiol Aging 18: 281–284

Eckert A, Oster M, Förstl H, Hennerici M, Müller WE (1997b) Impaired calcium regulation in subcortical vascular encephalopathy. Stroke 28: 1351–1356

Gelfand EW, Cheung RK, Grinstein S (1984) Role of membrane potential in the regulation of lectin-induced calcium uptake. J Cell Physiol 121: 533–539

Gibson GE, Toral-Barza L (1992) Cytosolic free calcium in lymphoblasts from young, aged and Alzheimer's subjects. Mech Ageing Dev 63: 1–9

Gottfries CG, Blennow K, Karlsson L, Wallin A (1994) The neurochemistry of vascular dementia. Dementia 5: 163–167

Grossmann A, Kukull WA, Jinneman JC, Birds TD, Villacres EC, Larson EB, Rabinovitch PS (1993) Intracellular calcium response is reduced in CD4+ lymphocytes in Alzheimer's disease and in older persons with Down's syndrome. Neurobiol Aging 14: 177–185

Hartmann H, Eckert A, Förstl H, Müller WE (1994) Similar age-related changes of free intracellular calcium in lymphocytes and central neurons: effects of Alzheimer's disease. Eur Arch Psychiatry Clin Neurosci 243: 218–223

Hartwig M (1995) Immune ageing and Alzheimer's disease. NeuroReport 6: 1274–1276

O'Flaherty JT, Rossi AG, Jacobson DP, Redman JF (1991) Roles of Ca^{2+} in human neutrophils responses to receptor agonists. Biochem J 278: 705–711

Peterson C, Ratan RR, Shelanski ML, Goldman JE (1986) Cytosolic free calcium and cell spreading decrease in fibroblasts from aged and Alzheimer donors. Proc Natl Acad Sci USA 83: 7999–8001

Tarkowski E, Naver H, Wallin BG, Blomstarnd C, Tarkowski A (1995) Lateralization of T-lymphocyte responses in patients with stroke. Stroke 26: 57–62

Weiss A, Littmann DR (1994) Signal transduction by lymphocyte antigen receptors. Cell 76: 263–274

Zweifach A, Lewis RS (1993) Mitogen-regulated Ca^{2+} current of T lymphocytes is activated by depletion of intracellular Ca^{2+} stores. Proc Natl Acad Sci USA 90: 6295–6299

Authors' address: Prof. Dr. W. E. Müller, Pharmakologisches Institut, Biozentrum der Universität Frankfurt, Marie-Curie-Strasse 9, D-60439 Frankfurt, Federal Republic of Germany

Free radicals in Alzheimer's dementia: currently available therapeutic strategies

M. Rösler, W. Retz, J. Thome, and **P. Riederer**

Psychiatric Department, University of Würzburg, Federal Republic of Germany

Summary. Substantial evidence now exists that oxidative stress may play an important role in the etiopathogenesis of DAT. The different sources of oxidative stress in DAT are suggesting several pharmacological opportunities for influencing the disease. It is possible to distinguish 2 major types of possible therapeutic agents according to their pharmacological point of attack.

1. Radical scavengers, agents directly interacting with free radicals. Candidates of this type are gingko biloba, vitamins A, C, E and estrogen.

2. Antioxidants, which are able to prevent or decrease the production of free radicals by use of specific neuropharmacological properties. Candidates are selegiline, a MAO-B inhibitor well established in the therapy of Parkinson's disease, and tenilsetam, which is believed to be an AGE-inhibitor.

Recent in vitro studies have demonstrated the efficacy of both types of therapeutic agents by preventing or delaying oxidative neural damage.

Some clinical data exist regarding the antidementive properties particularly in terms of gingko biloba, selegiline and vitamin E. The efficacy studies about these compounds seem to indicate a promising future strategy in the therapy of DAT. But it is too early to draw definite conclusions since it is well kown that all of our candidate substances do not act specifically as radical scavengers or antioxidants.

Introduction

The hypothesis that oxidative stress might play an important role within the framework of the etiopathogenesis of Alzheimer's disease (DAT) is currently the subject of intense discussion (Halliwell, 1992; Frölich and Riederer, 1995; Thome et al., 1996). This is a continuation of ideas that have already been discussed in connection with natural aging processes and other neurodegenerative diseases. According to all we know today, there is no uniform cause of oxidative stress in DAT. The production of free radicals can evidently be triggered or kept going by a series of pathomechanisms. In key words we can name the β-amyloid peptide, the neurofibrillary tangles, AGEs, leakage of electrons in the mitochondria, excitotoxicity, the imbalance in free radicals defence enzymes, etc. (Jenner, 1994; Smith et al., 1996).

In view of the variety of the possible causes one can imagine several therapeutic approaches towards reducing oxidative stress. It is possible to distinguish 2 types of substances to reduce oxidative stress:

— *Radical scavengers*: These are agents which interact directly with the free radicals and thus reduce oxidative stress. A considerable number of substances with radical scavenging properties is known and evaluated in pharmacological trials. From a clinical point of view, the following should be mentioned: gingko biloba, vitamin A, vitamin C, vitamin E, idebenone (see Gutzmann, this volume). Future candidates will be estrogens and iron chelators penetrating the blood-brain barrier.

— *Antioxidants*: On account of their pharmacological point of attack, these substances intervene in the process of the emergence of oxidative stress, prevent the production of free radicals or reduce them. The best known substance from this group is selegiline. A further drug with possible antioxidative effects in Alzheimer's dementia is tenilsetam. Future candidates may arrive from the group of antiphlogistics.

In the following, reports will be given on experiences with the therapeutic effects of gingko biloba, and vitamin E, C and A as examples for radical scavengers. Thereafter a synopsis of the clinical data with selegiline and tenilsetam will be presented.

Clinical experiences with gingko biloba

This is a standardized extract from leaves of gingko biloba (24% gingko flavone gycosides and 6% terpene lactones).

In the animal model neuroprotective properties could be demonstrated, for which its ability to trap toxic oxygen radicals and prevent pathological lipid peroxidation is primarily made responsible (Kleijnen and Knipschild, 1992; Gardes-Albert et al., 1995; Packer et al., 1995). Further modes of action are enhancement of cerebral metabolism and cerebral blood flow. Gingko biloba also possibly acts as an inhibitor of MAO-A and MAO-B (White et al., 1996).

The substance has been examined in various placebo-controlled double blind studies, most of which date from the period before the introduction of today's standards for the efficiency examination of antidementia drugs by the North American and European licensing authorities. By today's standards, a great deal of shortcomings and weakness make the interpretation of the results more difficult. The major point is the incommensurability of the diagnostic criteria used in these early studies to select patient with the international diagnostic systems (ICD-10, DSM-IV), which we use today. In accordance with traditions particularly in France and Germany, the syndromatic diagnosis of "organic psychosyndrome" has been made or the term of "cerebrovascular insufficiency" was used. The later is not comparable with the diagnosis of vascular dementia. With respect to this circumstances in most cases one cannot find out, whether the patients have suffered from Alzheimer's dementia (DAT), multi-infarct dementia (MID), age associated memory impairment (AAMI) or mild cognitive decline (MCD).

Herrschaft (1992) presented an overview of 15 placebo-controlled double blind studies (gingko biloba special extract EGb 761) with 931 patients from 1975 to 1992. The periods of observation varied from 4 weeks to one year. The most common diagnoses were cerebrovascular insufficiency and organic psychosyndrome. In 8 out of 11 studies with acceptable methodological standards, there were improvements in the global assessments of the patients or in various cognitive tests. Another overview (gingko biloba special extract LI 1370) was carried out by Hopfenmüller (1994). Here, 10 placebo-controlled double blind studies with a treatment duration of 6 to 12 weeks were analysed, and 8 or rather 6 studies were included separately in a meta-analysis. From the point of view of the total score of the individual symptoms (n = 696 patients) there were 7 studies with proof of a positive effect, with one negative study. With respect to the clinical global assessment, 5 positive and one negative study were counted.

Of the clinical studies mentioned here, that by Weitbrecht and Jansen (1986) and a more recent one by Hofferberth (1994) must be emphasised, because they are the only ones dealing exclusively with dementia of the Alzheimer type. Both trials with 40 and 60 patients respectively evaluated gingko biloba under placebo-controlled and double blind conditions. At the end of the 3 months period of observation, the global assessments, the neuropsychological test results, the ADL/IADL scales and the general psychopathology showed a significant improvement in the verum groups.

The most recent study about the efficacy of gingko biloba was performed by Kanowski et al. (1996). So far this is the most comprehensive randomised, double-blind, placebo-controlled and multicenter study, with 216 patients. Diagnostically, the patients suffered from mild to moderate DAT or MID. The treatment duration was 24 weeks. A global measure (CGIC), a neuropsychological test (SKT) and an ADL/IADL scale (NAB) served as primary outcome parameters. Depending on various response level criteria, significantly higher responder rates were found in the verum group than in the reference population after 24 weeks.

In a secondary statistical analysis the highest improvement rates were constantly found in the group of patients with Alzheimer dementia.

Summing up, it can be said that there is some evidence that gingko biloba may serve as an antidementive drug in the case of Alzheimer's disease.

Clinical experiences with alpha-tocopherol

Various in vitro experiments have shown that vitamin E can cancel out or reduce certain neurotoxic effects, presumably due to its ability to scavenge peroxyl radicals and to slow down pathological lipid peroxidation (Burton and Ingold, 1989; Meydani, 1995).

Clinical data with vitamin E have been obtained firstly from pharmacological studies in Parkinson's disease. No proof of efficacy could be established in the DATATOP study (Parkinson Study Group, 1993), even though in combination with vitamin C, a slowing of the progression of the disease was presumed in a pilot study (Fahn, 1992).

In a study focussing on Huntington's disease, efficacy modifying the course of the disease in its early stages was assumed (Peyser et al., 1995).

The Alzheimer's Disease Cooperative Study just published (Sano et al., 1997), which evaluated selegiline, vitamin E and a combination of both substances against a placebo, developed a new approach towards the definition of decisive primary outcome parameters. Within the framework of this 2-year study, the following study endpoints were defined among 341 patients with moderate DAT: occurrence of death, occurrence of institutionalization, loss of ability to perform at least 2 of 3 basic activities of daily living, occurrence of severe dementia defined as CDR 3. In all verum groups there was a distinct retardation in the progress of the disease, amounting to 230 days in the case of monotherapy with vitamin E. It is interesting to note that there were no additive effects in the combination treatment group with selegiline and vitamin E.

No further clinical studies on the effects of vitamin E in DAT are known.

Clinical experiences with vitamin C and provitamin A

The radical scavenging properties of vitamin C are well documented (Frei et al., 1989). In vitro experiments demonstrated neuroprotective properties (Bell et al., 1996). Only 2 clinical studies have been performed in Alzheimer dementia. One double-blind trial compared 3 drugs including ascorbic acid. Vitamin C was described to be inactive (Parnetti et al., 1995). The same was found to be true in a double-blind placebo controlled trial with vitamins B1, B2, B6 and C in 15 patients suffering from DAT and MID (Burns et al., 1989).

It is not known whether the antioxidative effects of beta carotene (Liebler, 1993; Hennekens et al., 1994) have positive effects in the case of Alzheimer's disease. Studies on this subject have evidently not been published.

Clinical experiences with selegiline

Selegiline is a MAO-B inhibitor, which prevents the formation of oxidative stress through the inhibition of oxidative deamination of biogenic amines. With selegiline one can observe dose-dependent mode of action (Sunderland et al., 1987; Martignoni et al., 1991). In doses up to 10 mg per day one can find MAO-B inhibition, in doses up to 40 mg inhibition of MAO-A + B is occuring. In low doses, special neuroprotective properties which are apparently independent of MAO-B inhibition have been observed (Koutsilieri et al., 1994).

In animal experiments a prolongation of active life has been described. The substance has an established position in the treatment of Parkinson's disease (Parkinson Study Group, 1993).

Favourable effects in Alzheimer's disease were first described by Tariot et al. (1987a,b). Since then a series of clinical studies have been conducted confirming this observation. In our search among relevant literature 16 studies since 1987 were found, which are listed in Table 1.

In 13 studies, beneficial effects could be achieved in at least one symptom domain of Alzheimer's dementia. The improvement in cognitive performance

Table 1. Pharmacological trials with selegiline — Responderstudies

Author	n	Dur	Design	GLOBAL	COG	ADL	BEHAV
Tariot et al. (1987a,b)	17	3 mo	double-blind placebo.	↑	↑	—	↑
Agnoli et al. (1990/1992)	20/10	3 mo/2 mo	double-blind placebo	—	↑	—	→
Piccinin et al. (1990)	20	6 mo	double-blind placebo, cross.	—	↑	—	—
Monteverde et al. (1990)	40	3 mo	single-blind selegiline vs. phosphatidylser.	—	↑	↑	—
Falsaperla et al. (1990)	40	3 mo	single-blind selegiline vs. oxiracetam	—	↑	↑	—
Campi et al. (1990)	40	3 mo	single-blind selegiline vs. l-acetylcarnitine	—	↑	↑	—
Mangoni et al. (1991)	119	3 mo	double-blind placebo	—	↑	↑	↑
Finali et al. (1991/1992)	19/22	6 mo	double-blind placebo, cross.	—	↑	—	—
Martignoni et al. (1991)	14	3 mo	double-blind placebo	—	↑	→	→
Schneider et al. (1991)	14	1 mo	open label pilotstudy	—	↑	—	↑
Goad et al. (1991)	8	2 mo	single-blind	—	→	—	→
Agnoli et al. (1990)	10	2 mo	double-blind placebo	—	↑	—	—
Burke et al. (1993a,b)	38	2/15 mo	double-blind placebo	→	→	→	(↑)
Schneider et al. (1993)	10	1 mo	double-blind placebo, cross. tacrine +/− selegeline	—	↑	—	—
Lawlor et al. (1997)	25	3 mo	double-blind placebo	—	(↑)	—	(↑)

↑ = sign. improvement, (↑) questionable improvement, → = unchanged, — = not tested. *GLOBAL* clinical global impression, *COG* cognitive test performance, *ADL* activities of daily living, *BEHAV* general psychopathology and behaviour

seemed relatively constant, even though 3 studies (Burke et al., 1993a,b; Goad et al., 1991; Lawlor et al., 1997) failed to demonstrate any efficacy.

The type of study mentioned here is designed to evaluate an improvement in symptomatology (responder studies), particularly in neuropsychological domains. Activities of daily living, behavioural symptoms and clinicians' global impression were assessed less frequently.

The above mentioned Alzheimer's Disease Cooperative Study (Sano et al., 1997) revealed evidence, that selegiline may slow the disease progression in DAT. On average, the slowing effect of selegiline amounted to 215 days over the observation period of 2 years.

In contrast to the short-term studies mentioned above, no positive changes were found in neuropsychological tests in any group (selegiline, vitamin E, combination therapy).

Summing up the data, the experiences provide growing evidence, that selegiline may serve as an antidementive agent.

Clinical experiences with the AGE inhibitor tenilsetam

Accumulation of AGEs in the brain is a feature of aging and degenerative diseases, in particular in Alzheimer's dementia. In this process, oxidative stress can occur in various ways (Münch et al., 1996). The substance tenilsetam, which like piracetam comes from the group of pyrrolidinone derivatives, inhibits protein crosslinking in vitro within the framework of AGE formation, and prevents the formation of stable, crosslinked amyloid (Münch et al., 1994).

In an open pilot study over 3 months of 12 patients with mild to moderate DAT, significant improvements were found, according to global assessments and to neuropsychological parameters (Ihl et al., 1989).

Conclusion

With reference to the present state of clinical studies there is substantial evidence that the treatment of Alzheimer's disease with vitamin E, selegiline, gingko biloba and idebenone (Gutzmann, this volume) may slow the progression of Alzheimer's disease. In a limited number of DAT patients an improvement of symptomatology may be observed. It seems conceivable, that other substances with antioxidative properties may also demonstrate beneficial effects. The relatively unknown substance tenilsetam has been mentioned here as an example. Results with antiphlogistic substances, oestrogens (Kawas et al., 1997) or new iron chelators are also of interest from the point of view of the hypothesis of oxidative stress in DAT.

The allmost all important question of whether the above-mentioned antidementive effects of the various compounds can be assigned unequivocally to the respective antioxidative properties cannot be answered with final certainty. All clinically tested substances, besides their ability to inhibit oxidative stress, have other active mechanisms which can influence the symptoms of Alzheimer's dementia. Unfortunately substances with a specifically antioxidative action are unknown until now. As a matter of principle, therefore, the possibility of mechanisms other than the antioxidative actions being involved in the antidementive effect cannot be ruled out.

On the other hand, the fact that very different radical scavengers and antioxidative agents with heterogeneous neurochemical points of attack are able to demonstrate similar effects can be seen as an indication that the reduction of oxidative stress will be one important point in the development of future strategies in DAT therapy.

Note added in proof

Further evidence that gingko biloba may have antidementive efficacy comes from a new multicentre study by LeBars et al. (1997) JAMA 278: 1327–1332.

References

Agnoli A, Martucci N, Fabbrini G, Buckley A, Fioravanti M (1990) Monoamine oxidase and dementia: treatment with an inhibitor of MAO-B activity. Dementia 1: 109–114

Agnoli A, Fabbrini G, Fioravanti M, Martucci N (1992) CBF and cognitive evaluation of Alzheimer type patients before and after MAO-B treatment: a pilot study. Eur Neuropharm 2: 31–35

Bell J, Beglan C, London E (1996) Interaction of ascorbic acid with the neurotoxic effects of NMDA and sodium nitroprusside. Life Sci 58: 367–371

Burke W, Ranno A, Roccaforte W, Wengel S, Bayer B, Willcockson N (1993a) L-deprenyl in the treatment of mild dementia of the Alzheimer type: preliminary results. J Am Geriatr Soc 41: 367–370

Burke W, Roccaforte W, Wengel S, Bayer B, Ranno A, Willcockson N (1993b) L-deprenyl in the treatment of mild dementia of the Alzheimer type: results of a 15-month trial. J Am Geriatr Soc 41: 1219–1225

Burns A, Marsh A, Bender D (1989) A trial of vitamin supplementation in senile dementia. Int J Ger Psychiat 4: 333–338

Burton G, Ingold K (1989) Vitamin E as an in vitro and vivo antioxidant. Ann NY Acad Sci 570: 7–21

Campi N, Todeschini GP, Scarzella L (1990) Selegiline versus l-acetylcarnitine in the treatment of Alzheimer-type dementia. Clin Ther 12: 306–3314

Frei B, England L, Ames B (1989) Ascorbate is an outstanding antioxidant in human blood plasma. Proc Natl Acad Sci 86: 6377–6381

Frölich I, Riederer P (1995) Free radical mechanisms in dementia of Alzheimer type and the potential for antioxidative treatment. Drug Res 45: 443–446

Falsaperla A, Monici Preti PA, Oliani C (1990) Selegiline versus oxiracetam in patients with Alzheimer's type dementia. Clin Ther 12: 376–384

Fahn S (1992) A pilot trial of high-dose alpha-tocopherol and ascorbate in early Parkinson's disease. Ann Neurol 32: 128–132

Finali G, Piccirilli M, Oliani C, Piccinin GL (1991) L-deprenyl therapy improves verbal memory in amnestic Alzheimer patients. Clin Neuropharm 14: 523–536

Finali G, Piccirilli M, Oliani C, Piccinin GL (1992) Alzheimer-type dementia and verbal memory performance: influence of selegiline therapy. Ital J Neurol Sci 13: 141–148

Gardes-Albert M, Khalil A, Fortun A, Bonnefont-Rousselot D, Delattre J, Droy-Lefaix MT (1995) Protective effect of Gingko biloba extract (Egb 761) against the lipid peroxidation of low-density lipoproteins initiated by ·OH and O_2· free radicals. In: Christen Y, Courtois Y, Droy-Lefaix MT (eds) Advances in gingko biloba research. Elsevier, Paris

Gerlach M, Riederer P, Youdim M (1995) Neuroprotective therapeutic strategies. Biochem Pharmacol 50: 1–16

Goad DL, Davis CM, Liem P, Fuselier CC, McCormack JR, Olsen KM (1991) The use of selegeline in Alzheimer's patients with behavior problems. J Clin Psychiat 52: 342–345

Gsell W, Conrad R, Hickethier M, Sofic E, Frölich L, Wichart I, Jellinger K, Moll G, Ransmayr G, Beckmann H, Riederer P (1965) Decreased catalase activity in brains of patients with dementia of Alzheimer type. J Neurochem 64: 1216–1223

Halliwell B (1992) Reactive oxygen species and the central nervous system. J Neurochem 59: 1609–1623

Hennekens C, Buring J, Peto R (1994) Antioxidant vitamins — benefits not yet proved. N Engl J Med 330: 1080–1081

Herrschaft H (1992) Zur klinischen Anwendung von Gingko biloba bei dementiellen Syndromen. Pharmazie in unserer Zeit 21: 266–275

Hofferberth B (1994) The efficacy of Egb 761 in patients with senile dementia of the Alzheimer type, a double blind, placebo-controlled study on different levels of investigation. Hum Psychopharmacol 9: 215–222

Hopfenmüller W (1994) Nachweis der therapeutischen Wirksamkeit eines Gingko biloba-Spezialextraktes. Drug Res 44: 1005–1013

Ihl R, Perisic I, Maurer K, Dierks T (1989) Effect of 3 months treatment with tenilsetam in patients suffering from dementia of Alzheimer type (DAT). J Neural Transm [PD-Sect] 1: 84–85

Jenner P (1994) Oxidative damage in neurodegenerative disease. Lancet 344: 796–798

Kanowski S, Herrmann WM, Staphan K, Wierich W, Hörr R (1996) Proof of efficacy of the Gingko biloba special extract Egb 761 in outpatients suffering from mild to moderate primary degenerative dementia of the Alzheimer Type or multi-infarct dementia. Pharmacopsychiatry 29: 47–56

Kawas C, Resnick S, Morrison A, Brookmeyer R, Corrada M, Zonderman A, Bacal C, Donnell Lingle D, Metter E (1997) A prospective study of estrogen replacement therapy and the risk of developing Alzheimer's disease: The Baltimore Longitudinal Study of Aging. Neurology 48: 1517–1521

Kleijnen J, Knipschild P (1992) Gingko biloba. Lancet 340: 1136–1139

Koutsilieri E, O'Callaghan JF, Chen TS, Riederer P, Rausch WD (1994) Selegiline enhances survival and neurite outgrowth of MPP^+-treated dopaminergic neurons. Eur J Pharmacol 269: R3–R4

Lawlor B, Aisen P, Green C, Fine E, Schmeidler J (1997) Selegiline in the treatment of behavioural disturbance in Alzheimer's disease. Int J Ger Psychiat 12: 319–322

Liebler D (1993) Antioxidant reactions of carotenoids. Ann NY Acad Sci 691: 20–31

Mangoni A, Grassi MP, Frattola L, Piolti R, Bassi S, Motta A, Marcone A, Smirne S (1991) Effects of a MAO-B inhibitor in the treatment of Alzheimer's disease. Eur Neurol 31: 100–107

Martignoni E, Bono G, Blandini F, Sinforiani E, Merlo P, Nappi G (1991) Monoamines and related metabolite levels in the cerebrospinal fluid of patients with dementia of Alzheimer's type. Influence of treatment with l-deprenyl. J Neural Transm [PD-Sect] 3: 15–25

Meydani M (1995) Vitamin E. Lancet 345: 170–174

Monteverde A, Gnemmi P, Rossi F, Monteverde A (1990) Selegiline in the treatment of mild to moderate Alzheimer-type dementia. Clin Ther 12: 315–322

Münch G, Taneli Y, Schraven E, Schindler U, Schinzel R, Palm D, Riederer P (1994) The cognition-enhancing drug tenilsetam is an inhibitor of protein crosslinking by advanced glycosylation. J Neural Transm [PD-Sect] 8: 193–208

Münch G, Simm A, Double KL, Riederer P (1996) Commentary: oxidative stress and advanced glycation endproducts — parts of a vicious circle of neurodegeneration. Alzheimer's Dis Rev 1: 71–74

Packer L, Haramaki N, Kawabata T, Marcocci L, Maitra I, Maguire JJ, Droy-Lefaix MT, Sebaki AH, Gardes-Albert M (1995) Gingko biloba extract (Egb 761): antioxidant action and prevention of oxidative stress-induced injury. In: Christen Y, Courtois Y, Droy-Lefaix MT (eds) Advances in Gingko biloba research, vol 4. Elsevier, Paris

Parkinson Study Group (1993) Effects of tocopherol and deprenyl on the progression of disability in early Parkinson's disease. N Engl J Med 328: 176–183

Parnetti L, Ambrosoli L, Abate G, Azzini C, Balestreri R, Bordin A, Crepaldi G, Christiani G, Cucinotta D (1995) Posatireline for the treatment of late onset Alzheimer's disease: a double-blind multicentre study vs citicoline and ascorbic acid. Acta Neurol Scand 92: 135–140

Peyser CE, Folstein M, Chase GA, Starkstein S, Brandt J, Cockrell JR, Bylsma F, Coyle JT, McHugh PR, Folstein SE (1995) Trial of d-α-Tocopherol in Huntington's disease. Am J Psychiatry 152: 1771–1775

Piccinin GL, Final G, Piccirilli M (1990) Neuropsychological effects of l-deprenyl in Alzheimer's type dementia. Clin Neuropharm 13: 147–163

Sano M, Ernesto C, Thomas R, Klauber M, Schafer K, Grundman M, Woodbury P, Growdon J, Cotman C, Pfreifer E, Schneider L, Thal L (1997) A controlled trial of selegiline, alpha-tocopherol, or both as treatment for Alzheimer's disease. N Engl J Med 336: 1216–1222

Schneider L, Pollo V, Zemansky M, Gleason R, Palmer R, Sloane B (1991) A pilot study of low-dose l-deprenyl in Alzheimer's disease. J Ger Psychiat Neurol 4: 143–148

Schneider L, Olin J, Pawluczyk S (1993) A double-blind crossover pilot study of l-deprenyl (selegiline) combined with cholinesterase inhibitor in Alzheimer's disease. Am J Psychiatry 150: 321–323

Smith MA, Sayre L, Perry G (1996) Is Alzheimer's a disease of oxidative stress? Alzheimer's Dis Rev 1: 63–67

Sunderland T, Tariot PN, Cohen RM, Newhouse PA, Mellow AM, Mueller EA, Murphy DL (1987) Dose-dependent effects of deprenyl on CSF metabolites in patients with Alzheimer's disease. Psychopharmacology 91: 293–296

Tariot P, Cohen R, Sunderland T, Newhouse P, Yount D, Mellow A, Weingartner H, Mueller E, Murphy D (1987) L-deprenyl in Alzheimer's disease. Arch Gen Psychiatry 44: 427–433

Tariot P, Sunderland T, Weingartner H, Murphy D, Welkowitz J, Thompson K, Cohen R (1987) Cognitive effects of l-deprenyl in Alzheimer's disease. Psychopharmacology 91: 489–495

Thome J, Gsell W, Rösler M, Kornhuber J, Frölich I, Hashimoto E, Zielke B, Wiesbeck G, Riederer P (1996) Oxidative stress associated parameters (lactoferrin, superoxide dismutase) in serum of patients with Alzheimer's disease. Life Sci 60: 13–19

Weitbrecht WU, Jansen W (1986) Primär degenerative Demenz: Therapie mit Gingko-biloba-Extrakt. Fortschr Med 104: 199–202

White HL, Scates P, Cooper BR (1996) Extracts of Gingko biloba leaves inhibit monoamine oxidase. Life Sci 58: 1315–1321

Authors' address: Dr. M. Rösler, Psychiatric Department, University of Würzburg, Füchsleinstrasse 15, D-97080 Würzburg, Federal Republic of Germany

Free radicals in Alzheimer's disease

W. Retz[1], **W. Gsell**[1], **G. Münch**[2], **M. Rösler**[1], and **P. Riederer**[1]

[1] Department of Psychiatry, and [2] Physiological Chemistry, Biocenter, University of Würzburg, Federal Republic of Germany

Summary. Alzheimer's disease is a neurodegenerative disorder comprising multisystem atrophies probably caused by multifactorial processes. The disease is characterized by typical neuropathology, impaired synaptic function and massive cell loss. The pathobiochemistry of this disorder involves oxidative stress, which accumulates free radicals leading to excessive lipid peroxidation and neuronal degeneration in certain brain regions. Moreover, radical induced disturbances of DNA, proteins and lipid membranes have been measured. The hypothesis has been proposed that cellular events involving oxidative stress may be one basic pathway leading to neurodegeneration in Alzheimer's disease. In this work we report evidence for increased oxidative stress and disturbed defense mechanisms in Alzheimer's disease, which may result in a self-propagating cascade of neurodegenerative events. Furthermore it is evident from experimental data, that aggregation of β-amyloid and β-amyloid toxicity is favourably caused by oxidative stress. Therefore, oxidative stress plays a key role in the conversion of soluble to unsoluble β-amyloid, suggesting that oxidative stress is primary to the β-amyloid cascade.

Alzheimer's disease represents the most common cause of senile dementia. However, since the first clinical and neuropathological description 90 years ago (Alzheimer, 1907) etiology and exact pathogenesis of this disease is still not clear. Pathological presentation of Alzheimers disease involves regionalized, transmitter-specific neuronal loss (Braak and Braak, 1991; Greenamyre and Maragos, 1993), synaptic pathology (Adams, 1991) and an accumulation of intracellular and extracellular protein aggregates presenting as neurofibrillary tangles and senile plaques respectively. These prominent neuropathological abnormalities have focused scientific interest on several independent parameters, which have been suggested to be responsible for these pathological changes, including hyperphosphorylation of cytoskeletal proteins (tau-protein), metabolism of β-amyloid and the β-amyloid precursor protein (APP) and the polymorphism of apolipoprotein E (APO-E). There is strong evidence that changes of brain glucose metabolism (Hoyer, 1996), mitochondrial disturbances (Wallace, 1992; Beal, 1996), excitotoxicity (Shaw, 1992), immunological processes (Bauer and Berger, 1993) and the biosynthesis of advanced glycation end products (AGEs) (Thome et al., 1996) might be primary responsible for Alzheimer's disease pathology. At present, there is no conclusive hypothesis to unify the enormous number of neuropathological and neurochemical findings. It has been concluded, that Alzheimer's disease might be a heterogenous disease (St George-Hyslop et al., 1990), with a wide spectrum of etiological factors, each of which is able to originate a cascade of pathological processes, leading to an at least uniform condition presenting clinically as dementia.

However, there is now a confluence of opinion that free radical oxidative stress plays a key role among the factors of this pathogenetic cascade of Alzheimer's disease (Benzi and Moretti, 1995). Oxygen free radicals are of particular interest, because of their interactions with almost all hypotheses about the pathogenesis of Alzheimer's disease, and the formation of unsoluble beta-amyloid in particular. Moreover, damage due to oxidative stress accumulates with age (Benzi et al., 1989) and age is the most important risk factor for Alzheimer's disease (Bachman et al., 1993).

Oxygen free radicals are formed as by-products of respiration and oxidative metabolism in all aerobic organisms. It is well established that the generation of radical molecules can lead to damage or destruction of a variety of tissues (McCord and Fridovich, 1988). Consequences of excessive reactive oxygen species are lipid peroxidation, oxidation of proteins and damage of DNA (Götz et al., 1994). It has been hypothesized, that normal aging is a result of permanent oxidative stress (Harman, 1956). Normal age-related radical damage is caused by environmental factors (chemicals, UV radiation, cosmic rays) and endogenous factors including the constant electron leakage in the mitochondrial respiratory chain (Zoccarato et al., 1988), the generation of superoxide and hydrogen peroxide by several enzyme systems, the formation of alkoxy and peroxy radicals from lipids, autooxidation and oxidative deamination of dopamine and the catalytic activity of iron (Götz et al., 1994). On the other hand detoxifying enzymes, e.g. glutathione peroxidase, gluthathione reductase, superoxide dismutase and catalase together with antioxidant mechanisms such as the glutathione system and vitamin E, C and A are involved in the defense system against radical injury (Halliwell and Gutteridge, 1984). An imbalance between the formation of oxygen free radicals due to a increased biosythesis or intake of toxins generating radicals and the protective mechanisms has been proposed as a major factor not only for normal aging, but also for pathological neurodegenerative processes and Alzheimer's disease in particular (Götz et al., 1994; Smith et al., 1995a).

Evidence of increased free radical production in Alzheimer's disease

Since there is much evidence that oxidative stress might be of significance in the etiopathogenesis of Alzheimer's disease, studies have been performed in the last years to prove this hypothesis and to demonstrate either an increase of free radical activity or a decrease of antioxidative defense in Alzheimer's disease. Zhou et al. (1995) demonstrated a 22% increased formation of free radicals following stimulation with $FeSO_4$ in postmortem frontal cortex from Alzheimer patients compared to age-matched normal controls, using electon paramagnetic resonance spectroscopy. The relevance of this finding for radical formation in vivo remained unclear. Direct evidence of increased radical production in Alzheimer's disease in vivo has never been demonstrated. However, own preliminary data from a challenge to estimate the free radical status in Alzheimer patients, determined as salicylate hydroxylation products after infusion of acetylsalicylic acid (Grootveld and Halliwell, 1986; Thome et al., 1997a), suggest an increase of overall free radical production in these patients in vivo (unpublished data).

Early investigations in postmortem brain tissue from Alzheimer patients and age-matched normal controls have shown changes of phospholipid metabolism suggestive for alterations of membrane function in Alzheimer's disease (Sofic et al., 1991; Nitsch et al., 1991, 1992), which may be due to free radical injury. In further studies regional alterations of a variety of markers of oxidative stress, e.g. lipid peroxidation (Table 1), oxidation of proteins and nucleic acids (Smith et al., 1991; Meccoci et al., 1994; Smith et al., 1996a), in Alzheimer's disease brains have been demonstrated. A selective increase of malondialdehyde, a product of lipid peroxidation was measured in the inferior temporal cortex of postmortem Alzheimer brain tissue (Palmer and Burns, 1994). Subbarao et al. (1990) found significantly elevated basal and iron-induced lipid peroxidation, which has been determined by the amount of thiobarbituric acid reactive substances (TBARS), in frontal cortex but not in cerebellum of Alzheimer's disease brains. Balazs and Leon (1994) also demonstrated increased TBARS concentration in multiple brain regions, significantly elevated in motor, sensory and occipital cortices. In other investigations of lipid peroxidation in Alzheimers disease, significant higher levels of TBARS compared to normal controls were found in several brain regions when tissues were stimulated with $FeSO_4$ and/or H_2O_2 (Hajimohammadreza and Brammer, 1990; Lovell et al., 1995). Andorn et al. (1990) described decreased $FeSO_4$ stimulation of TBARS in postmortem brain particular membrane fractions of Alzheimer's patients suggesting increased lipid peroxidation antemortem. However, it has been also argued that measurement of TBARS reflects susceptibility of brain tissue to oxygen-induced radical formation in vitro rather than products of lipid hydroperoxides performed in vivo (Götz et al., 1993).

Several studies have focused on iron (Fe) metabolism in Alzheimer's disease brains. Iron is a reactive agent that catalyses oxidation reactions and, depending on redox state, the generation of oxygen radicals via Fenton reaction (Halliwell and Gutteridge, 1984). Therefore, altered iron metabolism may cause neurodegenerative processes (Gerlach et al., 1994). Increased postmortem levels of total iron in Alzheimer's disease have been reported (Connor et al., 1992a; Good et al., 1992; Kala et al., 1996), but were not found in all investigations (Götz et al., 1992). In vivo evaluation of brain iron using magnetic resonance imaging revealed significantly higher iron content in caudate nucleus and globus pallidus of Alzheimer patients compared to normal

Table 1. Lipid peroxidation measured in several postmortem brain regions or serum from Alzheimer patients

Author	Parameter	Investigated compartment	Significant results
Ahlskog et al. (1995)	MDA	serum	no differences between Alzheimer patients and normal controls
Andorn et al. (1990)	TBARS	brain membrane fractions	decreased $FeSO_4$ stimulation of TBARS
Balazs and Leon (1994)	MDA	subcortical and cortical brain regions	significantly elevated concentration in motor, sensory and occipital cortex in AD
Hajimohammadreza and Brammer (1990)	MDA	brain regions	significant higher $FeSO_4/H_2O_2$ stimulated, but not basal MDA concentration in AD
Jaendel et al. (1989)	MDA	serum	no differences between AD and controls
Lovell et al. (1995)	TBARS	subcortical and cortical brain regions	significant elevation in hippocampus and pyriform cortex from AD patients compared to normal controls
Palmer and Burns (1994)	MDA	neocortical brain regions	significantly increased concentration in inferior temporal cortex from AD brains
Richardson (1993)	TBARS	brain cortex	significant elevation of TBARS in cortex of AD patients and further increase by iron
Subbarao et al. (1990)	TBARS	frontal cortex cerebellum	significant higher peroxidation in frontal cortex in AD compared to controls

AD Alzheimer's disease, *MDA* malondialdehyde, *TBARS* thiobarbituric acid reactive substances

controls, but not in frontal white matter and putamen (Bartzokis et al., 1994). The variance of results may be due, at least in part, to region-specific differences and discrimination of gray and white matter (Ehmann et al., 1986; Thompson et al., 1988). Further evidence for oxidative stress due to disruption of brain iron homeostasis comes from investigations of iron-regulatory proteins. In Alzheimer's disease, transferrin and ferritin have been found, beside their locatization in oligodendrocytes similar to normal brain, in astrocytes and in and close to amyloid plaques and neurofibrillary tangles (Grundke-Iqbal et al., 1990; Jellinger et al., 1990). Transferrin was found decreased in the white matter of various cortical regions, whereas ferritin and iron changes were inconsistent (Connor et al., 1992b). It has been speculated that defective binding of iron (and aluminium) to the transferrin C2 genetic subtype, which has been found significantly increased in Alzheimer's disease (van Rensburg et al., 1995) is of particular importance for radical-induced neuronal damage. Fleming and Joshi (1987) reported higher amounts of iron and aluminium in brain ferritin from Alzheimer patients. This together with reduced [³H]transferrin binding sites to hippocampus in Alzheimer's disease (Morris et al., 1994) may reflect decreased iron mobility in Alzheimer brains, responsible for locally enhanced free radical formation.

Lactoferrin, which is able to bind iron even at low pH values (4.0) and is involved in iron autoxidation has been found in an immunocyto-chemical study of Alzheimer diseased brains up-regulated in both neuronal and glial cells (Kawamata et al., 1993). Since lactoferrin may serve as an iron scavenger and complement inhibitor, this finding may be interpreted as defense reaction against oxidative stress in Alzheimer's disease (Halliwell and Gutteridge, 1984). However, lactoferrin measured in serum of Alzheimer's patients revealed no difference to normal controls (Thome et al., 1997b).

Further evidence for radical involvement in the pathogenesis of Alzheimer's disease comes from elevated aluminium levels (Delamarche, 1989; Ebrahim et al., 1989; Gautrin and Gauthier, 1989). Although data on aluminium content in Alzheimer brain tissue is a matter of controversy, data suggest aluminium accumulation at least in degenerating neurons (Markesberry and Ehmann, 1994). The most prominent aluminium contents occur within the neurofibrillary tangles (Good et al., 1992; Perl and Good, 1992). Even though neurotoxicity of aluminium is moderate, it increases iron cytotoxicity as a radical producing Fenton reagent (Gutteridge et al., 1985; Aruoma et al., 1989) and may hereby parcipitate in cross-linking of cytoskeletal proteins. Furthermore, in the presence of iron, aluminium induces a threefold increase of TBARS suggesting lipid peroxidation due to oxidative stress (Quinlan et al., 1988).

Moreover, decreased concentration of ceruloplasmin in gray and white matter from superior temporal gyrus in Alzheimer's disease has been reported (Connor et al., 1993). This loss of this copper binding and antioxidant protein is in line with the above mentioned findings of changes of reactive transition metals in brain tissue of Alzheimer patients, resulting in oxidative stress. Investigations of ceruloplasmin concentration in serum of Alzheimer patients showed no significant changes (Jeandel et al., 1989).

Another source of radical formation in chronic neurodegenerative disorders comes from central monoamine oxidase (MAO) activity (Riederer and Youdim, 1993; Götz et al., 1994). Several studies reported increased activities of MAO-B in the brain and platelets of patients suffering from dementia (Adolfsson et al., 1980; Oreland and Gottfries, 1986; Danielczyk et al., 1988; Fischer et al., 1994). In a 4 year follow up study, Götz et al. (1998) recently showed that MAO-B activity increases with severity of Alzheimer syndrome, probably due to advanced alterations of monoaminergic neu-rotransmitter systems in Alzheimer's disease. Therefore, the significance of MAO-B activity as an indirect source of oxidative stress may accelerate with disease progression.

Changes of antioxidative mechanisms in Alzheimer's disease

In order to prevent damage from lipids, proteins and DNA, neurons are equipped with several detoxifying enzyms and antioxidants. Whereas catalase (CAT), glutanthione peroxidase (GSH-px) and superoxid dismutase (SOD) prevent formation of reactive oxidants, non-enzymatic biological anti-oxidants, such as tocopherols, carotenoids, quinones, bilirubine, steroids, ascorbate, uric acid, glutathione (GSH) and cysteine, serve as free radical scavengers. There is evidence that not only free radical generation but also

Table 2. Studies of antioxidants and detoxifying enzymes in Alzheimer's disease (AD)

Author	Parameter	Investigated compartment	Significant results
Adams et al. (1991)	GSH, GSSG vitamin E	cortical and subcortical human brain regions	significant higher GSH levels in hippocampus, doubled midbrain vitamin E levels AD compared to controls
Balazs and Leon (1994)	SOD, CAT GSH	cortical and subcortical human brain regions	significant elevation of CAT in amygdala, SOD in occipital lobe compared to controls
Ceballos-Picot et al. (1996)	GSH-px	plasma erythrocytes	significant increase of plasma GSH-px activity in AD compared to controls
Chen et al. (1994)	SOD CAT GSH-px	cortical and subcortical human brain regions	significant lower SOD activity in frontal cortex, cerebellum and hippocampus from AD patients compared to controls
Gsell et al. (1995)	SOD CAT	cortical and subcortical human brain regions	significant reduction of CAT activity in parietotemporal cortex, basal ganglia and amygdala in AD compared to controls
Jeandel et al. (1989)	SOD GSH-px vitamin E, C, A	erythrocytes serum	significant decrease in GSH-px in erythro-cytes and serum vitamin E, C and A in AD patients compared to controls
Kish et al. (1986)	GSH-px	hippocampus, temporal and frontal cortex	no significant differences to normal controls
Lovell et al. (1995)	SOD, CAT GSH-px, GSSG-R	cortical and subcortical human brain regions	significant elevation of GSH-px, GSSG-R and CAT activity in hippocampus, amygdala (GSSG-R) and temporal cortex (CAT) of AD patients
Makar et al. (1995)	GSH	superior frontal gyrus cerebellum	significant increase in AD brains but not in normal controls

(continued)

defense mechanisms are altered in Alzheimer's disease. Changes of metal-binding proteins like ferritin, transferrin, lactoferrin and ceruloplasmin in Alzheimer's disease known so far, are described above.

Data about antioxidative enzymes in Alzheimer's disease, including post-mortem investigations of affected brain tissue, peripheral cells and serum concentrations, are conflicting (Table 2). It has been demonstrated that an unbalanced high activity of SOD occurs concomitantly with a decreased activity of CAT in basal ganglia, parietotemporal cortex and amygdala from Alzheimer patients, resulting in an increased level of H_2O_2 (Gsell et al., 1995). In contrast, significantly elevated activities of CAT in hippocampus and temporal cortex of Alzheimer patients are reported, together with an increase of GSH-px in hippocampus and GSSG-R activity in hippocampus and amygdala (Lovell et al., 1995). In hippocampus of Alzheimer patients also a significant higher level of GSH has been found compared to normal controls (Adams et al., 1991), whereas in frontal cortex and cerebellum an increase of GSH

Table 2. *Continued*

Margaglione et al. (1995)	radical generation	monocyte suspensions	normal free radical generation in monocytes of Ad patients
Marklund et al. (1985)	SOD	hypothalamus, hippocampus caudate nucleus, gyrus cinguli	no difference to normal controls
Metcalfe et al. (1989)	vitamin E	cortical human brain regions	no difference to normal controls
Perrin et al. (1990)	SOD CAT GSH-px	erythrocytes plasma	significant increase in erythrocyte SOD and CAT activity in AD compared to non-demented controls
Richardson (1993)	SOD CAT GSH-px	cortical and subcortical human brain regions	30% reduced SOD activity in frontal cortex, hippocampus and cerebellum of AD patients
Subbarao et al. (1990)	GSH	frontal cortex cerebellum	no difference between Alzheimer patients and normal controls
Thome et al. (1997)	SOD	serum	significant reduced SOD activity in AD compared to normal controls
Urakami et al. (1995)	SOD SODmRNA	serum, CSF, fibroblasts	significant higher SOD activity and SODmRNA in fibroblasts of AD patients
Zaman et al. (1992)	vitamin A, E carotenoids	serum	significant lower levels of vitamin A, E and beta-carotene in AD compared to controls
Zemlan et al. (1989)	SOD	fibroblast cell lines	30% elevated SOD activity in AD compared to normal controls

CAT catalase, *GSH* glutathione, *GSH-px* glutathione peroxidase, *GSSG* glutathione disulfide, *GSSG-R* glutathione reductase, *SOD* superoxide dismutase

with age has been described, which was not found in non-demented subjects (Makar et al., 1995). However, others did not find a significant difference of GSH concentration between Alzheimer brains and age-matched controls in these brain regions (Subbarao et al., 1990). Measures of other antioxidants like vitamin E (α-tocopherole) revealed doubled levels in the midbrain of Alzheimer patients compared to normal controls (Adams et al., 1991). Kish et al. (1986) did not find alterations of GSH-px in postmortem brains of demented patients compared to neurologically normal adults. Concerning studies of SOD, some, but not all investigators (Marklund et al., 1985; Gsell et al., 1995; Lovell et al., 1995), found decreased SOD activities in several regions from Alzheimer patient brains, e.g. hippocampus, frontal cortex and cerebellum (Richardson, 1993; Chen et al., 1994). Interestingly, there comes evidence from many studies suggesting regional differences of oxidative stress in Alzheimer brains, which can not be demonstrated in non-affected human brains (Marttila et al., 1988). Taken together, postmortem investigations in human brain strongly argue for changes of antioxidant defense mechanisms in Alzheimer's disease.

In some studies antioxidative enzyme activities in plasma/serum and periperal cells have been investigated (Table 3). In erythrocytes, normal (Sulkava et al., 1986; Perrin et al., 1990) and elevated GSH-px activities have been measured (Anneren et al., 1986). A significant increase of GSH-px was also found in plasma of Alzheimer patients (Ceballos-Picot et al., 1996). Jeandel et al. (1989) described a deficiency of SOD, GSH-px, vitamin E and C in serum of a subgroup of malnurished Alzheimer patients, suggesting that inadequate nutrition of patients suffering from dementia may contibute to pathogenesis. This may explain, why alterations of serum concentrations of antioxidative vitamins in Alzheimer's disease are not consistent (Zaman et al., 1992; Ahlskog et al., 1995). Ceballos-Picot et al. (1996) reported a significant elevation of plasma GSH-px activity in plasma of Alzheimer patients as compared to controls, but no differences of GSH-px, SOD and GSSG-R

Table 3. Changes of detoxifying enzyme activities in erythrocytes and serum/plasma levels of antioxidants in Alzheimer's disease

Author	SOD	CAT	GSH-px	A	Vitamins E	C
Ahlskog et al. (1995)					↔	
Anneren et al. (1986)			↑			
Ceballos-Picot et al. (1996)	↔		↑[#]			
Jeandel et al. (1989*)	↓		↓	↔	↓	↓
Perrin et al. (1990)	↑	↑	↔			
Sulkava et al. (1986)	↔		↔			
Thome et al. (1996)	↓					
Urakami et al. (1995)	↔					
Zaman et al. (1992)					↓	↓

CAT catalase, *GSH-px* glutathione peroxidase, *SOD* superoxide dismutase. *malnurished patients, [#]activity in plasma

activity has been found in erythrocytes. However, plasma as well as erythrocyte GSH-px activity were negatively correlated with age and no significant correlation with age was observed in controls. Activity of SOD determined in skin fibroblast cell lines from Alzheimer patients has been shown 30% higher when compared to normal euploid cell lines (Zemlan et al., 1989). Moreover, free radical generation in suspensions of monocytes from Alzheimer patients has been found neither quantitatively nor qualitatively different from normal controls (Margaglione et al., 1995). Although changes of peripheral markers of oxidative stress in Alzheimer's disease are not consistent and do not directly reflect free radical damage to the central nervous system, they do suggest that Alzheimer's pathology is associated with an imbalance between reactive oxygen species and the peripheral antioxidant opposing mechanisms.

Role of oxidative stress in Alzheimer's disease

Oxidative stress may not be the primary triggering event that starts the pathogenetic cascade of Alzheimer's disease, but in any case it is an important factor for disease progression. In addition to the imbalance between the formation and spread of oxygen free radicals and the antioxidant defenses, this hypothesis is supported by the observation that reactive oxygen species are involved in several components of the etiopathogenetic cascade of Alzheimer's disease, including

— formation and neurotoxicity of neurofibrillary tangles and amyloid plaques (Smith et al., 1996b)
— immunological processes (Bauer, 1994)
— mitochondrial dysfunction (Blass et al., 1990; Richardson, 1993)
— disturbed energy homeostasis (Beal, 1995; Hoyer, 1996)
— excitotoxicity (Mattson et al., 1992)
— apoptosis (Busciglio and Yankner, 1995; Greenlund et al., 1995)
— microglia activation (Colton and Gilbert, 1987)
— microvascular alterations (Kawai et al., 1993)
— advanced glycation (Smith et al., 1995b).

One of the most striking features of Alzheimer pathology is the formation and persistence of neurofibrillary tangles (NTF) and amyloid plaques. On the other hand, the mechanisms responsible for aggregation, unsolubility and posttranslational modifications of microtubular and amyloid precursor proteins are still not clear. In fact, microtubular proteins like the cytoskeletal proteins tau and neurofilaments, which normaly are soluble and suceptible to protease, are unsoluble in denaturants and resistant to protease in neurofibrillary tangles (Selkoe et al., 1982). Several posttranslational modifications of tau-protein and β-amyloid are known, e.g. phosphorylation, isomerization, racemization and crosslinking (Smith et al., 1995b). It has been argued that racemization, isomerization or aberrant protein processing might initialize deposition of protein aggregates, but cannot explain alone their observed insolubility. Therefore, non-enzymatic formation of Advanced Glycation Endproducts (AGEs) may play a key role for covalent crosslinking responsible for NTF and β-amyloid insolubility. AGEs are generated by reaction of sugar ketone or aldehyde group with the free amino group of a protein, peptide or amino acid via the Maillard reaction. While addition of reducing sugars to protein sidechain groups is non-oxidative, oxidative reactions are necessary to yield AGEs. Further, evolution of AGE modifications of proteins is accelerated by oxygen in a process called glycoxidation (Baynes, 1991). Therefore, oxidative stress in Alzheimer's disease as discribed above may contribute to AGE formation and the generation of unsolubable protein aggregates.

Some findings provide evidence that AGE formation and oxidative stress are involved in aggregation and stabilization of β-amyloid and NFT. Immuno-histochemical studies have shown that cerebral concentrations of AGEs are increased in Alzheimer's disease and were identified in NFT and amyloid plaques (Smith et al., 1994; Vitek et al., 1994). AGE-modified β-amyloid has been demonstrated to induce aggregates which act as "seeds" for further β-amyloid formation (Maggio et al., 1992). Yan et al. (1996) reported that binding of β-amyloid to an AGE-receptor activates microglia and promotes adherence to amyloid fibrils. It has further been shown that oxidation of β-amyloid by free radicals can generate insoluble protein aggregats (Dyrks et al., 1992) and tau filaments (Troncoso et al., 1993), which are not distinguishabel to those from Alzheimer NFT and senile plaques. In addition, elevation of the free radical scavenging enzyme superoxide dismutase (SOD) observed in fibroblast cell lines from Alzheimer patients supports the theory that paired helical filaments may be synthesized by free radical hydroxylation of proline residues in neurofibrillary precursor proteins (Zemlan et al., 1989).

On the other hand, AGEs induce further oxidative stress due to direct production of free radicals by chemical oxidation and degradation of AGEs (Mullarkey et al., 1990), AGE-receptor binding and activation of signaling pathways (Vlassara et al., 1995) and activation of microglia (McMillian et al., 1995). This might result in a self-propagating cascade of pathological events with oxidative stress as a crucial motor for a vicious circle of neurodegeneration. Therefore, reduction of oxidative stress suggests an interesting opportunity in pharmacological treatment of Alzheimer's disease (Frölich and Riederer, 1995; see also Rösler et al., this volume).

References

Adams IM (1991) Structural plasticity of synapses in Alzheimer's disease. Mol Neurobiol 5: 411–419

Adams JD, Klaidman LK, Odunze IN, Shen HC, Miller CA (1991) Alzheimer's disease and Parkinson's disease. Brain levels of glutathione, glutathione disulfide, and vitamin E. Mol Chem Neuropathol 14: 213–226

Adolfsson R, Gottfries C-G, Oreland L, Wiberg A, Winblad B (1980) Increased activity of brain and platelet monoamine oxidase in dementia of Alzheimer type. Life Sci 27: 1029–1034

Ahlskog JE, Uitti RJ, Low PA, Tyce GM, Nickander KK, Petersen RC, Kokmen E (1995) No evidence for systemic oxidant stress in Parkinson's or Alzheimer's disease. Mov Disord 10: 566–573

Alzheimer A (1907) Über eine eigenartige Erkrankung der Hirnrinde. Allg Z Psychiat 64: 146–148

Andorn AC, Britton RS, Bacon BR (1990) Evidence that lipid peroxidation and total iron are increased in Alzheimer's brain [abstract]. Neurobiol Aging 11: 316

Anneren G, Gardner A, Lundin T (1986) Increased glutathion peroxidase activity in erythrocytes in patients with Alzheimer's disease/senile dementia of Alzheimer's type. Acta Neurol Scand 73: 586–589

Aruoma OI, Halliwell B, Laughton MJ, Quinlan GJ, Gutteridge JMC (1989) The mechanism of initiation of lipid peroxidation. Evidence against a requirement for an iron(II)–iron(III) complex. Biochem J 258: 617–620

Bachman DL, Wolf PA, Linn RT, Knoefel JE, Cobb JL, Belanger AJ, White LR, D'Agostino RB (1993) Incidence of dementia and probable Alzheimer's disease in a general population: the Framingham Study. Neurology 43: 515–519

Balazs L, Leon M (1994) Evidence of an oxidative challenge in the Alzheimer's brain. Neurochem Res 19: 1131–1137

Bartzokis G, Sultzer D, Mintz J, Holt LE, Marx P, Phelan CK, Marder SR (1994) In vivo evaluation of brain iron in Alzheimer's disease and normal subjects using MRI. Biol Psychiatry 35: 480–487

Bauer J (1994) Die Alzheimer Krankheit. Neurobiologie, Psychosomatik, Diagnostik und Therapie. Schattauer, Stuttgart

Bauer J, Berger M (1993) Neuropathologie, Immunologie und psychobiologische Aspekte der Alzheimer Krankheit. Fortschr Neurol Psychiatr 61: 225–240

Banyes JW (1991) Role of oxidative stress in development of complications in diabetes. Diabetes 40: 405–412

Beal MF (1995) Aging, energy, and oxidative stress in neurodegenerative diseases. Ann Neurol 38: 357–366

Beal MF (1996) Mitochondria, free radicals, and neurodegeneration. Curr Opin Neurobiol 6: 661–666

Benzi G, Moretti A (1995) Are reactive oxygen species involved in Alzheimer's disease? Neurobiol Aging 16: 661–674

Benzi G, Marzatico F, Pastoris O, Villa RF (1989) Influence of oxidative stress on the age-linked alterations of the cerebral glutathione system. J Neurosci Res 26: 120–128

Blass JP, Baker AC, Ko L, Black RS (1990) Induction of Alzheimer antigen an uncoupler of oxidative phosphorylation. Arch Neurol 47: 864–869

Braak H, Braak E (1991) Neuropathological staging of Alzheimer-related changes. Acta Neuropathol 82: 239–259

Busciglio J, Yankner BA (1995) Apoptosis and increased generation of reactive oxygen species in Down's syndrome neurons in vitro. Nature 378: 776–779

Ceballos-Picot I, Merad-Boudia M, Nicole A, Thevenin M, Hellier G, Legrain S, Berr C (1996) Peripheral antioxidant enzyme activities and selenium in elderly subjects and in dementia of Alzheimer's type — place of the extracellular glutathion peroxidase. Free Radic Biol Med 20: 579–587

Chen L, Richardson JS, Caldwell JE, Ang LC (1994) Regional brain activity of free radical defense enzymes in autopsy samples from patients with Alzheimer's disease and from nondemented controls. Int J Neurosci 75: 83–90

Colton CA, Gilbert DL (1987) Production of superoxide anions by a CNS macrophage, the microglia. FEBS Lett 223: 284–288

Connor JR, Snyder BS, Beard JL, Fine RE, Mufson EJ (1992a) Regional distribution of iron and iron-regulatory proteins in the brain in aging and Alzheimer's disease. J Neurosci Res 31: 327–335

Connor JR, Menzies SL, St. Martin SM, Mufson EJ (1992b) A histochemical study of iron, transferrin, and ferritin in Alzheimer's diseased brains. Neurosci Res 31: 75–83

Connor JR, Tucker P, Johnson M, Snyder B (1993) Ceruloplasmin levels in the human superior temporal gyrus in aging and Alzheimer's disease. Neurosci Lett 159: 88–90

Danielczyk W, Streifler M, Konradi C, Riederer P, Moll G (1988) Platelet MAO-B activity and the psychopathology of Parkinson's disease, senile dementia and multiinfarct dementia. Acta Psychiatr Scand 78: 730–736

Delamarche C (1989) A homologous domain between the amyloid protein of Alzheimer's disease and the neuriofilament subunits. Biochimie 71: 853–856

Dyrks T, Dyrks E, Hartmann T, Masters C, Beyreuther KE (1992) Amyloidogenicity of β A4 and β A4-bearing amyloid protein precursor fragments by metal-catalyzed oxidation. J Biol Chem 267: 18210–18217

Ebrahim S, Schupf S, Silverman W, Zigman WB, Moretz RC, Wisniewski HM, Taylor E, Devakumar M, Lindegard B, Lindesay J, Grant DJ, McMurdo MET, Corrigan FM, Reynolds GP, Ward NI, Farrar G, Blair JA, Curran S, Hindmarch I, Steer C (1989) Aluminium and Alzheimer's disease. Lancet ii: 267–269

Ehmann WD, Markesbery WR, Alauddin M, Hossain TIM, Brubaker EH (1986) Brain trace elements in Alzheimer's disease. Neurotoxicology 7: 195–206

Fischer P, Götz ME, Ellinger B, Streifler M, Riederer P, Danielczyk W (1994) Platelet monoamine oxidase B activity and vitamin B12 in dementia. Biol Psychiat 35: 772–774

Fleming J, Joshi JG (1987) Ferritin: isolation of aluminium-ferritin complex from brain. Proc Natl Acad Sci 84: 7866–7870

Frölich L, Riederer P (1995) Free radical mechanisms in dementia of Alzheimer type and the potential for antioxidative treatment. Arzneimittelforschung 43: 443–446

Gautrin D, Gauthier S (1989) Alzheimer's disaese: environmental factors and etiologic hypothesis. Can J Neurol Sci 16: 375–387

Gerlach M, Ben Shachar D, Riederer P, Youdim MB (1994) Altered metabolism of iron as a cause of neurodegenerative diseases? J Neurochem 63: 793–807

Götz ME, Freyberger A, Hauer E, Burger R, Sofic E, Gsell W, Heckers S, Jellinger K, Hebenstreit G, Frölich L, Beckmann H, Riederer P (1992) Susceptibility of brains from patients with Alzheimer's disease to oxygen-stimulated lipid peroxidation and differential scanning calorimetry. Dementia 3: 213–222

Götz ME, Dirr A, Freyberger A, Burger R, Riederer P (1993) The thiobarbituric acid assay reflects susceptibility to oxygen-induced lipid peroxidation in vitro rather than levels of lipid hydroperoxides in vivo: a methodological approach. Neurochem Int 22: 255–262

Götz ME, Künig G, Riederer P, Youdim MBH (1994) Oxidative stress: free radical production in neuronal degeneration. Pharmac Ther 63: 37–122

Götz ME, Fischer P, Gsell W, Riederer P, Streifler M, Simanyi M, Müller F, Danielczyk W (1998) Platelet monoamine oxidase B activity in dementia: a 4 year follow up. Dementia 9: 74–77

Good PF, Perl DP, Bierer LM, Schmeidler J (1992) Selective accumulation of aluminium and iron in the neurofibrillary tangles of Alzheimer's disease: a laser microprobe (LAMMA) study. Ann Neurol 31: 286–292

Greenamyre JT, Maragos WF (1993) Neurotransmitter receptors in Alzheimer disease. Cerebrovasc Brain Metab Rev 5: 61–94

Greenlund LJ, Deckwerth TL, Johnson EM Jr (1995) Superoxide dismutase delays neuronal apoptosis: a role for reactive oxygen species in programmed neuronal death. Neuron 14: 303–315

Grootveld M, Halliwell B (1986) Aromatic hydroxylation as a potential measure of hydroxyl radical formation in vivo. Biochem J 237: 499–504

Grundke-Iqbal I, Fleming J, Tung YC, Lassmann H, Iqbal K, Joshi JG (1990) Ferritin is a component of the neuritic (senile) plaque in Alzheimer dementia. Acta Neuropathol (Berl) 81: 105–110

Gsell W, Conrad R, Hickethier M, Sofic E, Frölich L, Wichart I, Jellinger K, Moll G, Ransmayr G, Beckmann H, Riederer P (1995) Decreased catalase activity but unchanged superoxide dismutase activity in brain of patients with dementia of Alzheimer type. J Neurochem 64: 1216–1223

Gutteridge JM, Quinlan GJ, Clark I, Halliwell B (1985) Aluminium salts accelerate peroxidation of membrane lipids stimulated by iron salts. Biochim Biophys Acta 835: 441–447

Halliwell B, Gutteridge JM (1984) Oxygen toxicity, transition metals and disease. Biochem J 219: 1–14

Hajimohammadreza I, Brammer M (1990) Brain membrane fluidity and lipid peroxidation in Alzheimer's disease. Neurosci Lett 112: 333–337

Harman D (1956) Ageing: a theory based on free radical and rediation chemistry. J Gerontol 11: 298–300

Hoyer S (1996) Oxidative metabolism deficiencies in brains of patients with Alzheimer's disease. Acta Neuropathol Scand [Suppl] 165: 18–24

Jeandel C, Nicolas MB, Dubois F, Nabet-Belleville F, Penin F, Cuny G (1989) Lipid peroxidation and free radical scavengers in Alzheimer's disease. Gerontology 35: 275–282

Jellinger K, Paulus W, Grundke-Iqbal I, Riederer P, Youdim MB 1990) Brain iron and ferritin in Parkinson's and Alzheimer's diseases. J Neural Transm [PD-Sect] 2: 327–340

Kala SV, Hasinoff BB, Richardson JS (1996) Brain samples from Alzheimer's patients have elevated levels of loosely bound iron. Int J Neurosci 86: 263–269

Kawai M, Kalaria RN, Cras P, Siedlak SL, Velasco ME, Shelton ER, Chan HW, Greenberg BD, Perry G (1993) Degeneration of vascular muscle cells in cerebral amyloid angiopathy of Alzheimer's disease. Brain Res 623: 142–146

Kawamata T, Tooyama I, Yamada T, Walker DG, McGeer PL (1993) Lactotransferrin immunocytochemistry in Alzheimer and normal human brain. Am J Pathol 142: 1574–1585

Kish SJ, Morito CL, Hornykiewicz O (1986) Brain glutathione peroxidase in neuro-degenerative disorders. Neurochem Pathol 4: 23–28

Lovell MA, Ehmann WD, Butler SM, Markesbery WR (1995) Elevated thiobarbituric acid-reactive substances and antioxidant enzyme activity in the brain of Alzheimer's disease. Neurology 45: 1594–1601

Maggio JE, Stimson ER, Ghilardi JR, Allen CJ, Dahl CE, Whitcomb DC, Vigna SR, Vinters HV, Labenski ME, Mantyh PW (1992) Reversible in vitro growth of Alzheimer disease beta-amyloid plaques by deposition of labeled amyloid peptide. Proc Natl Acad Sci USA 89: 5462–5466

Makar TK, Cooper AJ, Tofel-Grehl B, Thaler HAT, Blass JP (1995) Carnitine, carnitine acetyltransferase, and glutathione in Alzheimer brain. Neurochem Res 20: 705–711

Margaglione M, Garofano R, Cirillo F, Ruocco A, Grandone E, Vecchione G, Milan G, di Minno G, de Blasi A, Postiglione A (1995) Cu/Zn superoxide dismutase in patients with non-familial Alzheimer's disease. Aging Milano 7: 49–54

Markesberry W, Ehmann WD (1994) In: Terry RD, Katzman R, Bick L (eds) Alzheimer's disease. Raven Press, New York, pp 353–367

Marklund SL, Adolffson R, Gottfries CG, Winblad B (1985) Superoxide isoenzymes in normal brains and in brains from patients with dementia of Alzheimer type. J Neurol Sci 67: 319–325

Marttila RJ, Röyttä M, Lorentz H, Rinne UK (1988) Oxygen toxicity protecting enzymes in the human brain. J Neural Transm 74: 87–95

Mattson MP, Cheng B, Davis D, Bryant K, Lieberburg I, Rydel RE (1992) β-amyloid peptides destabilize calcium homeostasis and render human cortical neurons vulnerable to excitotoxicity. J Neurosci 12: 379–389

McCord J, Fridovich I (1988) Superoxide dismutase: the first twenty years (1968–1988). Free Radic Biol Med 5: 363–369

McMillian M, Kong LY, Sawin SM, Wilson B, Das K, Hudson P, Hong JS, Bing G (1995) Selective killing of cholinergic neurons by microglial activation in basal forebrain mixed neuronal/glial cultures. Biochem Biophys Res Commun 215: 572–577

Metcalfe T, Bowen DM, Müller DP (1989) Vitamin E concentrations in human brain from patients with Alzheimer's disease, fetuses with Down's syndrome, cetenarians, and controls. Neurochem Res 14: 1209–1212

Meccoci P, MacGarvey MS, Beal MF (1994) Oxidative damage to mitochondrial DNA is increased in Alzheimer's disease. Ann Neurol 36: 747–751

Morris CM, Candy JM, Kerwin JM, Edwardson JA (1994) Transferrin receptors in the normal human hippocampus and in Alzheimer's disease. Neuropathol Appl Neurobiol 20: 473–477

Mullarkey CJ, Edelstein D, Brownlee M (1990) Free radical generation by early glycation products: a mechanism of accelerated atherogenesis in diabetes. Biochem Biophys Res Commun 173: 923–929

Nitsch RM, Pittas AG, Blusztajin JK, Slack BE, Growdon HJ (1991) Alterations of phospholipid metabolites in postmortem brain from patients with Alzheimer's disease. Ann NY Acad Sci 640: 110–113

Nitsch RM, Blusztajin JK, Pittas AG, Slack BE, Growdon JH, Wurtman RD (1992) Evidence for a membrane defect in Alzheimer disease brain. Proc Natl Acad Sci 89: 1671–1675

Oreland L, Gottfries CG (1986) Brain monoamine oxidase in aging and in dementia of Alzheimer type. Prog Neuropsychopharmacol Biol Psychiatry 10: 533–540

Palmer AM, Burns MA (1994) Selective increase in lipid peroxidation in the inferior temporal cortex in Alzheimer's disease. Brain Res 645: 338–342

Perl DP, Good PF (1992) Aluminium and the neurofibrillary tangle: results of tissue microprobe studies. Ciba Found Symp 169: 217–227

Perrin R, Briancon S, Jaendel C, Artur Y, Min A, Penin F, Siest G (1990) Blood activity of Cu/Zn superoxide dismutase, glutathione peroxidase and catalase in Alzheimer's disease: a case-control study. Gerontology 36: 306–313

Quinlan GJ, Halliwell B, Moorhouse CP, Gutteridge JMC (1988) Action of lead(II) and aluminium(III) ions on iron-stimulated lipid peroxidation in liposomes, erythrocytes and rat liver microsomal fractions. Biochim Biophys Acta 962: 196–200

Richardson JS (1993) Free radicals in the genesis of Alzheimer's disease. Ann NY Acad Sci 695: 73–76

Riederer P, Youdim MBH (1993) The therapeutic place and value of present and future MAO-B inhibitors — L-deprenyl as the gold standard. In: Szeleny I (ed) Inhibitors of monoamine oxidase B. Pharmacology and clinical use in neurodegenerative disorders. Birkhäuser, Basel, pp 327–338

Selkoe DJ, Ihara Y, Salazar F (1982) Alzheimer disease: insolubility of partially purified paired helical filaments in sodium dodecyl sulfate and urea. Science 215: 1243–1245

Shaw PJ (1992) Excitatory amino acid neurotransmission, excitotoxicity and excitotoxins. Curr Opin Neurol Neurosurg 5: 383–390

Smith CD, Corney JM, Starke-Reed PE, Oliver CN, Stadtman ER, Floyd RA, Markesbery WR (1991) Excess brain protein peroxidation and enzyme dysfunction in normal aging and Alzheimer's disease. Am J Pathol 145: 42–47

Smith MA, Taneda S, Richey PL, Yan S-D, Sayre LM, Monnier VM, Perry G (1994) Advanced Mallard reaction end products are associated with Alzheimer disease pathology. Proc Natl Acad Sci USA 91: 5710–5714

Smith MA, Sayre L, Perry G (1995a) Is Alzheimer's a disease of oxidative stress? Alz Dis Rev 1: 63–67

Smith MA, Sayre ML, Monnier VM, Perry G (1995b) Radical AGEing in Alzheimer's disease. Trends Neurosci 18: 172–176

Smith MA, Perry G, Richey PL, Sayre LM, Anderson VE, Beal MF, Kowall N (1996a) Oxidative damage in Alzheimer's. Nature 382: 120–121

Smith MA, Sayre ML, Monnier VM, Perry G (1996b) Oxidative posttranslational modifications in Alzheimer disease. A possible pathogenetic role in the formation of senile plaques and neurofibrillary tangles. Mol Chem Neuropathol 28: 41–48

Sofic E, Frölich L, Riederer P, Jellinger K, Heckers S, Beckmann H, Deinzer E, Pantucek F, Hebenstreit G, Ransmayr (1991) Biochemical membrane constituents and activities of alkaline and acid phosphatase and cathepsin in cortical and subcortical brain areas in dementia of the Alzheimer type. Dementia 2: 39–44

St George-Hyslop PH, Haines JL, Farrer, Polinsky R, van Broeckhoven C, Goate A, McLachlan DR, Orr H, Bruni HC (1990) Genetic linkage studies suggest that Alzheimer's disease is not a single homogeneous disorder. FAD Collaborative Study Group. Nature 347: 194–197

Subbarao KV, Richardson JS, Ang LC (1990) Autopsy samples of Alzheimer's cortex show increased lipid peroxidation in vitro. J Neurochem 55: 342–345

Sulkava R, Nordberg UR, Erkinjuntti T, Westermarck T (1986) Erythrocyte glutathione peroxidase and superoxide dismutase in Alzheimer's disease and other dementias. Acta Neurol Scand 73: 487–489

Thome J, Kornhuber J, Münch G, Schinzel R, Taneli Y, Zielke B, Rösler M, Riederer P (1996) Neue Hypothese zur Äthiopathogenese des Alzheimer-Syndroms — Advanced glycation end products (AGEs). Nervenarzt 67: 924–929

Thome J, Zhang J, Davids E, Foley P, Weijers H-G, Wiesbeck GA, Böning J, Riederer P, Gerlach M (1997a) Evidence for increased oxidative stress in alcohol-dependent patients provided by quantification of in vivo salicylate hydroxylation products. Alcohol Clin Exp Res 21: 82–85

Thome J, Gsell W, Rösler M, Kornhuber J, Frölich L, Hashimoto E, Zielke B, Wiesbeck GA, Riederer P (1997b) Oxidative-stress associated parameters (lactoferrin, superoxide dismutase) in serum of patients with Alzheimer's disease. Life Sci 60: 13–19

Thompson CM, Markesbery WR, Ehmann WD, Mao YX, Vance DE (1988) Regional brain trace-element studies in Alzheimer's disease. Neurotoxicology 9: 1–7

Troncoso JC, Costello A, Watson AL, Johnson GVW (1993) In vitro polymerization of oxidized tau into filaments. Brain Res 613: 313–316

Urakami K, Sato K, Okada A, Mura T, Shimomura T, Takenaka T, Wakutani Y, Oshima T, Adachi Y, Takahashi K et al. (1995) Cu, Zn superoxide dismutase in patients with dementia of the Alzheimer type. Acta Neurol Scand 91: 165–168

van Rensburg SJ, Carstens ME, Potocnik FC, van der Spuy G, van der Walt BJ, Taljaard JJ (1995) Transferrin C2 and Alzheimer's disease: another piece of the puzzle found? Med Hypotheses 44: 268–272

Vitek MP, Bhattacharya K, Glendening JM, Stopa E, Vlassara H, Bucala R, Manogue K, Cerami A (1994) Advanced glycation end products contribute to amyloidosis in Alzheimer disease. Proc Natl Acad Sci USA 91: 4766–4770

Vlassara H, Li YM, Imani F, Wojciechowicz D, Yang Z, Liu FT, Cerami A (1995) Identification of galectin-3 as a high-affinity binding protein for advanced glycation end products (AGE): a new member of the AGE-receptor complex. Mol Med 1: 634–646

Wallace DC (1992) Mitochondrial genetics: a paradigm for aging and degenerative diseases? Science 256: 628–632

Yan SD, Chen X, Fu J, Chen M, Zhu H, Roher A, Slattery T, Zhao L, Nagashima M, Morser J, Migheli A, Nawroth P, Stern D, Schmidt AM (1996) RAGE and amyloid-b peptide neurotoxicity in Alzheimer's disease. Nature 382: 685–691

Zaman Z, Roche S, Fielden P, Frost PG, Niriella DC, Cayley AC (1992) Plasma concentrations of vitamins A and E and carotenoids in Alzheimer's disease. Age Ageing 21: 91–94

Zemlan FP, Thienhaus OJ, Bosmann HB (1989) Superoxide dismutase activity in Alzheimer's disease: possible mechanism for paired helical filament formation. Brain Res 476: 160–162

Zhou Y, Richardson JS, Mombourquette MJ, Weil JA (1995) Free radical formation in autopsy samples of Alzheimer and control cortex. Neurosci Lett 195: 89–92

Zoccarato F, Cavallini L, Deana R, Alexandre A (1988) Pathways of hydrogen peroxide generation in guinea pig cerebral cortex mitochondria. Biochem Biophy Res Commun 154: 727–734

Authors' address: Dr. W. Retz, Psychiatric Department, University of Würzburg, Füchsleinstrasse 15, D-97080 Würzburg, Federal Republic of Germany

Simulation of cortical cholinergic deficits — a novel experimental approach to study pathogenetic aspects of Alzheimer's disease

V. Bigl and **R. Schliebs**

Paul Flechsig Institute for Brain Research, University of Leipzig, Leipzig,
Federal Republic of Germany

Summary. Cholinergic lesion paradigms have been used to study the role of the cholinergic system in cognitive function, and its implication in cognitive deficits that occur in Alzheimer's disease. In the last few years an increasing number of studies have applied neurotoxins including excitotoxins or cholinotoxins to produce reductions in cortical cholinergic activity. One of the most serious limitations of these lesion paradigms is the fact that the cytotoxins used are far from being selective to cholinergic cells. Recently, a monoclonal antibody to the low-affinity nerve growth factor (NGF) receptor, 192IgG, coupled to a cytotoxin, saporin, has been described as an efficient and selective immunotoxin for the NGF-receptor bearing cholinergic neurons in rat basal forebrain. Here we demonstrate the usefulness of 192IgG-saporin as a powerful tool for producing an animal model with selective and specific basal forebrain cholinergic lesions in rats which can be applied to simulate some neurochemical sequelae of Alzheimer's disease including cholinergic mechanisms in processing of the amyloid precursor protein, and could be of particular value to elaborate and to test therapeutical strategies compensating for the reduced cortical cholinergic input.

Introduction

The basal forebrain cholinergic system is known to play an important role in normal cognitive function, and cortical cholinergic dysfunction has been implicated in cognitive deficits that occur in Alzheimer's disease. This is emphasized by post mortem investigations demonstrating that the cholinergic projection from the nucleus basalis of Meynert to areas of the cerebral cortex is the pathway that is most early and severely affected in brains from Alzheimer patients. To characterize the role of the central cholinergic system in cortical information processing, learning and memory it requires adequate animal models to produce specific cholinergic deficits in vivo. This would allow for a detailed evaluation of the neurochemical, neuropathological, and behavioural sequela as well as functional implications of plastic repair mechanisms following cholinergic hypofunction, and provide information that cannot or only partially be obtained in humans. At present there is no adequate animal model available which could mimic all the biochemical, behavioural, and histopathological abnormalities as observed in patients with Alzheimer's disease. However, partial success can be achieved with experimental approaches representing partial parallelism between model and some human conditions (Fisher and Hanin, 1986). The value of such models is to delineate mechanisms underlying the pathological processes as well as to test for new potential therapeutic strategies. In the last few years an increasing number of studies have applied neurotoxins including excitotoxins or cholinotoxins by stereotaxic injection into the nucleus basalis of Meynert to produce reductions in cortical cholinergic activity. One of the most serious limitations of these lesion paradigms, however, is the fact that basal forebrain cholinergic neurons are always intermingled with populations of non-cholinergic cells and that the cytotoxins used are far from being selective to cholinergic cells. Recently, a novel approach for neuronal lesioning has been introduced by Wiley et al. (1991) by using immunotargeting of unspecific cytotoxins. Cholinergic neurons of the basal forebrain possess nerve growth factor (NGF) receptors whereas other neurons in this region including the cholinergic cells in the nearby striatum do not express detectable levels of NGF receptors (Gage et al., 1989; Yan and Johnson, 1989). It was demonstrated that a well-characterized monoclonal antibody to the low-affinity NGF receptor, 192IgG, accumulates bilaterally exclusively in cholinergic neurons of the basal forebrain following intracerebroventricular administration (Thomas et al., 1991). Employing these properties of 192IgG, a cholinergic immunotoxin was developed by chemical linking of 192IgG to the ribosome inactivating protein saporin (192IgG-saporin; Wiley, 1992).

This report describes the usefulness of this experimental approach to elucidate the mechanisms of how basal forebrain cholinergic cells affects cortical neurotransmission (Schliebs et al., 1996), as well as expression and processing of the cortical amyloid precursor protein. Further we demonstrate an example of how to use this model for proving therapeutical strategies.

192IgG-saporin — a useful tool to produce specific and selective basal forebrain cholinergic cell loss

Intracerebroventricular administration of 192IgG-saporin conjugate resulted in substantial reductions in the activity of choline acetyltransferase (ChAT) and acetylcholinesterase (AChE) in widespread areas of the cortex and hippocampus and in a nearly complete disappearance of ChAT-positive, NGF receptor-immunoreactive neurons in the medial septum, in both the vertical and horizontal limbs of the nucleus of the diagonal band of Broca and in the nucleus basalis magnocellularis, whereas cholinergic interneurons in the striatum are not affected (Berger-Sweeney et al., 1994; Book et al., 1992; Heckers et al., 1994; Roßner et al., 1994, 1995a–d). Moreover, a 40%-decrease in m2 muscarinic receptor mRNA in nuclei of the basal forebrain complex was observed after immunolesion, thus further emphasizing the loss of cholinergic cells (Roßner et al., 1995a). Non-cholinergic septal neurons containing parvalbumin and non-cholinergic substantia innominata neurons containing calbindin-D_{28K} or NADPH -diaphorase were not affected by 192IgG-saporin (Heckers et al., 1994). Similarly, the number of parvalbumin-containing GABAergic projection neurons in the septum-diagonal band of Broca complex and nucleus basalis of Meynert was not reduced following intraventricular 192IgG-saporin application (Roßner et al., 1995b; Leanza et al., 1995; Lee et al., 1994). Moreover, 192IgG-saporin did not destroy neurotensin, galanin, somatostatin, or neuropeptide neurons within the basal forebrain (Wenk et al., 1994). Corresponding to the topographic location of cholinergic neurons in the basal forebrain a dramatic increase in microglia has been demonstrated (Roßner et al., 1995b; Seeger et al., 1997), suggesting that the immunotoxin is lethal to cholinergic cells in the basal forebrain rather than suppressing the expression of cholinergic markers (e.g. ChAT) in these cells (Book et al., 1994).

It was found that 192IgG-saporin affects two neuronal groups outside of the basal forebrain which express p75NGF receptors: NGF-reactive cerebellar Purkinje cells after intraventricular injection and cholinergic striatal interneurons after injections into the substantia innominata (Heckers et al., 1994). There are ChAT-positive, but NGF-receptor negative neurons in the rat nucleus basalis-substantia innominata complex innervating the amygdala and parts of the rhinal paralimbic areas (Bickel and Kewitz, 1990; Woolf et al., 1989) which are spared or only partially affected by the immunotoxin (Heckers et al., 1994). Similarly, cholinergic neurons in the ventral pallidum and sublenticular substantia innominata not expressing p75NGF receptors are not affected by the immunotoxin.

Behavioural studies have shown that complete cholinergic lesion by 192IgG-saporin did not produce any deficit in the Morris water maze task (Torres et al., 1994). Despite the high depletion in cortical ChAT activity by 192IgG-saporin acquisition, performance of the delayed alternation or passive avoidance tasks were not impaired by the lesions suggesting that selective loss of cholinergic cells is not sufficient to produce functional impairments (Wenk et al., 1994). In contrast, other authors reported that intracerebral administration of 192IgG-saporin induced dose-dependent (ranging between 1 and 10 µg) impairments in the water maze task and passive avoidance retention, but only weak effects on locomotor activity (Leanza et al., 1995; Waite et al., 1995). Intracerebroventricular injections of 192IgG-saporin severely affected spatial and cued navigation (Berger-Sweeney et al., 1994, Nilsson et al., 1992). However, an almost 90% reduction in ChAT activity is needed to produce substantial behavioural deficits (Waite et al., 1995).

In conclusion, the detailed characterization of 192IgG-saporin suggests that cholinergic immunolesion by 192IgG-saporin exhibits a valuable tool to produce specific cholinergic deficits in rats, which can be used as model to study both the impact of reduced cortical cholinergic input on cortical neurotransmission and the efficiency of novel therapeutic strategies (see also Schliebs et al., 1996).

Effect of cholinergic immunolesion on cortical neurotransmission

Cholinergic degeneration is known to be a very early feature of Alzheimer's disease, and the question arose whether the changes in other neurotransmitter systems observed in brains from Alzheimer patients are consequences of cortical cholinergic deficits.

Receptor autoradiography for a number of receptor subtypes and AChE staining were performed in adjacent brain sections, which allows to simultanously detect the consequences of lesions on various parameters in a distinct cortical area, and thus provides an appropriate tool to reveal correlations between cortical cholinergic hypoactivity and lesion-induced adaptive response in distinct cholinoceptive target regions. NMDA receptor binding was markedly reduced in cortical regions displaying a reduced activity of acetylcholinesterase and high-affinity choline uptake sites as a consequence of cholinergic lesion, whereas AMPA and kainate binding sites were significantly increased in these regions (Roßner et al., 1995d). Muscimol binding to $GABA_A$ receptors was increased in the caudal portions of frontal and parietal cortices as well as occipital and temporal cortex as compared to the corresponding brain regions from vehicle-injected control rats. Binding levels of benzodiazepine receptors were not affected by the lesion in any of the cortical regions studied (Roßner et al., 1995d). α_1-adrenoceptor binding sites were not affected by cholinergic immunolesion in any of the cortical regions studied, whereas the levels of α_2- and β-adrenoceptor binding were decreased in a number of cortical regions and hippocampal formation after lesion. $5\text{-}HT_{2A}$-serotonin receptor binding was markedly reduced in cortical regions displaying a reduced activity of acetylcholinesterase, while $5\text{-}HT_{1A}$ receptor binding was found to be transiently reduced in some anterior cortical regions but not in the hippocampal areas following immunolesion (Heider et al., 1997).

The significantly increased $GABA_A$ but not benzodiazepine binding sites in the frontal and parietal cortices suggesting an up-regulation of postsynaptically localized $GABA_A$ receptors as an adaptive response to the reduced GABAergic input as measured by Gomeza et al. (1992). In a current study alterations in dendritic morphology of cortical neurons after basal forebrain lesions have been described (Wellman and Sengelaub, 1995) suggesting that the cholinergic input plays an important modulatory role in cortical function and plasticity. The changes in the number of cortical NMDA receptors following lesion could be considered as a loss and/or down-regulation of NMDA receptor sites. In contrast, the increased kainate and AMPA binding following lesion should be considered as up-regulation of receptor sites. Up-regulation of postsynaptic glutamate receptors is assumed to compensate for reduced presynaptic input. This would suggest that cholinergic terminals directly affect glutamate transmission on presynaptic glutamatergic elements. However, the radioligand used, MK-801, is assumed to bind to a site within the NMDA receptor ion-channel and thus can also be considered as a marker of the agonist-bound, open state of the channel (Seeburg, 1993). Therefore, the immunotoxin-induced decline in MK-801 binding also indicates a lower amount of glutamate bound to the NMDA receptor channel. This supports the suggestion that cholinergic hypofunction reduces cortical glutamatergic activity by less release of glutamate from presynaptic elements presumably due to enhanced inhibition by GABA. However, regardless of possible interpretations the immunotoxin-induced differential changes in glutamate and GABA receptor subtypes in cortical regions displaying reduced cholinergic activity clearly demonstrate that cortical glutamatergic and GABAergic markers are partially driven by cholinergic activity.

Reductions in the binding level of cortical receptors following lesion could be either due to a loss of receptor sites if located on degenerating terminals or due to a down-regulation of receptor function if there is any enhanced neuronal activity of the corresponding transmitter system (see e.g. Klein et al., 1989). Taking into account that the immunotoxin-induced loss of basal forebrain cholinergic neurons is accompanied by massive degeneration of cortical and hippocampal cholinergic terminals originating in the basal forebrain, the lesion-induced decreases in cortical and hippocampal α_2- and β-adrenoceptor as well 5-HT_{2A} receptor binding suggest a location of these receptor subtypes on cholinergic terminals (Heider et al., 1997). The lesion-induced decrease in α_2-, β- and 5-HT_{2A} receptor binding could also be considered as a receptor down-regulation and/or subsensitivity. Down-regulation of postsynaptic receptors is assumed to compensate for enhanced presynaptic input. Basal forebrain cholinergic cell loss may affect interactions of the cholinergic system with the serotonergic and noradrenergic neurotransmission which might result in a dysbalance and overactivation of the non-lesioned systems. Possible sites for such interactive processes could occur at the level of convergent projection areas of the two transmitter systems, or by direct contacts between cholinergic basal forebrain and serotonergic raphe nucleus and noradrenergic locus coeruleus neurons. It is well established that the basal forebrain cholinergic nuclei receive projections from the medial and dorsal raphe nuclei (Milner and Veznedaroglu, 1993; Törk, 1985). The loss of basal forebrain cholinergic neurons that are innervated by raphe nucleus serotonergic cells could result in an imbalance between cholinergic and serotonergic system leading to an enhancement of cortical serotonergic activity, which might explain a down-regulation or subsensitivity of postsynaptic serotonergic receptors. There is a noradrenergic modulation of cholinergic nucleus basalis neurons (Fort et al., 1995), presumably mediated by some locus coeruleus neurons which send collaterals to basal forebrain nuclei (Jones and Yang, 1985). Noradrenergic cells could thereby influence cortical activity by acting upon the cortically projecting cholinergic basal forebrain neurons.

Moreover, it is interesting to note that the same sort of alterations in NMDA, AMPA and kainate, α_2- and 5-HT_{2A} receptor subtypes observed in rat cortex following basal forebrain cholinergic immunolesion have been detected in cortical brain areas from patients with Alzheimer's disease (Nordberg, 1992; Kalaria and Andorn, 1991; see also Table 1), suggesting that the changes in cortical NMDA, AMPA, kainate as well as α_2- and 5-HT_{2A} receptor binding observed in these patients are secondary to the cholinergic deficits. The data available on β-adrenoceptors in cortical areas from Alzheimer brains are controversial demonstrating both increase and decrease

242 V. Bigl and R. Schliebs

Table 1. Receptor changes in cortical regions of brains from Alzheimer patients as compared to corresponding alterations in rat brain after cholinergic immunolesion by intracerebroventricular injection of 192IgG-saporin

Receptor type	Alzheimer brain*	Cholinergic immunolesion in rats
Glutamate receptor subtypes		
NMDA	decrease	decrease
AMPA	no change/increase	increase
Kainate	increase	increase
GABA receptor subtypes		
GABA$_A$	decrease	increased
GABA$_B$	decrease	n.d.
Benzodiazepine	no change	no change
Adrenoceptor subtypes		
Alpha-1 adrenoceptor	no change	no change
Alpha-2 adrenoceptor	no change	decrease
Beta-adrenoceptor	no change	decrease
Serotonergic receptor subtypes		
5-HT$_{1A}$	decrease	decrease (transiently)
5-HT$_{2A}$	decrease	decrease

*Data taken from Nordberg (1992)

in cortical and hippocampal β-receptor binding as compared to age-matched controls (Kalaria et al., 1989; Shimohama et al., 1987; for review, see Nordberg, 1992). Taken together, these findings support both an glutamatergic and aminergic strategy which might have therapeutic potential in treating Alzheimer's disease, and demonstrate that cholinergic immunolesion by 192IgG-saporin exhibits a valuable tool to produce specific cholinergic deficits in rats as a model to study the effect of treatment with various drugs.

Effect of cholinergic immunolesion on cortical expression and processing of amyloid precursor protein

Pathological processing of the amyloid precursor protein (APP) is associated with the production of βA4-amyloid, the main component of senile plaques and cerebrovascular deposits in Alzheimer's disease. Different pathways of APP processing have been suggested, including secretory cleavage of APP at the cell surface as well as internalization and lysosomal degradation. The non-amyloidogenic secretory pathway includes cleavage of APP by a putative alpha secretase within the beta amyloid sequence, which generates a water soluble 90–100 kDa secreted form (secretory APP, APPs), whereas the membrane-anchored C-terminal fragment of APP remains in the cell. From in vitro experiments it is known that APP processing is controlled by activation of various neurotransmitter receptors coupled to protein kinase C including M1-muscarinic acetylcholine receptors (see e.g. Kirazov et al., 1997). However, little is known on the situation in vivo. To elucidate the question whether reduced cortical cholinergic activity affects APP processing in vivo, cholinergic immunolesion was used to study cortical APP expression and processing in vivo by means of Western analysis and in situ hydbridization.

The membrane-bound APP detectable in tissue pellets was found to accumulate after immunolesion for two weeks by about 75% as compared to control. This increase in membrane-bound APP levels was complemented by a 50%-decrease in the level of the soluble secreted form of APP assayed in the corresponding supernatant of the tissue homogenates (Roßner et al., 1997). These changes in membrane-bound and secreted APP were found to strongly correlate to ChAT activity, thus clearly demonstrating a cholinergic regulation of APP processing in the cerebral cortex in vivo, which may play an important role for the pathogenesis of AD. Thus enhancement of cortical cholinergic neurotransmission by pharmacological manipulations may also interfere with cortical APP processing by favouring the non-amyloidogenic pathway.

In contrast to APP processing, cholinergic immunolesion did not affect the expression of APP751 and APP770 mRNA isoforms but resulted in slight reductions in the expression of APP695 mRNA in some cortical and basal forebrain regions (Apelt et al., 1997).

Usefulness of cholinergic immunolesion for testing therapeutical strategies to enhance cholinergic neurotransmission

Drugs to enhance cortical cholinergic neurotransmission are still the only therapeutic strategy to treat Alzheimer's disease. Specific and selective cholinergic lesion by 192IgG-saporin seems to represent an appropriate tool to test for novel therapeutic strategies to compensate for the reduced cholinergic activity.

To prove the capability of chronic nerve growth factor (NGF) treatment to induce recovery of cholinergic markers after partial lesion of rat basal forebrain cholinergic system, rats received intracerebroventricular transplants of Swiss 3T3 cells retrovirally transfected to secrete NGF (Roßner et al., 1996). Eight weeks after NGF treatment of immunolesioned rats, the activity of choline acetyltransferase, and the sodium-dependent high-affinity choline uptake in the parietal cortex and hippocampus have increased reaching corresponding values which are detectable in untreated control rats. Histochemistry revealed that the density of acetylcholinesterase-positive cells in the basal forebrain as well as fibers in cerebral cortex and hippocampus were reduced by up to 60% in immunolesioned rats, but was completely restored after chronic NGF treatment. The remaining cholinergic cells following partial immunolesion displayed a higher intracellular staining for NGF-like immunoreactivity and the cell size was increased by up to 25% as compared to unoperated controls (Roßner et al., 1996).

Our data on chronic NGF treatment of cholinergic immunolesioned rats suggest that NGF affects the remaining basal forebrain cholinergic cells by increasing both the size, activity of choline acetyltransferase activity and the accumulation of NGF through enhanced low-affinity NGF receptor density, and induces regenerative mechanisms in cholinoceptive target regions to restore cholinergic markers as well as to establish or remodel new synaptic contacts. The data further support the usefulness of a neurotrophic strategy to treat cholinergic deficits in dementing disorders like Alzheimer's disease and the capability of transfected cell lines to continouesly deliver trophic factors into lesioned nervous tissue.

Conclusions

We have demonstrated that changes in a number of cortical glutamate, GABA, adrenergic and serotonergic receptor subtypes observed in Alzheimer's brains can be simulated by 192IgG-saporin-induced basal forebrain cholinergic cell loss in rats, suggesting that alterations in non-cholinergic transmitter systems in Alzheimer's disease are secondary to the very early onset of cholinergic deficits. Moreover, cortical cholinergic dysfunction was shown to affect the processing of the amyloid precursor protein, a major step in the pathogenesis of Alzheimer's disease. Thus, this cholinergic immunotoxin represents a useful tool to mimic some neurochemical sequelae of Alzheimer's disease including cholinergic mechanisms in processing of the amyloid precursor protein, and could be of particular value to elaborate and to test therapeutical strategies compensating for the reduced cortical cholinergic input.

Acknowledgements

This work was granted by Schering AG and Bundesministerium für Bildung und Forschung, grant no. 0310666 to V.B.

References

Apelt J, Schliebs R, Beck M, Roßner S, Bigl V (1997) Expression of amyloid precursor protein mRNA isoforms in rat brain is differentially regulated during postnatal maturation and by cholinergic activity. Int J Dev Neurosci 15: 95–112
Berger-Sweeney J, Heckers S, Mesulam MM, Wiley RG, Lappi DA, Sharma M (1994) Differential effects on spatial navigation of immunotoxin-induced cholinergic lesions of the medial septal area and nucleus basalis magnocellularis. J Neurosci 14: 4507–4519
Bickel U, Kewitz H (1990) Colocalization of choline acetyltransferase and nerve growth factor receptor in the rat basal forebrain. Dementia 1: 146–150
Book AA, Wiley RG, Schweitzer JB (1992) Specificity of 192 IgG-saporin for NGF receptor-positive cholinergic basal forebrain neurons in the rat. Brain Res 590: 350–355

Book AA, Wiley RG, Schweitzer JB (1994) 192 IgG-saporin I. Specific lethality for cholinergic neurons in the basal forebrain of the rat. J Neuropathol Exp Neurol 53: 95–102

Fisher A, Hanin I (1986) Potential animal models for senile dementia of Alzheimer's type, with emphasis on AAF64A-induced cholinotoxicity. Annu Rev Pharmacol Toxicol 26: 161–181

Fort P, Khateb A, Pegna A, Mühlethaler M, Jones BE (1995) Noradrenergic modulation of cholinergic nucleus basalis neurons demonstrated by in vitro pharmacological and immunohistochemical evidence in the guinea-pig brain. Eur J Neurosci 7: 1502–1511

Gage FH, Batchelor P, Chen KS, Chin D, Deputy S, Rosenberg MB, Higgins GA, Koh S, Fischer W, Björklund A (1989) NGF-receptor expression and NGF-mediated cholinergic neuronal hypertrophy in the damaged adult neostriatum. Neuron 2: 1177–1184

Gomeza J, Aragón C, Giménez C (1992) High-affinity transport of choline and amino acid neurotransmitters in synaptosomes from brain regions after lesioning the nucleus basalis magnocellularis of young and aged rats. Neurochem Res 17: 345–350

Heckers S, Ohtake T, Wiley RG, Lappi DA, Geula C, Mesulam MM (1994) Complete and selective denervation of rat neocortex and hippocampus but not amygdala by an immunotoxin against the p75 NGF receptor. J Neurosci 14: 1271–1289

Heider M, Schliebs R, Roßner S, Bigl V (1997) Basal forebrain cholinergic immunolesion by 192IgG-saporin: evidence for a presynaptic location of subpopulations of α_2- and β-adrenergic as well as 5-HT$_{2A}$ receptors on cortical cholinergic terminals. Neurochem Res 22: 957–966

Jones BE, Yang TZ (1985) The efferent projections from the reticular formation and the locus coeruleus studies by anterograde and retrograde axonal transport in the rat. J Comp Neurol 242: 56–92

Kalaria RN, Andorn AC (1991) Adrenergic receptors in aging and Alzheimer's disease: decreased α_2-receptors demonstrated by [^{3}H]p-aminoclonidine binding in prefrontal cortex. Neurobiol Aging 12: 131–136

Kalaria RN, Andorn AC, Tabaton M, Whitehouse PJ, Harik SI, Unnerstall JR (1989) Adrenergic receptors in aging and Alzheimer's disease: increased β2-receptors in prefrontal cortex and hippocampus. J Neurochem 53: 1772–1781

Kirazov L, Löffler T, Schliebs R, Bigl V (1997) Glutamate-stimulated release of secretory amyloid precursor proteins from cortical rat brain slices. Neurochem Int 30: 557–563

Klein WL, Sullivan J, Skorupa A, Aguilar JS (1989) Plasticity of neuronal receptors. FASEB J 3: 2132–2140

Leanza G, Nilsson OG, Wiley RG, Björklund A (1995) Selective lesioning of the basal forebrain cholinergic system by intraventricular 192 IgG-saporin: behavioural, biochemical and stereological studies in the rat. Eur J Neurosci 7: 329–343

Lee MG, Chrobak JJ, Sik A, Wiley RG, Buzsáki G (1994) Hippocampal theta activity following selective lesion of the septal cholinergic system. Neuroscience 62: 1033–1047

Milner TA, Veznedaroglu E (1993) Serotonin-containing terminals synapse on septohippocampal neurons in the rat. J Neurosci Res 36: 260–271

Nilsson OG, Leanza G, Rosenblad C, Lappi DA, Wiley RG, Björklund A (1992) Spatial learning impairments in rats with selective immunolesion of the forebrain cholinergic system. Neuroreport 3: 1005–1008

Nordberg A (1992) Neuroreceptor changes in Alzheimer disease. Cerebrovasc Brain Met Rev 4: 303–328

Roßner S, Perez-Polo JR, Wiley RG, Schliebs R, Bigl V (1994) Differential expression of immediate early genes in distinct layers of rat cerebral cortex after selective immunolesion of the forebrain cholinergic system. J Neurosci Res 38: 282–293

Roßner S, Schliebs R, Perez-Polo JR, Wiley RG, Bigl V (1995a) Differential changes in cholinergic markers from selected brain regions after specific immunolesion of rat cholinergic basal forebrain system. J Neurosci Res 40: 31–43

Roßner S, Härtig W, Schliebs R, Brückner G, Brauer K, Perez-Polo JR, Wiley RG, Bigl V (1995b) 192IgG-saporin immunotoxin-induced loss of cholinergic cells differentially activates microglia in rat basal forebrain nuclei. J Neurosci Res 41: 335–346

Roßner S, Schliebs R, Härtig W, Bigl V (1995c) 192IgG-saporin-induced selective lesion of cholinergic basal forebrain system: neurochemical effects on cholinergic neurotransmission in rat cerebral cortex and hippocampus. Brain Res Bull 38: 371–381

Roßner S, Schliebs R, Bigl V (1995d) 192IgG-saporin-induced immunotoxic lesions of cholinergic basal forebrain system differentially affect glutamatergic and GABAergic markers in cortical rat brain regions. Brain Res 696: 165–176

Roßner S, Yu J, Pizzo D, Werrbach-Perez K, Schliebs R, Bigl V, Perez-Polo JR (1996) Effects of intraventricular transplantation of NGF-secreting cells on cholinergic basal forebrain neurons after partial immunolesion. J Neurosci Res 45: 40–56

Roßner S, Ueberham U, Yu J, Kirazov L, Schliebs R, Perez-Polo JR, Bigl V (1997) In vivo regulation of amyloid precursor protein secretion by cholinergic activity. Eur J Neurosci 9: 2125–2134

Schliebs R, Roßner S, Bigl V (1996) Immunolesion by 192IgG-saporin of rat basal forebrain cholinergic system: a useful tool to produce cortical cholinergic dysfunction. In: Klein J, Löffelholz K (eds) Cholinergic mechanisms: from molecular biology to clinical significance. Elsevier, Amsterdam, pp 253–264 (Prog Brain Res 109)

Seeburg PH (1993) The molecular biology of mammalian glutamate receptor channels. Trends Pharmacol Sci 14: 297–303

Seeger G, Härtig W, Roßner S, Schliebs R, Brückner G, Bigl V, Brauer K (1997) Electron microscopic evidence for microglial phagocytotic activity and cholinergic cell death after administration of the immunotoxin 192IgG-saporin in rat. J Neurosci Res 48: 465–476

Shimohama S, Taniguchi T, Fujiwara M, Kameyama M (1987) Changes in β-adrenergic receptor subtypes in Alzheimer-type dementia. J Neurochem 48: 1215–1221

Thomas LB, Book AA, Schweitzer JB (1991) Immunohistochemical detection of a monoclonal antibody directed against the NGF receptor in basal forebrain neurons following intraventricular injection. J Neurosci Meth 37: 37–45

Törk I (1985) Raphe nuclei and serotonin containing systems. In: Paxinos G (ed) The rat nervous system, vol 2. Hindbrain and spinal cord. Academic Press, Sydney, pp 43–78

Torres EM, Perry TA, Blokland A, Wilkinson LS, Wiley RG, Lappi DA, Dunnett SB (1994) Behavioural, histochemical and biochemical consequences of selective immunolesions in discrete regions of the basal forebrain cholinergic system. Neuroscience 63: 95–122

Waite JJ, Chen AD, Wardlow ML, Wiley RG, Lappi DA, Thal LJ (1995) 192 immunoglobulin G-saporin produces graded behavioral and biochemical changes accompanying the loss of cholinergic neurons in the basal forebrain and cerebellar Purkinje cells. Neuroscience 65: 463–476

Wellman CL, Sengelaub DR (1995) Alterations in dendritic morphology of frontal cortical neurons after basal forebrain lesions in adult and aged rats. Brain Res 669: 48–58

Wenk GL, Stoehr JD, Quintana G, Mobley S, Wiley RG (1994) Behavioral, biochemical, histological, and electrophysiological effects of 192 IgG-saporin injections into the basal forebrain of rats. J Neurosci 14: 5986–5995

Wiley RG (1992) Neural lesioning with ribosome- inactivating proteins: suicide transport and immunolesioning. Trends Neurosci 15: 285–290

Wiley RG, Oeltmann TN, Lappi DA (1991) Immunolesioning: selective destruction of neurons using immunotoxin to rat NGF receptor. Brain Res 562: 149–153

Woolf NJ, Gould E, Butcher LL (1989) Nerve growth factor receptor is associated with cholinergic neurons of the basal forebrain but not the pontomesencephalon. Neuroscience 30: 143–152

Yan Q, Johnson jr EM (1989) Immunohistochemical localization and biochemical characterization of nerve growth factor receptor in adult rat brain. J Comp Neurol 290: 585–598

Authors' address: Dr. R. Schliebs, Paul Flechsig Institute for Brain Research, University of Leipzig, Jahnallee 59, D-04109 Leipzig, Federal Republic of Germany

Neuronal anion exchange proteins in Alzheimer's disease pathology

**G. J. C. G. M. Bosman[1], K. Renkawek[2], F. P. A. Van Workum[2],
I. G. P. Bartholomeus[1], S. Marini[3], and W. J. De Grip[1]**

[1] Department of Biochemistry and [2] Research Laboratory of Morphological Neurology,
Institute of Neurology, Faculty of Medicine, University of Nijmegen, Nijmegen,
The Netherlands
[3] Department of Experimental Medicine and Biochemistry, University "Tor Vergata",
Rome, Italy

Summary. Anion exchange (AE) proteins are present in human neurons in the brain. Immunohistochemical data indicate that their apparent expression level increases with age, and especially with degeneration in Alzheimer's disease-affected brain areas. The increase in immunoreactivity is probably caused by changes in AE structure that lead to an increased accessibility of hitherto hidden epitopes. These epitopes correspond to regions in the membrane domain that are involved in generation of senescent cell-specific antigen from AE1 in aging erythrocytes. Elucidation of the molecular nature of these changes and the underlying mechanisms will lead to insight in the processes that govern aging- and degeneration-associated perturbation of membrane integrity. The functional consequences of changes in AE structure may range from acidosis and disturbance of cytoskeleton integrity to untimely or impaired recognition of neurons by microglia.

Introduction

Aging can be defined as a progressive, generalized impairment of function resulting in a loss of response to stress and in a growing risk of age-related diseases. There is a general consensus that there are only a few, possibly interrelated mechanisms that underly the different phenotypes associated with aging. One or a few basic aging processes may be coupled to the major geriatric disorders: neurodegenerative diseases such as Alzheimer's disease (AD), cardiovascular diseases, and late-onset cancer (Esser and Martin, 1995).

The physiological aging process of the human brain is largely unknown territory. The apparently gradual accumulation of aging-related phenomena (apparent neuronal cell and synapse loss, lipofuscin and corpora amylacea, amyloid plaques and neurofibrillary tangles, and an increase in number and reactivity of astrocytes (e.g. Price et al., 1991) still obviates any firm conclusion on primary events and causative mechanisms (Bosman and De Grip, 1996). This seriously hampers interpretation of the phenomena observed in the brains of patients suffering from aging-related neurodegenerative diseases such as AD. Together with the recently described increase in some apoptosis parameters in AD and Huntington's disease-affected brain areas (e.g. Su et al., 1994), the neuropsychological and the neuropathological characteristics indicate that an acceleration or disturbance of the normal neuronal aging and cell death processes lies at the bottom of these diseases.

A molecular understanding of the basics of the cellular aging process, and of the putative disturbances of this process in aging-related diseases such as AD, has been hampered by the absence of biomarkers of these processes. Recently, however, Anion Exchange (AE) proteins have moved into a central, and increasingly important, key position in the ubiquitous maintenance of cellular homeostasis. Simultaneously, AE proteins have emerged at a "hot spot" of advanced research on physiological and pathological cell death, especially of postmitotic cells such as erythrocytes, neurons, and cardiomyocytes. The AE proteins are responsible for chloride/bicarbonate exchange, which is instrumental in transport of carbon dioxide through the organism and in regulation of the intracellular pH in many cells. The cytoplasmic domain provides cell-specific, high-affinity binding sites for components such as ankyrin, glycolytic enzymes, hemoglobin, and carbonic anhydrase. Through these properties AE proteins are involved in the regulation of interaction between cell membrane and the cytoskeleton, and in the regulation of cell metabolism (Alper, 1991; Kay, 1993; Reithmeier, 1993; Tanner, 1993). AE functions are regulated by various signal transduction pathways (Harrison et al., 1991; Pucéat et al., 1993). Moreover, the cellular aging process accumulates in structural changes in AE1 that lead to immune recognition and removal of old and damaged cells (Kay, 1993). It is striking that the functional consequences of aging-related changes in AE expression and structure are all key events in the apoptosis process (e.g. Bursch et al., 1992). AE-connected symptoms of disturbed aging are sensitive markers for aging-related, systemic syndromes with organ-specific consequences, such as the non-familial form of Alzheimer's disease (Bosman et al., 1991), Down's syndrome (Bartosz et al., 1982; Bosman et al., 1993a), and cardiovascular diseases (Santos-Silva et al., 1995).

Our studies are aimed at characterization of expression and function of neuronal AE proteins as paradigms of basic cellular mechanisms of aging, and their connection with aging-related diseases such as Alzheimer's disease. Here we present some of the results of these studies.

Material and methods

Neuropathology and immunohistochemistry

Formalin-fixed, paraffin-embedded tissue from control and AD patients (up to 10h post mortem) was used for neuropathological examination and diagnosis as described before (e.g. Bosman et al., 1993b). Plaques and tangles were encountered only sporadically in the brains of control patients. Immunohistochemistry was performed on formaldehyde or paraformaldehyde/sublimate-fixed tissues. Sections were counterstained with hematoxylin. Control incubations contained pre-immune sera. Immunostaining was performed with the avidin-biotin-peroxidase technique (Bosman et al., 1993b).

Immunoblotting

Immunoblot analysis was performed on frozen tissue fractions from the same brains used for neuropathological and immunohistochemical analysis as described before (Bosman et al., 1993b).

Antisera

Antisera were poly- or monoclonal antibodies raised against purified fragments of human erythrocyte AE1 or against synthetic peptides representing various domains of AE1, based on the sequence of Tanner et al. (1988), and have been described before (Renkawek and Bosman, 1996; Bosman et al., 1996, 1997).

pH measurements

The contribution of the various ion transporters to the regulation of intracellular pH was determined with the fluorescent probe 2',7'-bis-(2-carboxyethyl)-5-(and-6)-carboxyfluorescein (Molecular Probes, Eugene, U.S.A.), following the procedures described before (Bosman et al., 1997).

Results and discussion

Neuronal degeneration in Alzheimer's disease is not accompanied by substantial alterations in neuronal anion exchange protein synthesis, but by alterations in membrane epitope accessibility

Previous immunohistochemical data, obtained with polyclonal antisera against the membrane domain of erythrocyte AE1, indicated an increase in expression level of AE proteins in Alzheimer's disease (AD)-affected brain areas, especially in large pyramidal neurons with morphological signs of degeneration (Bosman et al., 1993b). Recently, we could confirm and extend these findings: immunohistochemical analysis with monoclonal and anti-peptide polyclonal antibodies against epitopes of the membrane domain — which is highly conserved in the AE gene family — indicate an increased expression of one or more AE proteins in AD brain (Fig. 1; see also Bosman et al., 1996, 1997). On the other hand, antibodies specific for the — much more variable — cytoplasmic domains of AE1, AE2 and AE3 did not show an AD-related increase in immunoreaction. The results for AE1 are summarized in Table 1.

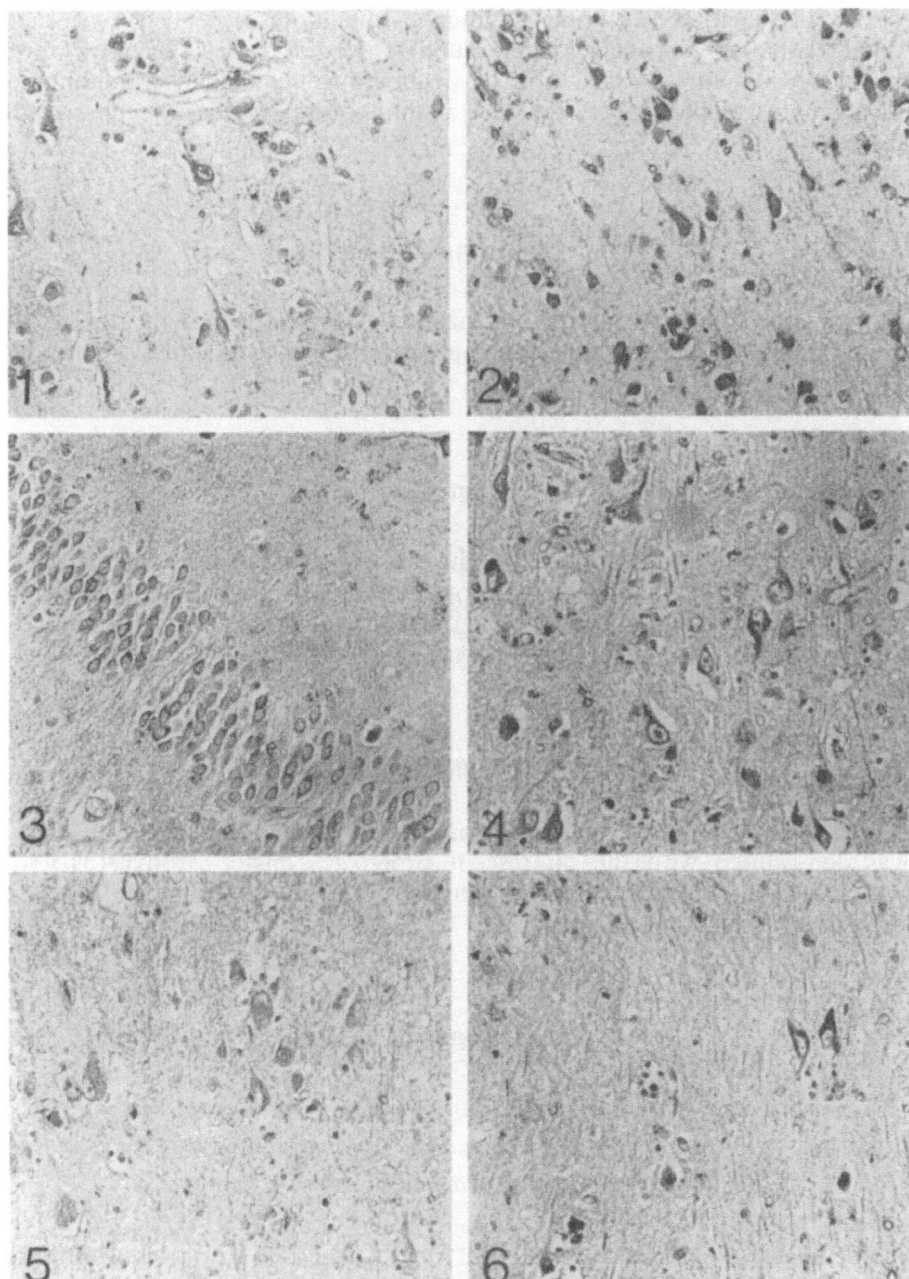

Fig. 1. Immunohistochemical analysis of Alzheimer and control brain tissue using antibodies specific for various epitopes of anion exchanger AE1. **1** control hippocampus, antiserum GB1B3 against residues 630–648. Immunoreactivity is restricted to the cytoplasm and axons of a few large pyramidal neurons; **2** Alzheimer hippocampus and **3** Alzheimer fascia dentata, both with antiserum GB1B3. Diffuse, strong immunoreactivity in all pyramidal cells; **4** Alzheimer hippocampus, antiserum GB2B3 against residues 620–637. Immunoreactivity in neuronal threads and degenerative neurons; **5** Alzheimer hippocampus, antiserum GB-AE02 against AE1 residues 566–569. Immunoreactivity lower than with GB1B3; **6** Alzheimer hippocampus, antibody B6 against residues 542–555. ×400

Table 1. Summary of semi-quantitative immunohisto-chemical analyses of control and Alzheimer hippocampal tissue with antisera against various epitopes of the anion exchange protein AE1[1]

Aminoacids	Control	Alzheimer
cyto	+ +	+ +
22–27	+ +	+ +
475–488	+	+
542–555	+ +	+ + +
562–565	+	+ + +
566–569	−/+	+
588–602	+	+ +
620–637	+/+ +	+ + +
628–642	+	+ +
630–648	+	+ +
650–658	+	+ +

[1] Antisera were poly- or monoclonal antibodies raised against purified fragments of human erythrocyte AE1 or against synthetic peptides representing various domains of AE1. Residue numbers are based on the sequence of Tanner et al. (1988), as described before (Renkawek and Bosman, 1996; Bosman et al., 1996, 1997). *Cyto*: a polyclonal antiserum raised against a fragment of the cytoplasmic domain of human erythrocyte AE1 (Bosman et al., 1996); −: no detectable immunoreaction (IR); +: weak IR in less than 25% of the cells; + +: IR in 25–50% of the cells; + + +: IR in more than 50% of the cells

Hippocampus, frontal and temporal cortex tissue were analyzed by immunoblotting, using the same antibodies as used for immunohistochemical analysis. The results of quantitative densitometric analysis of immunoblots do not show a significant AD-related increase in AE protein synthesis, but indicate an increase in the relative amount of the smaller immunoreactive proteins, suggesting increased breakdown of AE1 in AD-affected tissue. In addition, those antisera that mainly react with breakdown products of AE1 show the largest immunohistochemical differences between AD and control brains (Bosman et al., 1997). Some antisera also react with corpora amylacea, small particles thought to be the physiological endproducts of neuronal membrane degradation in the brain, and present in increased concentrations in AD brains (Renkawek and Bosman , 1995). This supports our working hypothesis that neuron degeneration and specific AE epitope expression are related. More specifically, together these findings confirm the hypothesis that changes in the conformation of AE1, in a manner that is similar to that in aging erythrocytes, occurs in the membranes of neurons in AD-affected brain areas. Such changes seem to especially affect the conformation of the regions 538–554 and 620–637 of AE1, that are both predicted to be at the interface of membrane and extracellular environment (Wood, 1992). In the native protein, these regions are in close proximity with the 788–827 sequence (Okubo et al., 1994), the other region implicated in recognition of old cells by the immune system (Kay, 1993). It is noteworthy that these regions are cryptic in normal erythrocytes, but become exposed in P. falciparum (malaria)-infected cells, and may be involved in their sequestration (Guthrie et al., 1995).

In order to further distinguish between the possible causes for these earlier findings (increased transcription and/or translation, increased expression of alternatively spliced isoforms, increased accessibility of membrane epitopes, or reduction in turnover rate), we measured AE expression at the mRNA level. For this purpose, we developed a method for semi-quantitative measurement of AE-mRNA levels in human brain tissue, using the reverse transcriptase-polymerase chain reaction (RT-PCR), oligonucleotide primers coding for regions of the membrane domains of the various AE proteins, and suitable primers for actin mRNA in order to obtain internal standard signals. Our results do not indicate an increase in AD-affected hippocampus, but rather a decrease in AE1 mRNA levels as compared with controls (Bosman et al., 1996). Quantification of the other AE mRNAs is in progress.

Degeneration-related breakdown of neuronal AE proteins will disturb regulation of intracellular pH, and interaction between plasma membrane and cytoskeleton

AE proteins take up a central position in the cellular homeostasis network: regulation of intracellular pH, interaction between cytoskeleton and plasma membrane (control of cell shape and plasticity), regulation of cell metabolism by binding of glycolytic enzymes, and generation of a neoantigen that acts as a signal by which the immune system recognizes dying and damaged cells (Kay, 1993; Tanner, 1993). These functions have been thoroughly characterized for AE1 in erythrocytes, but only fragmentarily for AE proteins in other cells. In order to obtain a comprehensive picture of these functions in neuronal cells, by which we will be able to estimate the consequences of AE breakdown on neuronal homeostasis and survival, we started to characterize AE functions in neuronal cells.

So far, the only protein known to function as a link between cytoskeleton and membrane AE proteins, is ankyrin. Ankyrin isoforms have been described for (rat and mouse) brain (Bennett, 1991), and have been found to bind to AE1 in rat brain (Kay et al., 1991). Since the cellular localization of ankyrin in the human brain had not yet been determined, we used antibodies against the conserved and the variable domains of erythrocyte ankyrin (a gift of Dr. J. C. Pinder, University of London, UK) for immunohistochemical and immunoblot analysis of control and AD-affected frontal and temporal cortex, hippocampus, and cerebellum. According to our immunohistochemical data, ankyrin-related proteins are present in neurons (including Purkinje cells) as well as in astrocytes (Bosman et al., 1997). In some, but not all neurons, ankyrin immunoreactivity coincided with AE immunoreactivity. We performed an extensive semi-quantitative analysis, but the interindividual variation was too large to allow any conclusions on differences between AD and control brains. This variation is probably due to the extreme sensitivity of ankyrin to degradation, which may occur even during the shortest possible (3 hours) post mortem delay (J. C. Pinder, personal communication). This was also indicated by immunoblot analysis, that showed mainly immunoreactive bands that were smaller than the intact ankyrin molecule. These data seem to present the first evidence for the presence of ankyrin proteins in the human brain (Bosman et al., 1997).

AE proteins are all involved in regulation of intracellular pH (pHi). This function can be determined only *in vitro*. We and others have found that AE proteins are present in human neuronal cell lines of various origins and neurotransmitter profiles (Goodman et al., 1994; Havenga et al., 1994). We measured the contribution of AE-mediated chloride/bicarbonate exchange to pHi maintenance of neuronal cells, using a spectrophotofluorometric method and the intracellular probe BCECF. AE-mediated anion transport across the plasma membrane was found to be essential in maintenance of neuronal pHi (Bosman et al., 1995, 1996). This conclusion was recently confirmed by others (Bettendorff et al., 1995). In a complementary approach, we addressed the presence of and pHi regulation by AE proteins in primary hippocampal cultures of newborn rats. Immunohistochemical analysis again showed the presence of AE proteins mainly in neurons, with only a weak reaction in astrocytes. In agreement with this observation, cultures enriched in astrocytes could recover from acidosis by the sole activity of the sodium/proton antiporter. In cultures enriched in neurons, AE-mediated chloride/bicarbonate exchange was necessary for maintenance of pHi (Bosman et al., 1997).

Conclusions

All available data indicate that AD-related neurodegeneration is not characterized by an increased synthesis of AE proteins, or by the synthesis of altered AE proteins, but by structural changes in selected regions of the membrane domain. These regions share epitopes with those that are implicated in senescent cell antigen formation in aging erythrocytes. This confirms our hypothesis that aging- and degeneration-specific mechanisms leading to alterations in AE protein processing and/or conformation are shared by erythrocytes and neurons. The functional studies show that AE proteins are involved in regulation of intraneuronal pH, and probably also in the interaction between cytoskeleton and neuronal membrane. Disturbance of these functions, as may occur in AD-related degeneration, may compromise cell integrity, and lead to degeneration and cell death, and to elimination of cells by activated, phagocytic, microglia. The important roles of intracellular pH and the membrane/cytoskeleton integrity in apoptosis and necrosis, now also implicated in the AD etiology, place the AE gene family in a "hot spot" of present biomedical research.

References

Alper SL (1991) The band 3-related anion exchanger (AE) gene family. Annu Rev Physiol 53: 549–564

Bartosz G, Soszynski M, Kedziora J (1982) Aging of the erythrocyte. VI. Accelerated red cell membrane aging in Down's syndrome. Cell Biol Int Rep 6: 73–77

Bennett V (1992) Ankyrins. J Biol Chem 267: 8703–8706

Bettendorff L, Margineanu I, Wins P, Grisar T (1995) An atypical anion transporter functioning at acid pH in neurobalstoma cells. Biochem Biophys Res Commun 207: 375–381

Bosman GJCGM, De Grip WJ (1996) Neuronal aging and Alzheimer's disease. Adv Cell Aging Gerontol 1: 157–168

Bosman GJCGM, Bartholomeus IGP, De Man AJM, et al (1991) Erythrocyte membrane characteristics indicate abnormal cellular aging in patients with Alzheimer's disease. Neurobiol Aging 12: 13–18

Bosman GJCGM, Visser FE, De Man AJM, et al (1993a) Erythrocyte membrane changes in individuals with Down's syndrome in various stages of Alzheimer-type dementia. Neurobiol Aging 14: 223–228

Bosman GJCGM, Van Workum FPA, Renkawek K, et al (1993b) Proteins immunologically related to erythrocyte anion transporter band 3 are altered in brain areas affected by Alzheimer's disease. Acta Neuropathol 86: 353–359

Bosman GJCGM, Vollaard CH, De Grip WJ (1995) Maintenance of neuronal homeostasis: the role of anion exchange proteins in regulation of intracellular pH. Eur J Neurosci 8: 115

Bosman GJCGM, Engbersen A, Vollaard CH, et al (1996) Implications of aging- and degeneration-related changes in anion exchange proteins for the maintenance of neuronal homeostasis. Cell Mol Biol 42: 905–918

Bosman GJCGM, Renkawek K, Van Workum FPA, et al (1997) Involvement of neuronal anion exchange proteins in cell death in Alzheimer's diseas. Gerontol 43: 67–78

Bosman GJCGM, Albers-Reijnen A, Renkawek K, De Grip WJ (1997) Anion exchange proteins and regulation of intracellular pH in cultured rat astrocytes and neurons. NeuroReport 8: 427–430

Bursch W, Oberhammer F, Schulte-Hermann R (1992) Cell death by apoptosis and its protective role against disease. Trends Pharmacol Sci 13: 245–251

Esser K, Martin GM (1995) Molecular aspects of aging. John Wiley & Sons, New York

Goodman JR, Gamble D, Kay MMB (1994) Distribution and function of multiple anion transporter proteins in brain tumor cell lines in relation to glucose transport. Brain Res Bull 33: 411–417

Guthrie N, Crandall IE, Marini S, et al (1995) Monoclonal antibodies that react with human band 3 residues 542–555 recognize different conformations of this protein in uninfected and Plasmodium falciparum infected erythrocytes. Mol Cell Biochem 144: 117–123

Havenga MJE, Bosman GJCGM, Appelhans H, De Grip WJ (1994) Expression of the anion exchanger (AE) gene family in human brain. Identification of a new AE protein: AE0. Mol Brain Res 25: 97–104

Harrison ML, Rathinavelu P, Arese P, et al (1991) Role of band 3 tyrosine phosphorylation in the regulation of erythrocyte glycolysis. J Biol Chem 266: 3106–4111

Kay MMB (1993) Generation of senenescent cell antigen on old cells initiates IgG binding to a neoantigen. Cell Mol Biol 39: 131–153

Kay MMB, Hughes J, Zagon I, Lin F (1991) Brain membrane protein band 3 performs the same functions as erythrocyte band 3. Proc Natl Acad Sci USA 88: 2778–2782

Okubo K, Kang D, Hamasaki N, Jennings ML (1994) Red blood cell band 3 Lysine 539 and Lysine 851 react with the same H2DIDS molecule. J Biol Chem 269: 1918–1926

Price JL, Davis PB, Morris JC, White DL (1991) The distribution of tangles, plaques and related immunohistochemical markers in healthy aging and Alzheimer's disease. Neurobiol Aging 12: 295–312

Pucéat M, Cassoly R, Vassort G (1993) Purinergic stimulation induces a tyrosine phosphorylation of a band 3-like protein in isolated rat cardiac cells. J Physiol 459: 226P

Reithmeier RAF (1993) The erythrocyte anion transporter (band 3). Curr Opin Struct Biol 3: 515–523

Renkawek K, Bosman GJGCM (1995) Anion exchange proteins are a component of corpora amylacea in Alzheimer disease brain. NeuroReport 6: 929–932

Santos-Silva A, Castro EM, Teixeira NA, et al (1995) Altered erythrocyte membrane band 3 profile as a marker in patients at risk for cardiovascular disease. Atherosclerosis 116: 199–209

Su JH, Anderson AJ, Cummings BJ, Cotman CW (1994) Immunohistochemical evidence for apoptosis in Alzheimer's disease. NeuroReport 5: 2529–2533

Tanner MJA (1993) Molecular and cellular biology of the erythrocyte anion exchanger (AE1). Semin Hematol 30: 34–57

Wood PG (1992) The anion exchange proteins: homology and secondary structure. Prog Cell Res 2: 325–352

Authors' address: G. Bosman, Ph.D., Department of Biochemistry, Faculty of Medicine, University of Nijmegen, P.O. Box 9101, NL-6500 HB, Nijmegen, The Netherlands

Lymphocytes as cell model to study apoptosis in Alzheimer's disease: vulnerability to programmed cell death appears to be altered

A. Eckert[1,5], **C. W. Cotman**[3], **R. Zerfass**[2], **M. Hennerici**[4], and **W. E. Müller**[1,5]

Departments of [1]Psychopharmacology and [2]Psychiatry, Central Institute of Mental Health, J5, Mannheim, Federal Republic of Germany
[3]Institute for Brain Aging and Dementia, University of California, Irvine, CA, USA
[4]Neurological Clinic, Klinikum Mannheim of the University of Heidelberg, Mannheim, and [5]Department of Pharmacology, Biocenter, University of Frankfurt, Frankfurt, Federal Republic of Germany

Summary. Recent evidence indicates that programmed cell death (apoptosis) may contribute to neuronal death in Alzheimer's disease (AD). *In situ* data derived from post mortem brain tissue indicate that DNA fragmentation which represents an important and typical apoptotic feature is markedly increased in brain cells of AD patients compared to controls. Furthermore, *in vitro* studies demonstrate that the peptide β-amyloid (Aβ) and its fragments induce apoptosis in neuronal cell cultures. One possible mechanism initiating apoptosis could be free radical generation by the peptide leading to oxidative stress. In a wide range of cell types common morphological and molecular events occur during apoptosis and several genes appear to be involved. Particularly in lymphocytes, apoptosis plays an important physiological role. Our data demonstrate that similar oxidative stressors induce apoptosis in mature human lymphoctes as in neurons. In addition, first evidence indicates that susceptibility to apoptosis is altered in lymphocytes from AD patients compared to non-demented controls. Our preliminary findings suggest that changes of the individual sensitivity to undergo cellular apoptosis are already detectable in lymphocytes from AD patients, probably as a consequence of genetic as well as other risk factors. Therefore, this biochemical marker might have the potential for identifying individuals at risk of the diseases.

Introduction

Several lines of evidence point to programmed cell death (PCD) having a primary role in neuronal dysfunction and cell loss in Alzheimer's disease (AD) (Cotman et al., 1994, 1995). Apoptotic cell death is characterized by cell shrinkage, cell surface blebbing, chromatin condensation, and DNA fragmentation with maintenance of cell membrane integrity. A series of different stimuli can trigger the apoptotic pathway. Recent studies indicate that β-amyloid (Aβ), the primary component of neuritic plaques that are a hallmark of AD, places neurons at risk for injury, damages neuronal processes, and is one of the stimuli that initiates cell death by apoptosis (Pike et al., 1993; Loo et al., 1993; Forloni et al., 1993; Watt et al., 1993). Aβ can also affect signal transduction processes in neuronal and non-neuronal cells (Eckert et al., 1993, 1995) and thereby might reprogram the microenvironment of the brain in the course of aging and neurodegeneration by enhancing its vulnerability for apoptosis. Evidence has been mounting for a role for free radicals in Aβ-induced toxicity (Hensley et al., 1994) increasing reactive oxygen species within cells (Mark et al., 1996), intracellular peroxide levels (Behl et al., 1994), and lipid oxidation (Butterfield et al., 1994). A similar apoptotic cell suicide pathway has been detected in cultured cortical neurons after brief exposure to direct oxidative damage (H_2O_2) (Whittemore et al., 1994). Furthermore, post mortem brain tissue from AD patients show extensive DNA damage in some neurons, nuclear morphology and especially DNA fragmentation consistent with apoptosis (Su et al., 1994; Lassmann et al., 1995). In a wide range of cell types, common morphological and molecular events occur during apoptosis and several common genes appear to be involved (Cotman et al., 1994). Excessive cell death can result from acquired or genetic conditions that enhance the accumulation of signals that induce apoptosis or that decrease the threshold at which such events induce PCD. Particularly in lymphocytes, apoptosis plays an important physiological role.

In the present study, we could demonstrate that the same agents (oxidative stressors) that induce PCD in neuronal cells are also active in mature human lymphocytes. Based on the hypothesis that genetic defects leading to an enhanced vulnerability for apoptosis in AD brains are similarly expressed in other human cells, the lymphocytes represent a valuable and most accessible peripheral system to study mechanisms of the apoptotic program in individual humans and specifically in AD patients.

Methods

Subjects

To study the induction of apoptosis in human mature lymphocytes, lymphocytes from young healthy controls (age <35 years) were investigated.

Study with patients: The experiments were performed using blood cells from 10 patients (5 men and 5 women) with "probable" (n = 6) or "possible" (n = 4) AD according to the NINCDS-ADRDA criteria. The mean age was 74.2 ± 7.9 years (range 59 to 83 years). The majority of cases exhibited moderate dementia. The clinical dementia ratings (CDR) ranged from mild to severe (CDR = 0.5 − 3.0).

Blood cells from 9 non-demented individuals of similar age (mean age 70.6 ± 6.1 years, range 63 to 79 years, 5 men and 4 women) were used as controls.

Lymphocyte separation and culture conditions

Peripheral blood lymphocytes were separated from heparinized blood by centrifugation on Ficoll-Hypaque for $400 \times g$ for 40 min as previously described (Eckert et al., 1993).

After depletion of monocytes, cells were investigated directly ("native cells") or after short-term culture ("predisposed cells") as indicated. For short-term culture, lymphocytes were resuspended in RPMI-1640 (Dutch Modification, Sigma, Germany) supplemented with 5% heat-inactivated fetal bovine serum, 100 U of penicillin/ml and 0.1 mg streptomycin/ml. The lymphocyte suspension was adjusted to 5×10^5 cells/ml and treated with 5 μg/ml concanavalin A for 48 h, washed with 10 mg/ml α-methylmannoside, and cultured again for 48 h with 50 units of human recombinant interleukin-2 (IL-2; Boehringer Mannheim, Germany) according to the method of Zheng et al. (1995) to predispose to apoptosis. Cells were washed with normal RPMI-1640, transfered into 24-well plates (5×10^5 cells/well), and incubated with different stimuli to induce apoptosis.

Quantitative measurement of cell death

Cell Death Detection ELISA^{PLUS}: The detection of histone-associated DNA fragments in one immunoassay demonstrating the internucleosomal degradation of genomic DNA during apoptosis was used. The assay is based on the quantitative sandwich-enzyme-immunoassay principle using mouse monoclonal antibodies directed against DNA and histones, respectively. This allows the specific determination of mono- and oligonucleosomes in the cytoplasmic fraction of cell lysates. Cytoplasmic fractions (lysates) and cell-culture-supernatants (5×10^4 cells/200 μl) were collected at different incubation times, frozen at $-80°C$ for one week, then analyzed in the ELISA (correspond to 5×10^3 cell equivalents). Following the protocol for cytochemistry (Boehringer Mannheim, Germany) the Cell Death Detection ELISA^{PLUS} was used visualizing the retained amount of POD photometrically with ABTS. Absorption values of each ELISA were standardized to the positive controls (Positive Control = 1.0).

DNA labeling assay using flow cytometry: DNA labeling was performed with propidium iodide (PI) and flow cytometric analysis. The method was essentially that described by Nicoletti et al. (1991). In brief, the 200 g centrifuged cell pellet was gently resuspended in 1.2 ml hypotonic fluochrome solution of PI 50 μg/ml in 0.1% sodium citrate plus 0.1% Triton X-100. After 20 hours in the dark at 4°C, the samples were applied to FACScan (Becton Dickinson, CA, USA). The lower DNA content of cells with less PI staining than that of G_1 cells have been considered apoptotic ("sub-G_1 peaks" = "A_0" cells, marked with M_1 in the figures).

Results

Induction of apoptosis in mature human lymphocytes

Lymphocytes, which were predisposed to apoptosis by treatment with Il-2 according to the method of Zheng et al. (1995), were incubated for 24 hours with different agents leading to oxidative damage. In contrast to freshly prepared native cells, short term lymphocyte cultures showed a high portion of cells undergoing spontaneous apoptosis (control, 10.2% apoptotic

262 A. Eckert et al.

cells) (Fig. 1). Freshly prepared lymphocytes usially show only about 1% apoptotic cells. Furthermore, cells incubated with aggregated Aβ1–42 (25 μmol/l) for 24h exhibit a similar portion of apoptotic cells (30.5%) as lymphocytes briefly treated with direct oxidative stressors as hydrogen peroxide (H_2O_2, 1 mmol/l; 33.3% apoptotic cells) or t-Butyl-hydroperoxide (B-H_2O_2, 4 mmol/l; 27.0% apoptotic cells) respectively (Fig. 1). Treatment with soluble Aβ1–42 at the same concentration was considerable less effective (data not shown). Preaggregated Aβ23–35 at an equal concentration (25 μmol/l) and high order protein assembly (Pike et al., 1993), however, is also less effective after this incubation period. The portion of apoptotic cells was not different in Aβ25–35 treated cells compared to control cells (control: 10.2% vs. Aβ25–35: 12.1%) (Fig. 1). As far as we know, these data are the first results that Aβ can also induce an apoptotic pathway in peripheral cells.

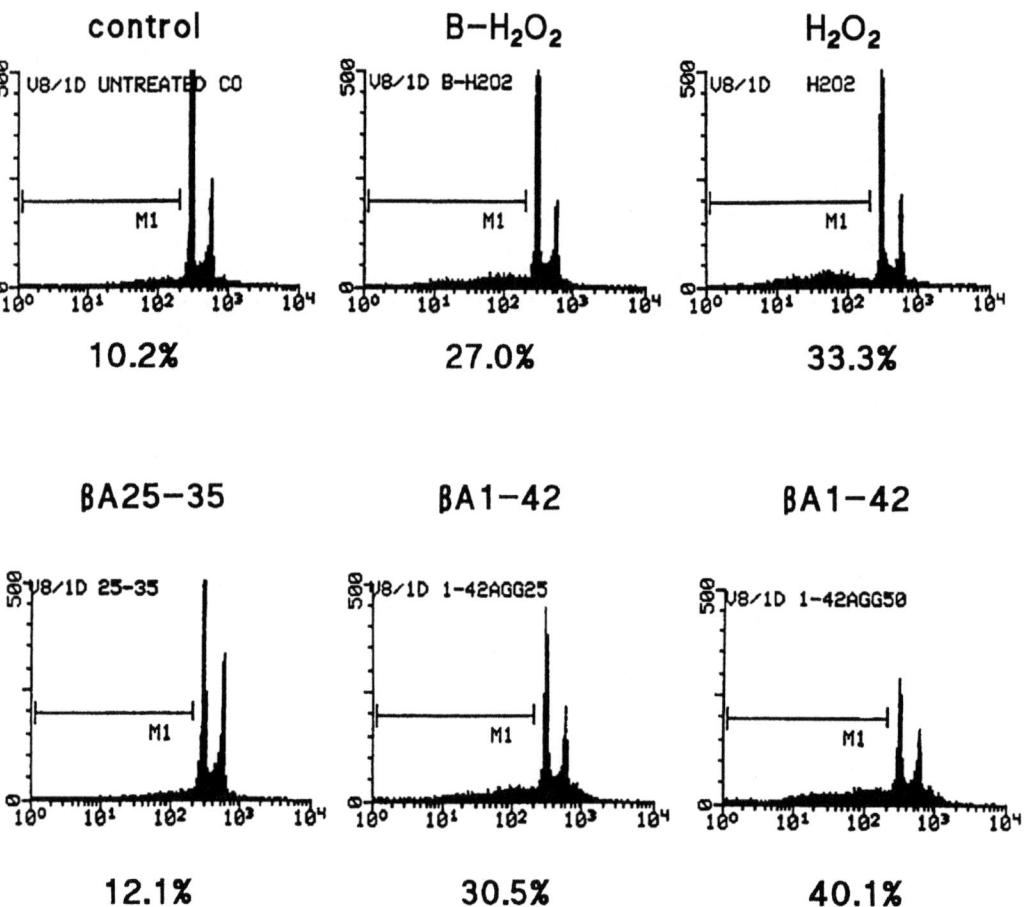

Fig. 1. Representative DNA histograms of human short-term cultered lymphocytes of young individuals incubated for 24 hours in the absence of stimuli (Control) or in the presence of aggregated βA25–35 (25 μmol/l) or aggregated βA1–42 (25 and 50 μmol/l respectively). Lymphocytes were briefly exposed to H_2O_2 (1 mmol/l) or to B-H_2O_2 (4 mmol/l) for 30 min followed by further incubation in normal buffer for 24 hours. Values represent the portion of apoptotic cells (M_1 fraction = A_0 cells)

According with recent findings (Barbieri et al., 1994), when lymphocytes were incubated with 2-deoxy-D-ribose (d-Rib, 50 mmol/l) for 24 and 48 hours (Fig. 2), a marked increase in cells undergoing apoptosis analyzed by flow cytometry was seen. The percentage of apoptotic cells in the control incubation was similar after 24 hours and after 48 hours (24 h: 9.6 ± 1.2% vs. 48 h: 9.4 ± 2.2%; n = 3 − 4). Enhancement of the apoptotic cell fraction became evident 24 hours after addition of d-Rib and increased slightly in a time-dependent manner (24 h: 30.1 ± 8.9% vs. 48 h: 36.4 ± 7.2%, n = 3 − 4).

The time-dependent detection of cytoplasmic histone-associated DNA fragments (mono- and oliginucleosomes) after incubation of lymphocytes with d-Rib (50 mmol/l) (Fig. 3) confirms our flow cytometric findings (Fig. 2). These method allows the detection of early events in DNA fragmentat-

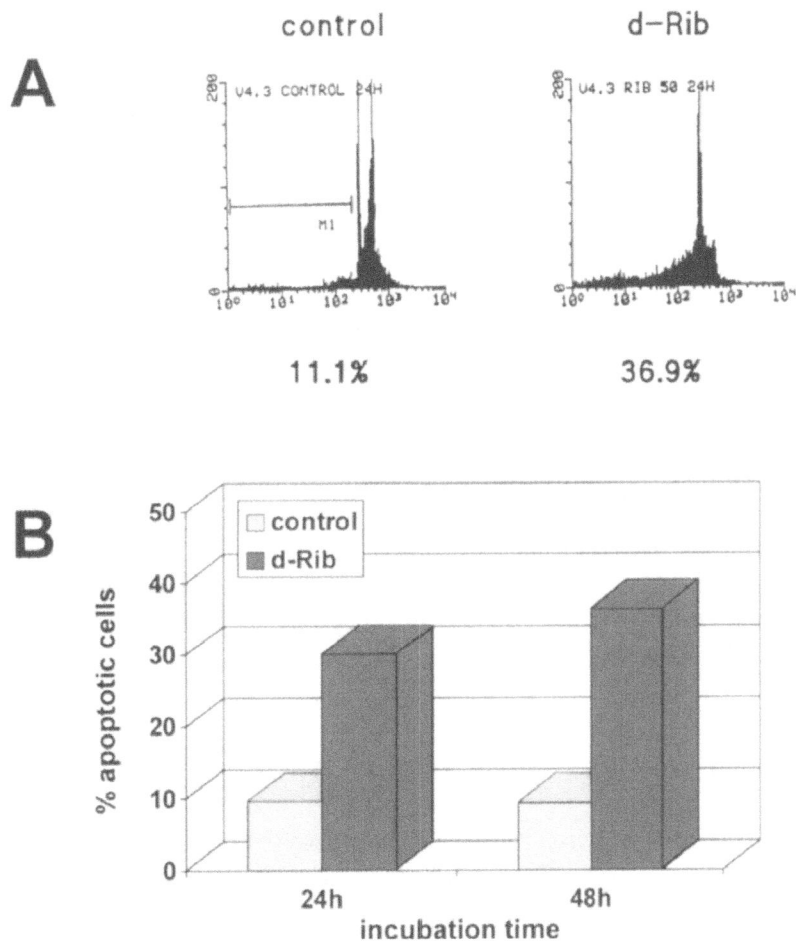

Fig. 2. A Representative DNA histograms of human short-term cultered lymphocytes of young individuals incubated for 24 hours in the absence of stimuli (Control) or in the presence of 2-deoxy-D-ribose (d-Rib, 50 mmol/l). Values represent the portion of apoptotic cells (M_1 fraction = A_0 cells). B Increase in apoptotic cells after treatment of lymphocytes with d-Rib (50 mmol/l) for 24 and 48 hours compared to control cells quantitated by flow cytometry. Data are means (n = 3 − 4)

264 A. Eckert et al.

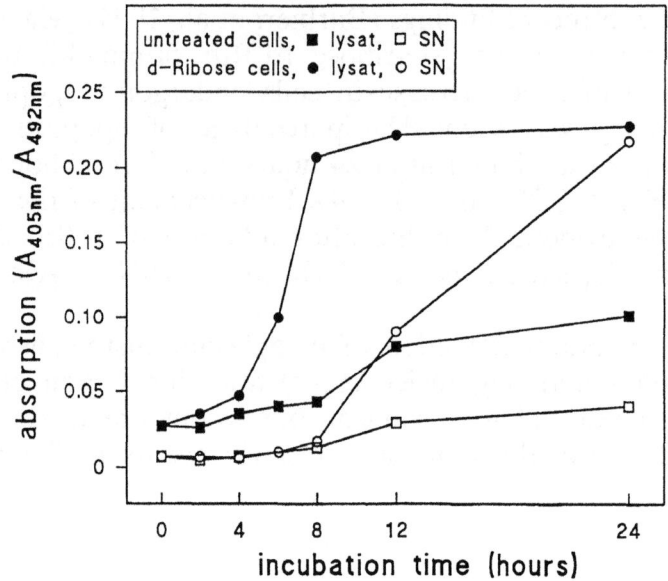

Fig. 3. Kinetics of 2-deoxy-D-ribose-induced apoptotic cell death in human lymphocytes (young healthy control). Cells were incubated either in the presence of d-Rib (50 mmol/l) or in the absence of d-Rib for 2 to 24 hours at 37°C. After the times indicated, supernatant (=SN) and cells (cytoplasmic fraction = lysat) were removed and tested by CDD ELISA[PLUS]

ion within cells. Four hours after incubation with d-Rib, nucleosomes became detectable in the cytoplasm of apoptotic cells. The maximum level was reached after 8–12 hours (Fig. 3). In contrast, no nucleosomes were detected in the supernatant during the first 8 hours after cell death induction indicating that DNA fragmentation occured prior to plasma membrane lysis discriminating between apoptosis and necrosis (Fig. 3). Membrane integrety is a typical feature for apoptosis. Therefore, low molecular weight DNA which is increased in apoptosis is found only within cell. As apoptosis proceeds in vitro, however, cells develop secondary necrosis characterized among other things by cells lysis (Watt et al., 1994) and the appearance of DNA fragments in the supernatant.

Apoptotic features in lymphocytes from AD patients and from controls

Based on our findings in mature lymphocytes from healthy controls, it was of great interest to look for AD-related alterations in apoptosis. Therefore, we investigated basal susceptibility to apoptosis in lymphocytes from AD patients and aged non-demented control subjects. Freshly isolated native lymphocytes from AD patients showed significantly enhanced basal levels of DNA fragmentation when compared to aged non-demented controls (p = 0.01) (Fig. 4). Thereby, lymphocytes from AD patients exhibited a twofold increase in absorption values than the lymphocytes from control subjects (mean values of absorption: AD 0.18

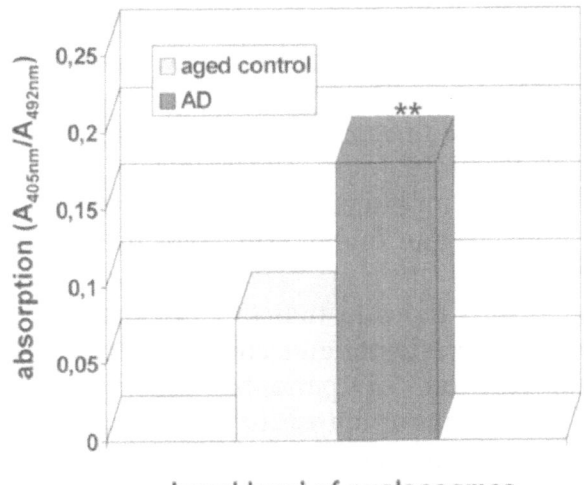

Fig. 4. Basal levels of nucleosomes in quiescent lymphocytes from AD patients (n = 10) and from aged non-demented controls (n = 9) quantitated by CDD ELISA[PLUS]. Data are mean values of each group. Apoptotic nucleosomes were significantly enhanced in lymphocytes from AD patients compared to controls (**p $\leq$ 0.01, ANOVA)

$\pm$ 0.11; controls 0.08 $\pm$ 0.03) indicating enhanced spontaneous apoptosis in AD.

Discussion

Our present report demonstrates that agents inducing oxidative stress can initiate apoptosis in mature human lymphocytes. Under normal conditions, mature human lymphocytes appear to be relatively insensitive to apoptosis (Barbieri et al., 1994; Zheng et al., 1995), but can be primed to apoptosis by mitogens and interleukin 2 (IL-2) treatment (Leonardo, 1991; Zheng et al., 1995). How mature cell selects between death or proliferation and life respectively is not completely understood. IL-2 seems to be a critical determinant of the choice between these two fates (Leonardo, 1991) and may participate in a feedback regulatory mechanism for cell proliferation by predisposing mature lymphocytes to apoptosis. Damaging agents can directly induce apoptosis in mature lymphocytes, but preactivation of cells facilitates this pathway or is even generally required in some cases (Zheng et al., 1995). In contrast to spontaneous apoptosis, the active generation of a death signal which initiates a signal transduction event triggering PCD is thus called activation-induced cell death (Cotman et al., 1994, 1995). In lymphocytes predisposed to apoptosis, Aβ1–42 exhibited about a four times higher efficacy than Aβ25–35 at equal concentrations confirming findings in neuronal cells (Loo et al., 1993; Watt et al., 1994) as well as in cerebrovascular smooth muscle cells (Davis-Salinas et al., 1994). In addition, direct oxidative stress (H_2O_2, t-Butyl-hydroperoxide) induced apoptosis in peripheral lymphoctes. The same oxidative insults induce cell death via apoptosis in cultured rat cortical neurons

(Whittemore et al., 1994). Consistent with findings of Barbieri et al. (1994), 2-deoxy-D-ribose, a sugar with high reducing activity provoking oxidative stress (Barbieri et al., 1994), also induced apoptosis in these cells.

As far as we know, the present data are the first findings demonstrating that the same agents that initiate programmed cell death in neurons are also active in mature human lymphocytes. Therefore, the lymphocyte provides a powerful model to investigate ongoing mechnisms in apoptosis in man and especially during disease.

Moreover, our results indicate that the susceptibility to apoptosis is altered in lymphocytes from AD patients compared to non-demented controls. Quiescent lymphocytes from AD patients already show enhanced levels of cells undergoing spontaneous apoptosis to an abnormally high extent (Eckert et al., 1996, 1998). The findings of elevated apoptotic features in the brain (Su et al., 1994; Lassmann et al., 1995) and in peripheral blood cells of AD patients appears to be remarkable. Obviously, genetic and other risk factors relevant for the disease lead to a similar pattern of apoptotic cell death not only in brain cells, but also in peripheral lymphocytes.

Acknowledgments

This study was supported by grants from the Deutsche Forschungsgemeinschaft, SFB 258, project K5, the Forschungsfond Fakultät Mannheim, and a Boehringer Ingelheim Fonds fellowship to A.E.

References

Barbieri D, Grassilli E, Salvioli S, Franceschini MG, Franchini A, Bellesia E, Salomoni P, Negro P, Capri M, Tojano L, Franceschi C (1994) D-ribose and deoxy-D-ribose induce apoptosis in human quiescent peripheral blood mononuclear cells. Biochem Biophys Res Commun 201: 1109–1116

Behl C, Davis JB, Lesley R, Schubert D (1994) Hydrogen peroxide mediates amyloid β protein toxicity. Cell 77: 817–827

Butterfield DA, Hensley K, Harris M, Mattson M, Carney J (1994) β-Amyloid peptide free radical fragments initiate synaptosomal lipoperoxidation in a sequence-specific fashion: implications to Alzheimer's disease. Biochem Biophys Res Commun 200: 710–715

Cotman CW, Anderson A (1995) A potential role for apoptosis in neurodegeneration and Alzheimer's disease. Mol Neurobiol 10: 19–45

Cotman CW, Whittemoore ER, Watt JA, Anderson AJ, Loo DT (1994) Possible role of apoptosis in Alzheimer's disease. Ann NY Acad Sci 747: 36–49

Davis-Salinas J, Saporito-Irwin SM, Cotman CW, van Norstrand WE (1995) Amyloid β-protein induces its own production in cultured degenerating cerebrovascular smooth muscle cells. J Neurochem 65: 931–934

Eckert A, Hartmann H, Müller WE (1993) β-Amyloid protein enhances the mitogen-induced calcium response in circulating human lymphocytes. FEBS Lett 330: 49–52

Eckert A, Förstl H, Hartmann H, Czech C, Mönning U, Beyreuther K, Müller WE (1995) The amplifying effect of β-amyloid on cellular calcium signalling is reduced in Alzheimer's disease. Neuroreport 6: 1199–1202

Eckert A, Cotman CW, Zerfass R, Hennerici M, Müller WE (1996) Vulnerability of lymphocytes against programmed cell death in Alzheimer's disease. Soc Neurosci 22: 827

Eckert A, Cotman CW, Zerfass R, Hennerici M, Müller WE (1998) Enhanced vulnerability to apoptotic cell death in sporadic Alzheimer's disease. Neuroreport (in press)

Forloni G, Chiesa R, Smiroldo S, Verga L, Salmona M, Tagliavini F, Angeretti N (1993) Apoptosis mediated neurotoxicity induced by chronic application of β amyloid fragment 25–35. Neuroreport 4: 523–526

Hensley K, Carney JM, Mattson MP, Aksenova M, Harris M, Wu JF, Floyd RA, Butterfield DA (1994) A model for β-amyloid aggregation and neurotoxicity based on free radical generation by the peptide: relevance to Alzheimer disease. Proc Natl Acad Sci USA 9: 3270–3274

Lassmann H, Bancher C, Breitschopf H, Wegiel J, Bobinski M, Jellinger K, Wisniewski HM (1995) Cell death in Alzheimer's disease evaluated by DNA fragmentation in situ. Acta Neuropathol 89: 35–41

Leonardo MJ (1991) Interleukin-2 programs mouse αβ T lymphocytes for apoptosis. Nature 353: 858–861

Loo DT, Copani A, Pike CJ, Whittemoore ER, Walencewicz AJ, Cotman CW (1993) Apoptosis is induced by β-amyloid in cultured central nervous system neurons. Proc Natl Acad Sci USA 90: 7951–7955

Mark RJ, Blanc EM, Mattson MP (1996) Amyloid β-peptide and oxidative cellular injury in Alzheimer's disease. Mol Neurobiol 12: 211–224

Nicoletti I, Migliorati G, Pagliacci MC, Grignani F, Riccardi C (1991) A rapid and simple method for measuring thymocyte apoptosis by propidium iodide staining and flow cytometry. J Immunol Meth 139: 271–279

Pike CJ, Burdick D, Walencewicz A, Glabe CG, Cotman CW (1993) Neurodegeneration induced by β-amyloid peptides in vitro: the role of peptide assembly state. J Neurosci 13: 1676–1687

Su JH, Anderson AJ, Cummings BJ, Cotman CW (1994) Immunohistochemical evidence for apoptosis in Alzheimer's disease. Neuroreport 5: 2529–2533

Watt JA, Pike CJ, Wassermann AJ, Cotman CW (1994) Ultrastructural analysis of β-amyloid-induced apoptosis in cultured hippocampal neurons. Brain Res 661: 147–156

Whittemore ER, Loo DT, Cotman CW (1994) Exposure to hydrogen peroxide induces cell death via apoptosis in cultured rat cortical neurons. Neuroreport 5: 1485–1488

Zheng L, Fisher G, Miller RE, Peschon J, Lynch DH, Leonardo MJ (1995) Induction of apoptosis in mature T cells by tumor necrosis factor. Nature 377: 348–351

Authors' address: Dr. A. Eckert, Pharmakologisches Institut, Biozentrum der Universität Frankfurt, Marie-Curie-Strasse 9, D-60439 Frankfurt, Federal Republic of Germany

Potential link between interleukin-6 and arachidonic acid metabolism in Alzheimer's disease

B. L. Fiebich, M. Hüll, K. Lieb, G. Schumann, M. Berger, and **J. Bauer**

Department of Psychiatry, University of Freiburg Medical School, Freiburg,
Federal Republic of Germany

Summary. Prostaglandins (PGs) and cytokines, such as interleukin-1 (IL-1) and interleukin-6 (IL-6), have been implicated in the etiopathology of various inflammatory and degenerative disorders, including Alzheimer's disease (AD). Previously, we detected the presence of IL-6 in cortices of AD patients. On the other hand, non-steroidal antiinflammatory drugs (NSAIDs), potent inhibitors of prostaglandin synthesis, have been shown to be beneficial in the treatment of AD. Until now, it remained unclear whether and how these two observations were functionally connected. Here, we show that PGs are able to induce IL-6 synthesis in a human astrocytoma cell line. PGE_1 and PGE_2, but not PGD_2 and $PGF_{2\alpha}$, led to a rapid and transient induction of astrocytic IL-6 mRNA, followed by IL-6 protein synthesis. Furthermore, PGE_2 potentiated IL-1β-induced IL-6 mRNA synthesis. These results suggest a possible link between the release of PGs from activated microglia and the astrocytic synthesis of IL-6, which itself may affect neuronal cells, as hypothesized for Alzheimer's disease. Finally we demonstrate that microglia are a strong source of PGE_2 synthesis indicating that these cells may act as the origin of the pathogenic cascade.

Abbreviations

AD Alzheimer's disease, *COX* cyclooxygenase, *IL-1* interleukin-1, *IL-6* interleukin-6, *NSAID* non-steroidal antiinflammatory drug, *PG* prostaglandin, *SDS* sodium dodecyl sulfate, *SSC* standard saline citrate, *TCA* trichloracetic acid.

Introduction

Prostaglandins are important for several central nervous functions, including control of the sleep-wake cycle (Hayaishi, 1991), the generation of fever (Stiit, 1991), and the transmission of pain (Horiguchi et al., 1986). In pathological situations prostaglandin formation increases dramatically. Elevated levels of prostaglandines have been observed in multiple sclerosis, AIDS-associated dementia and other neurodegenerative disorders (Chen et al., 1986; Fretland, 1992). Moreover increased synthesis of PGE_2 has been found in an animal model of scrapie (Williams et al., 1994; Brown et al., 1996).

A key enzyme in the synthesis of PGs is cyclooxygenase (COX), also referred to as prostaglandin H synthase. COX occurs in two isoforms, a constitutive COX-1 and an inducible COX-2 [for review, see Pairet et al. (1996)]. In the rat brain, COX-2 has been localized in cortical neuronal and glial cells (Yamagata et al., 1993; Breder et al., 1995) and is induced in microglial and astrocytic cultures in response to lipopolysaccharide (LPS), various cytokines and adenosine (Sawada et al., 1993; Schettini et al., 1994; Minghetti et al., 1995; Molina-Holgado et al., 1995; Fiebich et al., 1996; Bauer et al., 1997). Thus, the synthesis of PGs can be expected to occur in neurons, and after inflammatory activation in microglial and astroglial cells.

Inhibition of the enzymatic activity of COX is the main target of nonsteroidal antiinflammatory drugs (NSAIDs). Recent data suggest that NSAIDs may be beneficial not only for the treatment of various inflammatory disorders, but also for the treatment of Alzheimer's disease (AD) (Rogers et al., 1993; Breitner et al., 1995). In addition, previous use of NSAIDs has found to be inversely associated with the risk of AD (Breitner, 1996).

The cytokine interleukin-6 (IL-6) is involved in the pathology of a variety of CNS disorders, including AD (Bauer et al., 1991; Wood et al., 1993; Huell et al., 1995). Transgenic mice bearing an additional IL-6 gene under the control of the brain-specific GFAP promotor display massive neurodegeneration including alteration of the dendritic organization, gliosis, and loss of cholinergic innervation of the hippocampus (Campbell et al., 1993; Chiang et al., 1994). Until now it remained unclear whether the presence of IL-6 in the cortices of AD patients and the beneficial effects of NSAIDs in AD point to a functional connection between cytokine activation and arachidonic acid (AA) metabolism. Therefore, we investigated whether PGs are able to induce IL-6 synthesis in a well established in vitro model, the human astrocytoma cell line U373 MG (Fiebich et al., 1996a; Lieb et al., 1996). This cell line has been shown to share characteristics with primary rat astrocytes such as the expression of GFAP and the synthesis of IL-6 in response to IL-1β-treatment. In addition, we wanted to clarify the potential cellular source of PG synthesis. For this reason, we studied PGE_2 synthesis in microglial cells.

Materials and methods

Materials

IL-1β was purchased from Boehringer (Mannheim, FRG); PGD_2, PGE_1, PGE_2 and $PGF_{2\alpha}$ were from Sigma (Deisenhofen, Germany) and rabbit polyclonal antibodies raised against human IL-6 from Biozol (Eching, Germany) and Genzyme (Cambridge, MA,

USA). LPS (Salmonella typhimurium) was from SEBAK (Aidenbach, FRG). The NSAIDs meloxicam, indomethacin, diclofenac and ibuprofen were a generous gift from Drs. Pairet and Trummlitz and Prof. Engelhardt (Boehringer-Ingelheim Research Laboratories, Biberach/Riss, FRG). The cDNA probe for IL-6 was a generous gift from T. Hirano (Institute for Molecular and Cellular Biology, Osaka University, Japan).

Methods

Cell culture

The human astrocytoma cell line U373 MG was obtained from the American Type Culture Collection (Rockville, USA) and was grown in MEM-Earle's medium (Seromed, Berlin, Germany) containing 10% fetal calf serum, L-glutamine, antibiotics, vitamins, amino acids, and pyruvate. For total RNA extraction, cells were plated in 10 cm dishes (Falcon, 10^5 cells/dish in 10 ml culture medium) and for immunoprecipitation, 6-well plates (Falcon, 10^4 cells/well in 1 ml culture medium). Cultures were grown for 5 to 6 days at 37°C in 5% CO_2. The medium was changed one day before treatment for RNA extraction and directly prior to stimulation for IL-6-protein detection. Cells were stimulated 18 h for immunoprecipitation, 2 h for immunocytochemistry and 1 h for RNA extraction, unless otherwise indicated. Primary glial cultures were established from cerebral cortices of one-day neonatal Wistar rats as described (Gebicke-Haerter et al., 1989; Keller et al., 1985). Briefly, forebrains were minced and gently dissociated by repeated pipetting in Hanks's balanced salt solution (HBSS). Cells were collected by centrifugation, resuspended in DMEM containing 10% FCS and antibiotics and cultured on 10 cm cell culture dishes (Falcon, 5×10^5 cells/plate) in 5% CO_2 at 37°C. Media were prepared taking extreme care to avoid LPS contamination. Floating migroglia were harvested from 10–14 day mixed primary cultures and reseeded into cell culture plates (24 wells).

RNA extraction and northern analysis

Total RNA was extracted using an RNA extraction kit (Qiagen, Hilden, Germany) according to the manufacturer's protocols. Total RNA (10 μg per lane) was separated by agarose-formaldehyde gel electrophoresis, blotted onto positively charged Nylon membranes (Pharmacia, Freiburg), and cross-linked by exposure to 120°C for 30 min. The filters were prehybridized in 50% formamide, 0.25 M sodium-phosphate buffer, pH 7.2, 0.25 M NaCl, 10 mM EDTA, 20 μg/ml salmon sperm DNA and 7% SDS at 43°C for 2 h. cDNA probes were labeled with 50 μCi [^{32}P]dCTP (Amersham & Buchler, Braunschweig, Germany) using a random priming kit from Stratagene (Heidelberg, Germany). Unincorporated nucleotides were removed using a nucleotide removal kit from Qiagen. Overnight hybridization was performed at 43°C, adding the radiolabeled probe to the prehybridization buffer. Membranes were washed in $2 \times SSC/0.1\%$ SDS (3×20 min) at 60°C and exposed to Kodak XAR film at −80°C for adequate periods of time. For rehybridization, probes were removed by boiling the filter at 95°C in distilled water. Experiments were done at least in triplicate.

Immunoprecipitation

Cells were stimulated in methionine-free RPMI 1640 medium, supplemented with 0.01% heat-inactivated (56°C, 30 min) fetal calf serum, penicillin (100 U/ml), streptomycin

(100 mg/ml), 2 mM L-glutamine (all from Gibco, Karlsruhe, Germany) and [^{35}S]-methionine (100 μCi/ml; Amersham, Braunschweig, Germany). Culture supernatants were collected after 18 h, clarified by centrifugation at 1,600 × g, and passed through 0.45 μ-filters. Total de novo protein synthesis in the different supernatants was determined as TCA-precipitable cpm from 20-μl-aliquots. The culture supernatants were diluted in 2 volumes of TNET immunoprecipitation buffer (20 mM Tris-HCl, pH 7.5, 140 mM NaCl, 5 mM EDTA, 1% Triton X-100; 0.1 mM PMSF, 20 mg/ml soybean trypsin inhibitor, 4 mM leupeptin, and 4 mM antipain) and precleared with 10 mg Protein-A-Sepharose (Pharmacia, Freiburg, Germany). Immune adsorption of IL-6 in culture supernatants was performed by rotating 1 ml of diluted supernatant (equivalent to 2 × 10^6 TCA-precipitable cpm) with a saturating amount (10 μl) of specific rabbit antiserum and an excess (7 mg) of Protein-A-Sepharose overnight at 4°C. The Sepharose beads were washed twice in TNET and twice in 50 mM sodium phosphate buffer (pH 7.5) to remove nonadsorbent proteins. The proteins were released from the beads by heating at 95°C (5 min) in sample buffer (100 mM Tris-HCl, ph 6.8; 10% mercaptoethanol; 5% SDS and 10% glycerin) and separated on 15% SDS-polyacrylamide slab gels. The gels were dried and developed by autoradigraphy.

Determination of prostaglandin E$_2$ (PGE$_2$)

Microglial cells (5 × 10^5 cells/well) were preincubated with various inhibitors for 30 min. Thereafter, cells were treated with the different stimuli for 24 h. Culture supernatants were harvested, centrifuged 10 min at 10,000 × g and levels of PGE$_2$ in the media were measured by EIA (Immunotech, Hamburg, FRG) according to the manufacturer's instructions. Experiments were carried out in triplicate, typical data are shown.

Results

PGE$_1$ and PGE$_2$, but not PGD$_2$ or PGF$_{2\alpha}$, induce IL-6 mRNA in U373 MG cells

Different PGs were investigated for their ability to induce increased IL-6 mRNA levels in U373 MG human astroglioma cells. Only PGE$_1$ and PGE$_2$ were found to induce IL-6 mRNA expression, whereas PGD$_2$ and PGF$_{2\alpha}$ had no effect (Fig. 1a, upper panel). Expression of the β-actin gene was used as a control for standardization in all lanes (Fig. 1a, lower panel). Since PGE$_1$ and PGE$_2$ had similar effects, we used PGE$_2$ for all further experiments. PGE$_2$-induced IL-6 mRNA expression in U373 MG cells correlates with the de novo synthesis of IL-6 protein as shown by immunoprecipitation (Fig. 1b). Unstimulated cells only marginally synthesized IL-6 (Fig. 1b, lane 1), whereas PGE$_2$ strongly induced IL-6 protein synthesis. Two forms of newly synthesized IL-6 were detectable, an unglycosylated form with a molecular weight of about 23 kD and a glycosylated form with a molecular weight of about 26 kDa (Fig. 1b, lane 2).

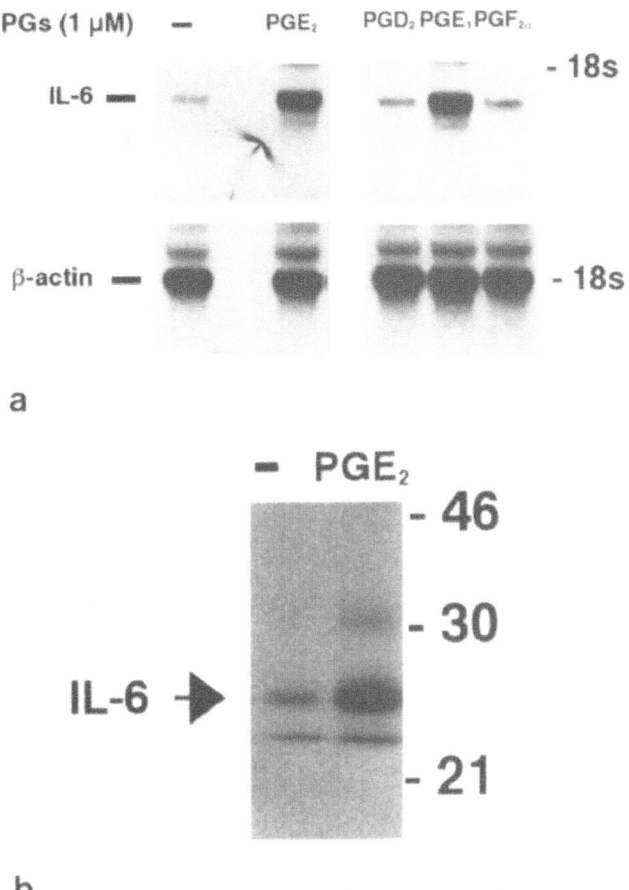

a

b

Fig. 1. a Induction of IL-6 mRNA by PGE_1 or PGE_2, but not by PGD_2 or $PGF_{2\alpha}$. After stimulation with different PGs (1 h, 1 μM each), total RNA was isolated and subjected to northern analysis. After hybridization with an IL-6 cDNA (upper panel), filters were hybridized with a β-actin cDNA for standardization (lower panel). **b** PGE_2-induced IL-6 protein synthesis in astrocytoma cells. Astrocytoma cells were cultured and radioactively labeled in methionine-free medium in the absence or presence of PGE_2 (1 μM) for 18 h. Supernatants were harvested and equal amounts of incorporated radioactivity were subjected to immunoprecipitation with an IL-6 specifc antibody. Immunoprecipitates were loaded on a 12% SDS-PAGE and visualized by autoradiography

Rapid and transient induction of IL-6 mRNA and IL-6 protein synthesis by
PGE_2 in U373 MG cells

Induction of IL-6 mRNA by PGE_2 was time and dose dependent. Increased IL-6 mRNA levels were found 30 min after PGE_2 treatment and maximal mRNA levels were achieved 1 h after stimulation. After 2 h of stimulation with PGE_2, IL-6 mRNA levels declined to baseline level at about 6 h after stimulation (Fig. 2a). Induction of IL-6 mRNA expression became detectable upon 0.01 μM PGE_2 and about ninty percent of maximal expression was achieved upon stimulation with 1 μM PGE_2. Maximum IL-6 mRNA levels were obtained using 10 μM PGE_2 (Fig. 2b) Expression of the β-actin gene was used as a control for standardization (Figs. 2a and b, lower panels).

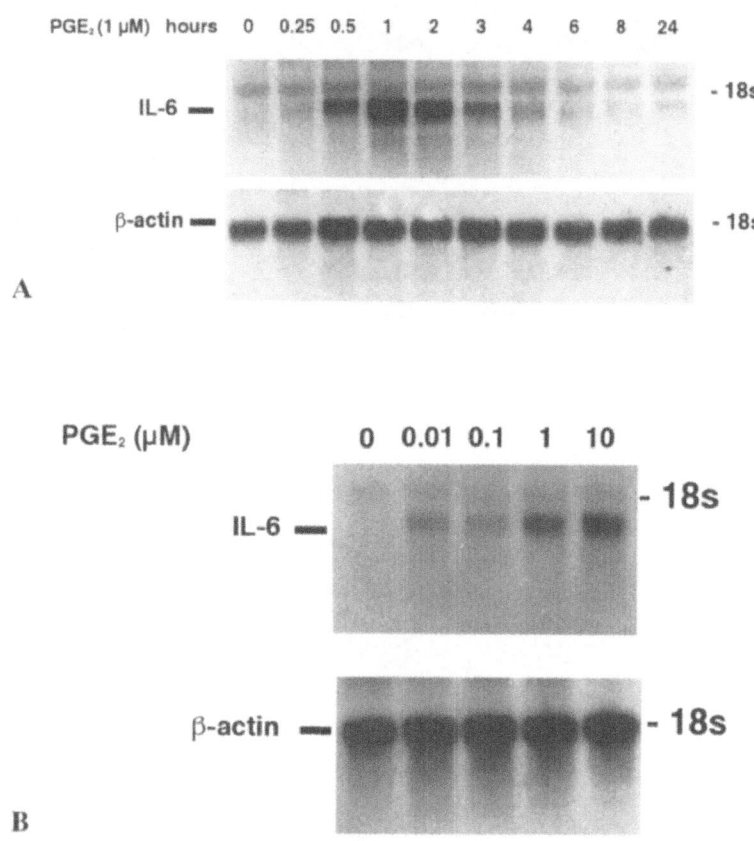

Fig. 2. Time-kinetics (**A**) and dose-dependency (**B**) of IL-6 mRNA induction by PGE_2 in human astrocytoma cells. Astrocytoma cells were stimulated (A) with $1\,\mu M$ PGE_2 for different periods of time and (B) for 1 h with different concentrations of PGE_2 (0.01 to $10\,\mu$). Total RNA was isolated and subjected to northern analysis. After hybridization with an IL-6 cDNA (upper panel), filters were hybridized with a β-actin cDNA for standardization (lower panel)

PGE_2 potentiate IL-1β-induced IL-6 mRNA expression

1 U/ml IL-1β alone induced only small amounts of IL-6 mRNA after 4 h (Fig. 3). PGE_2 potentiated the IL-1β-induced IL-6 mRNA expression more than two-fold compared to the effect of IL-1β alone (Fig. 3).

Activated microglia release PGE_2, inhibition by several NSAIDs

In order to clarify the potential source of prostaglandins in the brain, we analyzed the effects of microglia activation by LPS on the release of prostaglandin E_2 (PGE_2). As determined by a specific immunoassay, lipopolysaccharide strongly activated PGE_2 formation (Fig. 4) which is in line with data from other reports (Minghetti et al., 1996; Slepko et al., 1996). The use of the NSAIDs indomethacin, diclofenac, ibuprofen and meloxicam totally abolished the endotoxin-induced PGE_2 release (Fig. 4).

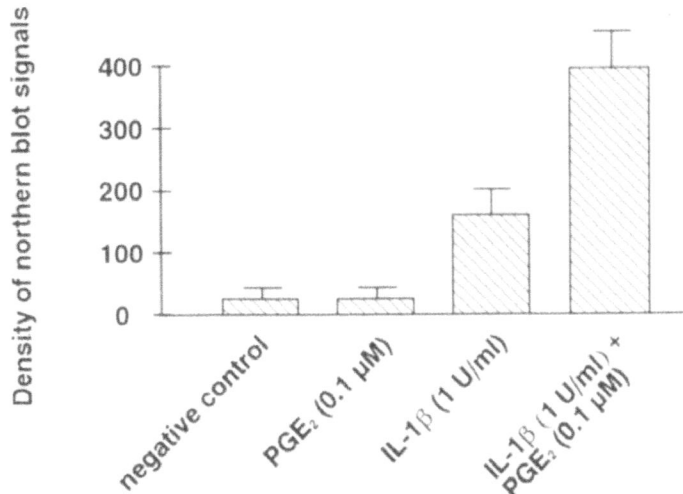

Fig. 3. Enhancement of IL-1β-induced IL-6 mRNA expression by PGE_2. Cells were unstimulated, stimulated with IL-1β (1 U/ml) or PGE_2 (0.1 μM) alone or in combination for 4 h. After stimulation, total RNA was isolated and subjected to northern analysis. After hybridization with an IL-6 cDNA, filters were hybridized with a β-actin cDNA for standardization. Density of IL-6 signals was measured densitometrically (Biometra ScanPack2). The β-actin signal was used for standardization

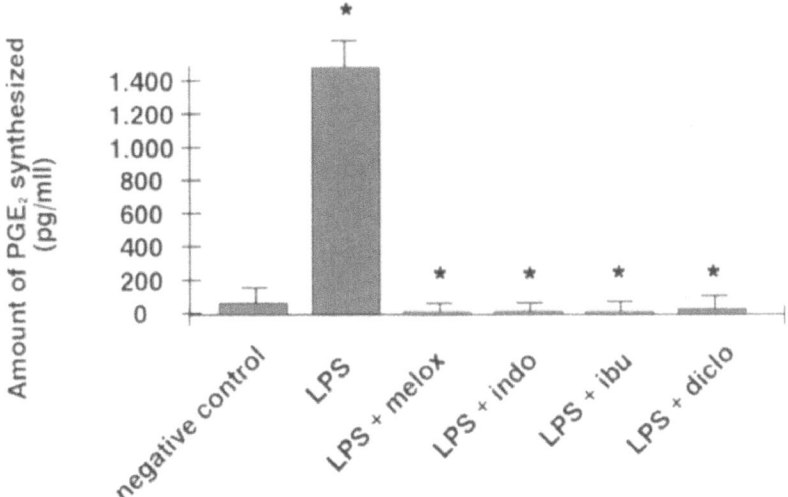

Fig. 4. Activated microglia synthesize PGE_2. Microglial cultures were treated with medium alone (control) or stimulated with lipopolysaccharide (100 ng/ml) in the presence of meloxicam (0.1 μM) (Melox), indomethacin (0.1 μM) (Indo), diclofenac (0.1 μM) (Diclo) or ibuprofen (0.1 μM) (Ibu). After stimulation for 24 h, supernatants were harvested and analyzed for PGE_2 using a specific immunoassay. Data are mean ± SD (bars) given as pg/ml PGE_2; *$p < 0.05$ (unpaired Wilcoxon test)

Discussion

We show that PGE_1 and PGE_2 induce increased IL-6 mRNA levels and IL-6 protein synthesis in human astroglioma cells. Other PGs such as PGD_2 or $PGF_{2\alpha}$ failed to induce IL-6 mRNA expression. We demonstrate

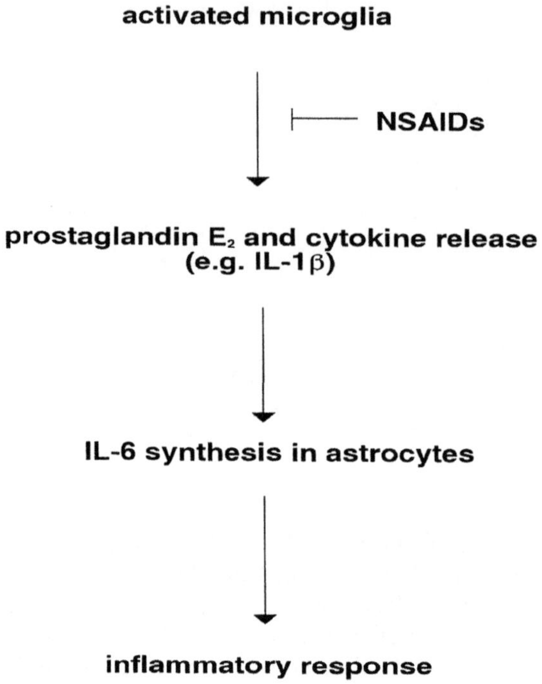

activated microglia

|—— **NSAIDs**

**prostaglandin E$_2$ and cytokine release
(e.g. IL-1β)**

IL-6 synthesis in astrocytes

inflammatory response

Fig. 5. Hypothetic model of the link between the arachidonic acid metabolism and IL-6 synthesis. Activated microglia relase prostaglandins, which induce IL-6 synthesis in astrocytes. Release of IL-6 is followed by an inflammatory response

that activated microglia produce PGE$_2$ and that this production is inhibited by several NSAIDs. Since we are in addition able to show that NSAIDs are potent inhibitors of PGE$_2$ synthesis in microglia, it appears likely that NSAIDs exert their therapeutical benefit in Alzheimer's disease by the inhibition of PG synthesis in microglial cells.

Acknowledgements

We would like to thank K. Gyufko for skillful technical assistance. This study was supported in part by grants of the Deutsche Forschungsgemeinschaft (SFB505/B1, DFG Fi 683/1-1 and Li 643/2-1).

References

Bauer J, Strauss S, Schreiter-Gasser U, Ganter U, Schlegel P, Witt I, Volk B, Berger M (1991) Interleukin-6 and alpha2-macroglobulin indicate an acute-phase state in Alzheimer's disease cortices. FEBS Lett 285: 111–114
Bauer MKA, Lieb K, Schulze-Osthoff K, Berger M, Gebicke-Haerter PJ, Bauer J, Fiebich BL (1997) Expression and regulation of cyclooxygenase-2 in rat microglia. Eur J Biochem 243: 726–731
Breder CD, Dewitt D, Kraig RP (1995) Characterization of inducible cyclooxygenase in rat brain. J Comp Neurol 355: 296–315

Breitner JCS (1996) The role of anti-inflammatory drugs in the prevention and treatment of Alzheimer's disease. Annu Rev Med 47: 401–411

Breitner JCS, Welsh KA, Helms MJ, Gaskell PC, Gau BA, Roses AD, Pericak-Vance MA, Saunders AM (1995) Delayed onset of Alzheimer's disease with nonsteroidal anti-inflammatory and histamine H2 blocking drugs. Neurobiol Aging 16: 523–530

Brown DR, Schmidt B, Kretzschmar HA (1996) Role of microglia and host prion protein in neurotoxicity of a prion protein fragment. Nature 380: 345–347

Campbell IL, Abrahman CR, Masliah E, Kemper P, Inglis JD, Oldstone MB, Mucke L (1993) Neurologic disease induced in transgenic mice by cerebral overexpression of interleukin 6. Proc Natl Acad Sci USA 90: 10061–10065

Chen ST, Hsu CY, Hogan EL, Halushka PV, Linet OI, Yatsu FM (1986) Thromboxane, prostacyclin, and leukotrienes in cerebral ischemia. Neurology 36: 466–470

Chiang CS, Stalder A, Samimi A, Campbell IL (1994) Reactive gliosis as a consequence of interleukin-6 expression in the brain: studies in transgenic mice. Dev Neurosci 16: 212–221

Fiebich BL, Biber K, Gyufko K, Berger R, Bauer J, Van Calker D (1996a) Adenosine A_{2b} receptors mediate an increase in interleukin (IL)-6 mRNA and IL-6 protein synthesis in human astroglioma cells. J Neurochem 66: 1426–1431

Fiebich BL, Biber K, Lieb K, Van Calker D, Berger M, Bauer J, Gebicke-Haerter PJ (1996b) Cyclooxygenase-2 expression in rat microglia is induced by adenosine A_{2a}-receptors. Glia 18: 152–160

Fretland DJ (1992) Potential role of prostaglandins and leukotrienes in multiple sclerosis and experimental allergic encephalomyelitis. Prostaglandins Leukot Essent Fatty Acids 45: 249–257

Gebicke-Haerter PJ, Bauer J, Schobert A, Northoff H (1989) Lipopolysaccharide-free conditions in primary astrocyte cultures allow growth and isolation of microglial cells. J Neurosci 9: 183–194

Hayaishi O (1991) Molecular mechanism of sleep wake regulation: roles of prostaglandins D_2 and E_2. FASEB J 5: 25–75

Horiguchi S, Ueno R, Hyodo M, Hayaishi O (1986) Alterations in nociception after intracisternal administraction of prostaglandin D2, E2 or F2 to conscious mice. Eur J Pharmacol 122: 173–179

Huell M, Strauss S, Volk B, Berger M, Bauer J (1995) Interleukin-6 is present in early stages of plaque formation and is restricted to brains of Alzheimer's disease patients. Acta Neuropathol 89: 544–551

Keller M, Jackisch R, Seregi A, Hertting G (1985) Comparison of prostanoid forming capacity of neuronal and astroglia cells in primary culture. Neurochem Int 7: 655–665

Lieb K, Kaltschmidt C, Kaltschmidt K, Baeuerle PA, Berger M, Bauer J, Fiebich BL (1996) Interleukin-1β uses common and distinct signaling pathways for induction of the interleukin-6 and tumor necrosis factor α genes in the human astrocytoma cell line U373. J Neurochem 66: 1496–1503

Minghetti L, Levi G (1995) Induction of prostanoid biosynthesis by bacterial lipopolysaccharide and isoproterenol in rat microglial cultures. J Neurochem 65: 2690–2698

Minghetti L, Polazzi E, Nicolini A, Créminon C, Levi G (1996) Interferon-gamma and nitric oxide down-regulate lipopolysaccharide-induced prostanoid production in cultured rat microglial cells by inhibiting cyclooxygenase-2 expression. J Neurochem 66: 1963–1970

Molina-Holgado F, Lledó A, Guaza C (1995) Evidence for cyclooxygenase activation by nitric oxide in astrocytes. Glia 15: 167–172

Pairet M, Engelhardt G (1996) Distinct isoforms (COX-1 and COX-2) of cyclooxygenase: possible physiological and therapeutic implications. Fundam Clin Pharmacol 10: 1–15

Rogers J, Kirby LC, Hempelman SR, Berry DL, McGeer PL, Kaszniak AW, Zalinski J, Cofield M, Mansukhani L, Wilson P (1993) Clinical trial of indomethacin in Alzheimer's disease. Neurology 43: 1609–1611

Sawada M, Suzumura A, Ohno K, Marunouchi T (1993) Regulation of astrocyte proliferation by prostaglandin E2 and the alpha subtype of protein kinase C. Brain Res 613: 67–73

Schettini G, Grimaldi M, Navarra P, Pozzoli G, Reichlin S, Preziosi P (1994) Regulation of interleukin 6 production by cAMP-protein kinase-A pathway in rat cortical astrocytes. Pharmacol Res 30: 13–24

Slepko N, Levi G (1996) Progressive activation of adult microglial cells in vitro. Glia 16: 241–246

Stiit JT (1991) Differential sensitivity in the sites of fever production by prostaglandin-E_1 within the hypothalamus of the rat. J Physiol 432: 99–110

Williams AE, Van Dam AM, Man-A-Hing WK, Berkenbosch F, Eikelenboom P, Fraser H (1994) Cytokines, prostaglandins and lipocortin-1 are present in the brains of scrapie-infected mice. Brain Res 654: 200–206

Wood JA, Wood PL, Ryan R, Graff Radford NR, Pilapil C, Robitaille Y, Quirion R (1993) Cytokine indices in Alzheimer's temporal cortex: no changes in mature IL-1 beta or IL-1RA but increases in the associated acute phase proteins IL-6, alpha 2-macroglobulin and C-reactive protein. Brain Res 629: 245–252

Yamagata K, Andreasson KI, Kaufmann WE, Barnes CA, Worley PF (1993) Expression of a mitogen-inducible cyclooxygenase in brain neurons: regulation by synaptic activity and glucocorticoids. Neuron 11: 371–386

Authors' address: Prof. Dr. J. Bauer, University of Freiburg Medical School, Department of Psychiatry, Hauptstrasse 5, D-79104 Freiburg, Federal Republic of Germany

Neurotrophin binding to the p75 neurotrophin receptor is necessary but not sufficient to mediate NGF-effects on APP secretion in PC-12 cells

S. Roßner[1], U. Ueberham[1], R. Schliebs[1], J. R. Perez-Polo[2], and V. Bigl[1]

[1] Department of Neurochemistry, Paul Flechsig Institute for Brain Research, Leipzig, Federal Republic of Germany
[2] Department HBC&G, University of Texas Medical Branch, Galveston, TX, USA

Summary. In the present study the pheochromocytoma cell line (PC-12) was used as a model system to determine the role of the two neurotrophin receptors in the regulation of amyloid precursor protein (APP) secretion by nerve growth factor (NGF). To stimulate TrkA and/or p75^{NTR} signaling in PC-12 cells, we used NGF, brain-derived neurotrophic factor (BDNF), and NGF in the presence of an excess of BDNF or the monoclonal antibody 192IgG, to block p75^{NTR} binding to NGF. Our results demonstrate that NGF stimulates APP secretion in a dose dependent fashion with maximum effects at 10 ng/ml, known to saturate high-affinity NGF binding sites. Treatment of PC-12 cells with varying concentrations of BDNF, 1–1,000 ng/ml, did not alter APP secretion, suggesting that binding to p75^{NTR} alone is not sufficient to affect APP secretion. When blocking NGF binding to p75^{NTR} with BDNF or 192IgG, on the other hand, NGF effects on APP secretion were abolished. These findings suggest that in cells expressing p75^{NTR} and TrkA receptors, binding of NGF to the p75^{NTR} is required to mediate NGF effects on APP secretion. Our data are also consistent with a proposed function of the p75^{NTR} in receptor recruitment and "presentation" of NGF to receptors.

Introduction

Nerve growth factor (NGF) is a neurotrophic factor that regulates developmental survival, differentiation and cholinergic activity of basal forebrain cholinergic neurons. Since these neurons undergo severe degeneration in the course of Alzheimer's disease (AD), the therapeutic use of NGF has been suggested to treat AD patients. However, NGF affects not only synthesis of cholinergic marker enzymes but also elevates amyloid precursor protein (APP) synthesis and release (Fukuyama et al., 1993; Ohyagi and Tabira, 1993; Smith et al., 1991; Yamada et al., 1991). Because increased expression and abnormal processing of APP have been closely associated with the pathogenesis of AD, it is of particular interest to identify the neurotrophin receptor that mediates neurotrophin actions on APP metabolism.

To elucidate any interaction between neurotrophin signaling pathways and APP processing in more detail, the pheochromocytoma cell line (PC-12) was used as a model system. Like cholinergic neurons of the basal forebrain, PC-12 cells express both TrkA and p75 neurotrophin receptors (p75^{NTR}) and also a significant level of APP.

The specificity of neurotrophin action derives in part from binding to specific high-affinity receptors that bind neurotrophins with a K_D of 10^{-11} M (Dechant et al., 1994). For example, NGF binds to TrkA, brain-derived neurotrophic factor (BDNF) to TrkB, and neurotrophin-3 to TrkC and with lesser affinity to TrkA (Ip et al., 1993; Kaplan et al., 1991). Cognate ligand binding to Trk receptors activates several signaling pathways, including those depending on p21^{Ras}, mitogen-activated protein kinases, phospholipase C$_\gamma$, and phosphatidylinositol 3-kinase (Muroya et al., 1992; Peraldi et al., 1993; Soltoff et al., 1992; Vetter et al., 1991).

On the other hand, all known neurotrophins bind to the p75^{NTR} with similar affinity (10^{-9} M) but different kinetics (Rodriguez-Tebar et al., 1992). The p75^{NTR} is likely to play a role in recruitment of NGF and its presentation to high-affinity receptors that modulate Trk signaling (Verdi et al., 1994). Also, neurotrophin binding to p75^{NTR} is known to activate sphingomyelinase (Dobrowsky et al., 1994), NKϰB (Carter et al., 1996) and a p75^{NTR}-associated protein kinase (Canossa et al., 1996).

In order to identify which neurotrophin receptors regulate APP secretion, we stimulated p75^{NTR}- and TrkA-containing PC-12 cells with NGF and we blocked NGF binding to p75^{NTR} by the addition of excess BDNF or of the monoclonal antibody 192IgG to the culture medium. Additionally, in order to stimulate p75^{NTR} alone, PC-12 cells were treated with varying concentrations of BDNF. After treatment of cells for 48 hours, APP secreted into the culture medium was measured by Western blot analysis.

Material and methods

Materials

Human recombinant BDNF was generously donated by Dr. R. Lindsay (Regeneron, New York, NY). Renin-free mouse β-NGF (2.5S) was purified from adult male submandibular glands as previously described (Taglialatela et al., 1990).

Cell culture

Rat pheochromocytoma PC-12 cells were a gift of Dr. L. A. Greene (Columbia University, New York, NY). PC-12 cells were cultured in RPMI 1640 cell culture medium (Gibco BRL, Eggenstein, Germany) supplemented with 10% horse serum and 5% fetal calf serum (Gibco BRL, Eggenstein, Germany) at 37°C under 5% CO_2 atmosphere. Before any treatment, cells were subcultured and allowed to attach overnight.

Treatment of cells

PC-12 cells were treated with varying concentrations of NGF and BDNF (ranging from 1 to 1,000 ng/ml culture medium) for 48 hours. Additionally, cells were incubated with 20 ng/ml NGF in the presence of a 70-fold excess of the monoclonal antibody 192IgG against the p75[NTR] or a 50-fold excess of BDNF, to suppress NGF binding to the p75[NTR]. Blocking reagents were added 30 minutes before the addition of NGF.

Western Blots

At the end of an experiment the medium was collected and concentrated by filtration through microconcentrators (Microcon 100, Amicon, Inc. Beverly, MA). Aliquots of concentrated medium were loaded on a 6% SDS-acrylamide/bisacrylamide gel and separated by electrophoresis at 200V for 90 minutes. Proteins were blotted onto nitrocellulose membranes (Schleicher&Schuell, Dassel, Germany), blocked overnight in 4% BSA in TBST (TBST/BSA) and then incubated with primary mouse anti APP antibodies that recognize an N-terminal fragment (22C11, Boehringer Mannheim, Mannheim, Germany, 1:500) in the same medium. After three washes in TBST, nitrocellulose membranes were incubated with digoxygenin-tagged goat anti mouse antibodies in TBST-BSA (1:2,000), washed again three times in TBST and incubated with alkaline phosphatase conjugated anti digoxygenin Fab fragments (Boehringer Mannheim, Mannheim, Germany, 1:500) in TBST/BSA. Nitrocellulose membranes were washed twice in TBST, preincubated in alkaline phosphatase buffer (100 mM Tris, 100 mM NaCl, 5 mM $MgCl_2$, pH 9.5) and the presence of the marker enzyme was visualized by incubating nitrocellulose membranes with 5-bromo-4-chloro-3-indolyl phosphate (BCIP, 1.65 mg/10 ml, Sigma, St. Louis, MO) and Tetranitro blue tetrazolium (TNBT, 3.3 mg/10 ml, Sigma, St. Louis, MO) in alkaline phosphatase buffer.

Results

In the first set of experiments, the dose-response characteristics of NGF and BDNF regulation of APP secretion in PC-12 cells were assessed. NGF treatment increased APP secretion into the culture medium at concentrations as low as 1 ng/ml by 65%. A maximum effect (increase of APP secretion by 110%) was observed at 10 ng NGF/ml culture medium. Further increases in NGF concentrations had no effect on APP secretion (Table 1).

BDNF, which binds to the p75[NTR] but not to the TrkA receptors, had no effect on APP secretion at any of the concentrations used, ranging from 1 to 1,000 ng/ml culture medium (Table 1).

When NGF binding to p75[NTR] was blocked by adding a 50-fold excess of BDNF 30 minutes before the addition of NGF to the culture medium, NGF effects on APP secretion were abolished. Additionally, the addition of a 70-fold excess of the monoclonal antibody 192IgG against the p75[NTR] prior to the addition of NGF also completely abolished NGF effects on APP-secretion (Table 1).

Discussion

The aim of this study was to identify which neurotrophin receptors regulate the secretion of APP. We used a cell line that posseses both, the neurotrophin-

Table 1. Effects of neurotrophin treatment on APP secretion

Ligand/concentration	APP-Secretion (% of control)
NGF 1 ng/ml	165.2 ± 19.6*
10 ng/ml	209.0 ± 21.3*
20 ng/ml	284.0 ± 55.7*
100 ng/ml	214.6 ± 23.9*
1,000 ng/ml	206.7 ± 18.4*
BDNF 1 ng/ml	103.2 ± 14.3
10 ng/ml	109.7 ± 17.7
100 ng/ml	74.2 ± 19.4
1,000 ng/ml	71.0 ± 21.6
NGF (20 ng/ml) + BDNF (1,000 ng/ml)	173.7 ± 28.8*·§
NGF (20 ng/ml) + anti p75^{NTR} (20 µg/ml)	94.2 ± 5.2
NGF (20 ng/ml) + anti NGF (25 µg/ml)	114.4 ± 18.2

*$P < 0.05$ versus untreated control; §$P < 0.05$ versus 20 ng/ml NGF

binding p75^{NTR} and the more NGF specific TrkA. NGF binds to both, p75^{NTR} and to TrkA receptors, and is known to increase APP secretion and the ratio of APP695 to APP751/770 mRNA in PC-12 cells (Fukuyama et al., 1993; Ohyagi and Tabira, 1993; Smith et al., 1991; Yamada et al., 1991) as well as to stimulate APP release from rat hippocampal explants (Clarris et al., 1994). NGF deprivation, on the contrary, reduces the ratio of APP695 to APP751/770 (Smith et al., 1993). The effects of exogenously applied NGF on APP metabolism are less well understood. While Mobley et al. (1988) observed increased APP mRNA levels in the developing hamster brain after NGF administration, others report no effects of NGF treatment on APP mRNA levels and APP in rat brain (Forloni et al., 1993; Neve et al., 1996).

In order to determine the role of the neurotrophin receptors in the regulation of APP metabolism, we treated PC-12 cells with varying concentrations of neurotrophins and blocking agents and measured APP secretion into the culture medium. NGF treatment of PC-12 cells for 48 hours increased APP secretion at concentrations known to saturate high-affinity NGF binding sites, suggesting a significant role for TrkA, a conclusion further supported by the observation that further increases in NGF concentration in the culture medium likely to increase p75^{NTR} occupancy did not increase APP secretion further.

BDNF binds to p75^{NTR} but not to TrkA receptors. The finding that treatment of PC-12 cells with BDNF at concentrations between 1 and 1,000 ng/ml culture medium did not alter APP secretion also suggests that p75^{NTR}-associated signaling in the presence of TrkA does not affect APP secretion. However, BDNF alone does not activate NFκB or increase ceramide levels in Schwann cells prepared from sciatic nerve of postnatal day 2 rats or mouse PCNA cells that only display p75^{NTR} (Carter et al., 1996), and BDNF does not induce the p75^{NTR}-mediated cell death of cultured oligodendrocytes (Casaccia-Bonnefil et al., 1996). However, binding of any of the neurotrophins to p75^{NTR} in T9 glioma cells or NIH3T3 cells can activate sphingomyelinase and ceramide production (Dobrowsky et al., 1995). Also, BDNF can rescue serumless PC-12 cells from apoptotic cell death only when TrkA is suppressed (Taglialatela et al., 1996). This is consistent with there being two distinct signaling pathways activated by binding of NGF to p75^{NTR} alone or to associated p75^{NTR}-TrkA on cell surfaces. Thus, it is not clear which signaling pathway is activated by BDNF binding to p75^{NTR} alone under our experimental conditions. To overcome these problems, treatment of PC-12 cells with substances that mimic the effects of downstream second messengers such as C2-ceramide might be an appropriate tool.

When blocking NGF binding to the p75^{NTR} by either 192IgG or an excess of BDNF, NGF effects on APP secretion were greatly reduced. This is consistent with the observation that the disruption of NGF binding to the p75^{NTR} reduces NGF binding to TrkA on PC-12 cells (Barker and Shooter, 1994) and provides further evidence for a specifying role for TrkA activation with regard to neurotrophin effects on APP metabolism via p75^{NTR} alone or p75^{NTR} and TrkA interactions. Involvement of p75^{NTR} regulation of APP is also consistent with the hypothesis that the p75^{NTR} signal transduction pathway acts via NFϰB because there is an NFϰB site in the APP promoter (Grilli et al., 1995). In the present study we did not determine the effects of exclusive stimulation of TrkA and we could not ascertain whether BDNF treatment initiated the p75^{NTR}-associated signaling mechanisms under our experimental conditions. Our results do suggest that neurotrophin binding to p75^{NTR} alone may be sufficient to mediate neurotrophin effects on APP metabolism in PC-12 cells and that blockade of NGF binding to p75^{NTR} abolishes NGF effects on APP secretion, consistent with a role of the p75 neurotrophin receptor in the regulation of APP.

References

Barker PA, Shooter EM (1994) Disruption of NGF binding to the low affinity neurotrophin receptor p75^{LNTR} reduces NGF binding to TrkA on PC12 cells. Neuron 13: 203–215

Canossa M, Twiss JL, Verity AN, Shooter EM (1996) p75^{NGFR} and TrkA receptors collaborate to rapidly activate a p75^{NGFR}-associated protein kinase. EMBO J 15: 3369–3376

Carter BD, Kaltschmidt C, Kaltschmidt B, Offebhäuser N, Böhm-Matthaei, Baeuerle P, Barde Y-A (1996) Selective activation of NF-ϰB by nerve growth factor through the neurotrophin receptor p75. Science 272: 542–545

Cassacia-Bonnefil P, Carter B, Dobrowsky R, Chao M (1996) Death of oligodendrocytes mediated by the interaction of nerve growth factor with its receptor p75. Nature 383: 716–719

Clarris HJ, Nurcombe V, Small DH, Beyreuther K, Masters CL (1994) Secretion of nerve growth factor from septum stimulates neurite outgrowth and release of the amyloid protein precursor of Alzheimer's disease from hippocampal explants. J Neurosci Res 38: 248–258

Dechant G, Rodriguez-Tebar A, Barde YA (1994) Neurotrophin receptors. Prog Neurobiol 42: 347–352

Dobrowsky RT, Jenkins GM, Hannan YA (1995) Neurotrophins induce sphingomyelin-modulation by coexpression of p75(NTR) with Trk receptors. J Biol Chem 270: 22135–22142

Forloni G, Delbo R, Angeretti N, Smiroldo S, Gabellini N, Vantini G (1993) Nerve growth factor does not influence the expression of beta amyloid precursor protein messenger RNA in rat brain — in vivo and in vitro studies. Brain Res 620: 292–296

Fukuyama R, Chandrasekaran K, Rapoport SI (1993) Nerve growth factor-induced neuronal differentiation is accompanied by differential induction and localization of the amyloid precursor protein (APP) in PC12-cells and variant PC12S-cells. Mol Brain Res 17: 17–22

Grilli M, Ribola M, Alberici A, Valerio A, Memo M, Spano P (1995) Identification and characterization of a kappa B/Rel binding site in the regulatory region of the amyloid precursor protein gene. J Biol Chem 270: 26774–26777

Ip NY, Stitt TN, Tapley P, Klein R, Glass DJ, Fandl J, Greene LA, Barbacid M, Yancopoulos GD (1993) Similarities and differences in the way neurotrophins interact with the Trk receptors in neuronal and nonneuronal cells. Neuron 10: 137–149

Kaplan DR, Hempstead BL, Martin-Zanca D, Chao MV, Parada LF (1991) The trk proto-oncogene product: a signal transducing receptor for NGF. Science 252: 554–558

Mobley WC, Neve RL, Prusiner SB, McKinley MP (1988) Nerve growth factor increases mRNA levels for the prion protein and the β-amyloid precursor protein in the developing hamster brain. Proc Natl Acad Sci USA 85: 9811–9815

Muroya K, Hattori S, Nakamura S (1992) Nerve growth factor induces rapid accumulation of the GTP-bound form of p21ras in rat pheochromocytoma PC12 cells. Oncogene 7: 277–281

Neve RL, Valletta JS, Li Y, Ventosa-Michelman M, Holtzman DM, Mobley WC (1996) A comprehensive study of the spatiotemporal pattern of β-amyloid precursor protein mRNA and protein in the rat brain: lack of modulation by exogenously applied nerve growth factor. Mol Brain Res 39: 185–197

Ohyagi Y, Tabira T (1993) Effect of growth factors and cytokines on expression of amyloid beta protein precursor messenger RNAs in cultured neural cells. Mol Brain Res 18: 127–132

Peraldi P, Scimeca JC, Filloux C, Van Obberghen E (1993) Regulation of extracellular signal-regulated protein kinase-1 (ERK-1; pp44/mitogen -activated protein kinase) by epidermal growth factor and nerve growth factor in PC12 cells: implication of ERK1 inhibitory activieties. Endocrinology 132: 2578–2585

Rodriguez-Tebar A, Dechant G, Gotz R, Barde YA (1992) Binding of neurotrophin-3 to its neuronal receptors and interactions with nerve growth factor and brain-derived neurotrophic factor. EMBO J 11: 917–922

Smith CJ, Wion D, Brachet P (1991) Nerve growth factor-induced neuronal differentiation is accompanied by differential splicing of beta-amyloid precursor messenger RNAs in the PC12 cell line. Mol Brain Res 10: 351–354

Smith CJ, Johnson EM, Osborne P, Freeman RS, Neveu I, Brachet P (1993) NGF deprivation and neuronal degeneration trigger altered beta-amyloid precursor protein gene-expression in the rat superior cervical ganglia in vivo and in vitro. Mol Brain Res 17: 328–334

Soltoff SP, Rabin SL, Cantley LC, Kaplan DR (1992) Nerve growth factor promotes the activation of phosphatidylinositol 3-kinase and its association with the trk tyrosine kinase. J Biol Chem 267: 17472–17477

Taglialatela G, Angelucci L, Ramacci M, Foreman PJ, Perez-Polo JR (1990) ^{125}I-β-nerve growth factor binding is reduced in rat brain after stress exposure. J Neurosci Res 25: 331–335

Taglialatela G, Hibbert C, Hutton LA, Werrbach-Perez K, Perez-Polo JR (1996) Suppression of p140[trkA] does not abolish nerve growth factor-mediated rescue of serum-free PC12 cells. J Neurochem 66: 1826–1835

Verdi JM, Birren SJ, Ibanez CF, Persson H, Kaplan DR, Benedetti M, Chao MV, Anderson DJ (1994) p75LNGFR regulates Trk signal transduction and NGF-induced neuronal differentiation in MAH cells. Neuron 12: 733–745

Vetter ML, Martin-Zanca D, Parada LF, Bishop JM, Kaplan DR (1991) Nerve growth factor rapidly stimulates tyrosine phosphorylation of phospholipase C-gamma 1 by a kinase activity associated with the product of the trk protooncogene. Proc Natl Acad Sci USA 88: 5650–5654

Yamada T, Araki E, Izumi R, Goto I, Sasaki H, Sakaki Y (1991) Expression of Alzheimer amyloid-beta protein precursor gene in neuronal cells. Gerontology 37: 24–30

Authors' address: S. Roßner, Ph.D., Paul Flechsig Institute for Brain Research, Department of Neurochemistry, Jahnallee 59, D-04109 Leipzig, Federal Republic of Germany

Aromatic alcohols as neuroprotectants

M. Uhr, B. Moosmann, and **C. Behl**

Max-Planck-Institute of Psychiatry, Munich, Federal Republic of Germany

Summary. Free radicals and oxidative stress-induced neuronal cell death have been implicated in various neurological disorders including neuro-degenerative diseases. We have recently shown that estrogens can protect neurons against oxidative stress due to their antioxidant potential. Here, we report that also other aromatic alcohols with intact phenolic groups and different phenol derivatives can protect neurons against oxidative cell death as induced by glutamate and hydrogen peroxide. Starting with melatonin, in this study, we degraded the chemical structure step by step and tested various aromatic alcohols as well as phenol derivatives for their potential antioxidant activity. We found that aromatic alcohols with intact phenolic groups protect neurons effectively against oxidative damage and cell death and that this neuroprotective activity is independent of the time the compound is added before the toxin. Methylation of the phenolic hydroxyl group led to a decrease or loss in neuroprotection. Moreover, the tested compounds directly inhibited peroxidation reactions suggesting that the neuroprotection is mediated by antioxidant properties. Our result may have some impact on the design of future drugs for the antioxidant treatment or prevention of oxidative stress-associated pathological conditions.

Introduction

Oxidative stress describes the imbalance between free radical generation and various enzymatic and non-enzymatic antioxidant defense systems. It is believed that oxidative stress may directly contribute to a variety of pathological changes including atherosclerosis and several neurodegenerative disorders, including Alzheimer's disease (for review: Halliwell and Gutteridge, 1989; Coyle and Puttfarcken, 1993). Brain cells are at a particular risk to be damaged by oxidative stress because they have a high rate of oxygen consumption. Moreover, neuronal membranes have a high content of polyunsaturated fatty acids that are susceptible to lipid peroxidation reactions.

The most prominent excitatory amino acid glutamate can be cytotoxic to neurons in vitro and in vivo (Choi, 1992; Murphy et al., 1989). It has been shown in various experimental paradigms of glutamate toxicity that this excitotoxin can induce the generation of several reactive oxygen species in neurons indicating a general role of free radicals in glutamate toxicity (for review: Coyle and Puttfarcken, 1993). In clonal hippocampal cells (HT22), glutamate induces a rapid increase in the level of intracellular peroxides, mainly hydrogen peroxide, and finally oxidative cell death in a glutamate receptor independent manner (Davis and Maher, 1994). Peroxides and especially hydrogen peroxides are precursor molecules of highly reactive hydroxyl radicals, which can directly attack unsaturated carbohydrate side chains of the membrane's lipid molecules leading to peroxidation (for review: Halliwell and Gutteridge, 1989; Halliwell et al., 1992).

In the search for novel and potent antioxidant compounds for neurons, we used glutamate and hydrogen peroxide-induced cell death in primary cortical neurons from rat and in HT22 cells as toxicity paradigms. Several different antioxidants have already been described to prevent oxidative stress-induced neuronal cell death including N-acetyl-5-methoxytryptamine (melatonin) (Lezoualc'h et al., 1996) and 17-β estradiol (Behl et al., 1995). More recently, we were able to describe that the presence of the free C3 hydroxyl group of the estrogen molecule's A ring, which represents a phenolic group, is the only structural prerequisite that is necessary for the antioxidative and neuroprotective effect of this particular aromatic alcohol (Behl et al., 1997). Employing liver microsomes, it has previously been demonstrated that natural phenolic compounds may potentially prevent damage caused by peroxidation reactions (Sugioka et al., 1987; Nakano et al., 1987; Liu et al., 1992).

The purpose of the present study was to investigate whether the antioxidant activity of phenolic groups as present in estrogen does also afford neuroprotective potential to other aromatic alcohols. Therefore, we studied a whole panel of various aromatic alcohols and some of their derivatives for their activity to prevent glutamate and hydrogen peroxide-induced cell death as well as lipid peroxidation reactions in neuronal cells.

Results

In Fig. 1, the chemical structures of some of the aromatic alcohols, their derivatives and their precursor (phenol), which were tested in the present study for their potential neuroprotective activities, are shown. Firstly, the effect of selected aromatic alcohols on the survival of HT22 cells incubated with various concentrations of glutamate was investigated. A 24-h incubation of HT22 cells with glutamate increased the fraction of dead cells as detected by the staining with the fluorescence dye propidium iodide indicative of dead cells (Behl et al., 1995). When the cultures were pretreated with aromatic alcohols containing an intact phenolic hydroxyl group, almost no signs of cell damage or cell death could be observed. Otherwise, the tested compounds had considerable structural differences. In stark contrast, when the phenolic hydroxyl group was modified, such as by methylation, no prevention of glutamate-induced cell death could be observed (data not shown).

In a second set of experiments, the whole array of aromatic compounds and their derivatives, shown in Fig. 1, were tested within the glutamate and

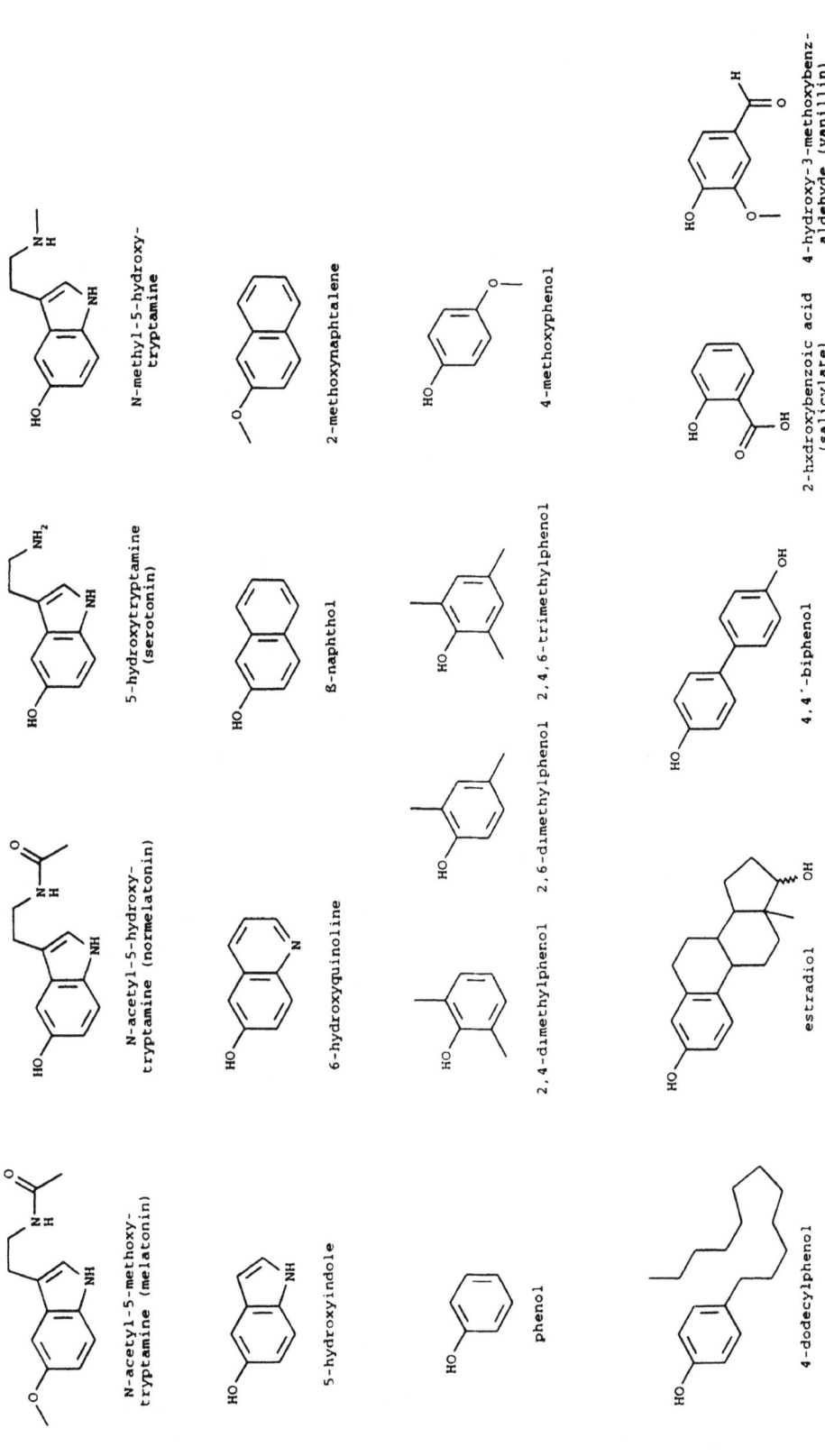

Fig. 1. Molecular structures of various aromatic alcohols and their derivatives. Different compounds that were tested for potential neuroprotective antioxidant activity are shown

the hydrogen peroxide toxicity paradigm. This time, cell survival was quantified by the MTT test (Behl et al., 1992). As shown in Table 1, 4-dodecylphenol and 4,4′-biphenol were highly protective against glutamate at concentrations as low as 5 μM. Various indole derivatives had to be used at concentrations of around 20 μM in order to be protective. Also β-naphthol was highly protective at 20 μM, but its ether-modified derivative, 2-methoxynaphthalene, did not protect the cells against glutamate toxicity. An almost identical pattern of protective activity of these various tested compounds could be observed employing 250 μM hydrogen peroxide as oxidative challenge for HT22 cells (Table 1). But not only clonal hippocampal cells could be protected by the various aromatic alcohols. Also the survival of primary cortical neurons was significantly increased after preincubation with N-acetyl-5-hydroxytryptamine (normelatonin), 5-hydroxytryptamine (serotonin), 5-hydroxy-indole, 4,4′-biphenol and 17-β estradiol before the challenge with hydrogen peroxide (Table 2). In a kinetic study, we could observe that the protective activity of these aromatic compounds was completely independent from the time the various aromatic alcohols were added before the toxin. The protective effect of the compounds was identical when added 22 h before or 1 h before or even together with the toxin. In contrast, the addition of the potentially protective chemicals after toxin addition led to a complete loss of the protective effect of the compounds (data not shown).

In order to investigate whether the neuroprotective compounds can directly inhibit lipid peroxidation reactions which may cause cell lysis and, therefore, cell death, we employed two cell-free lipid peroxidation assays. One assay was the measurement of in vitro lipid peroxidation by a single photon counting-chemiluminescence assay (Reiber et al., 1994). The other assay was the detection of end-products of lipid peroxidation represented by the measurement of thiobarbituric acid reactive substances (TBARS) (Fukunaga et al., 1995). As shown in Table 3, with both assays we found that at 100 μM normelatonin and β-naphthol prevented lipid peroxidation reactions to a similar extent like 17-β estradiol. Melatonin and 2-methoxynaphthalene did not prevent lipid peroxidation. On the basis of these results, we concluded that compounds that can be directly neuroprotective in cellular models of oxidative stress-induced neuronal cell death can act as potent direct inhibitors of lipid peroxidation reactions.

Discussion

In the present study we show that different aromatic alcohols can prevent oxidative cell death of neurons as induced by the excitatory amino acid glutamate and hydrogen peroxide, the precursor of hydroxyl radicals. The phenolic compounds 4-dodecylphenol, 4,4′-biphenol, 5-hydroxyindole, serotonin, N-methyl-5-hydroxytryptamine and normelatonin were as effective in neuroprotection as 17-β estradiol at μM concentrations. Interestingly, 6-hydroxyquinoline, β-naphthol and also different methylphenols can also protect neurons against oxidative challenges and oxidative cell death. Apart from

Table 1. Protection of clonal hippocampal HT22 cells against oxidative cell death by various aromatic alcohols

Control 20 mM glut. Alone ($250\,\mu$M H_2O_2 alone)	100 2 ± 4 (6 ± 5)		
20 mM glut. ($250\,\mu$M H_2O_2) treatment after 3 h (16 h) preincubation with	$5\,\mu$M	$20\,\mu$M	$200\,\mu$M
N-acetyl-5-hydroxytryptamine	$9 \pm 3^*$ $(17 \pm 2^{**})$	$18 \pm 6^{**}$ $(66 \pm 9^{**})$	$89 \pm 5^{**}$ $(87 \pm 7^{**})$
N-acetyl-5-methoxytryptamine	5 ± 3 (13 ± 4)	9 ± 5 $(21 \pm 6^*)$	$25 \pm 7^{**}$ $(43 \pm 10^{**})$
5-hydroxytryptamine	8 ± 6 $(28 \pm 5^{**})$	$28 \pm 4^{**}$ $(81 \pm 7^{**})$	$72 \pm 6^{**}$ $(79 \pm 5^{**})$
N-methyl-5-hydroxytryptamine	6 ± 5 $(16 \pm 4^*)$	$15 \pm 6^{**}$ $(68 \pm 9^{**})$	$79 \pm 8^{**}$ $(76 \pm 4^{**})$
5-hydroxyindole	$14 \pm 7^*$ $(41 \pm 8^{**})$	$80 \pm 5^{**}$ $(77 \pm 9^{**})$	$95 \pm 4^{**}$ $(96 \pm 10^{**})$
6-hydroxyquinoline	4 ± 3 $(20 \pm 3^{**})$	$22 \pm 7^{**}$ $(29 \pm 7^{**})$	$90 \pm 5^{**}$ $(45 \pm 6^{**})$
β-naphthol	3 ± 3 (13 ± 4)	$42 \pm 10^{**}$ $(27 \pm 6^{**})$	$88 \pm 10^{**}$ $(34 \pm 4^{**})$
2-methoxynaphthalene	4 ± 4 (7 ± 4)	4 ± 5 (14 ± 6)	5 ± 3 $(15 \pm 4^*)$
phenol	2 ± 3 (6 ± 5)	6 ± 4 (9 ± 6)	$60 \pm 6^{**}$ $(19 \pm 4^*)$
2,4-dimethylphenol	3 ± 2 (14 ± 6)	$66 \pm 6^{**}$ $(50 \pm 8^{**})$	$59 \pm 5^{**}$ $(72 \pm 4^{**})$
2,6-dimethylphenol	6 ± 4 $(24 \pm 6^{**})$	$53 \pm 7^{**}$ $(67 \pm 6^{**})$	$66 \pm 5^{**}$ $(74 \pm 9^{**})$
2,4,6-trimethylphenol	$11 \pm 6^*$ $(49 \pm 7^{**})$	$69 \pm 8^{**}$ $(66 \pm 8^{**})$	$64 \pm 4^{**}$ $(71 \pm 5^{**})$
4-methoxyphenol	7 ± 4 $(24 \pm 7^{**})$	$28 \pm 8^{**}$ $(76 \pm 6^{**})$	$84 \pm 5^{**}$ $(75 \pm 5^{**})$
4-dodecylphenol	$58 \pm 14^{**}$ $(40 \pm 4^{**})$	$89 \pm 7^{**}$ $(66 \pm 5^{**})$	n.d.
17-β estradiol	$30 \pm 8^{**}$ $(32 \pm 9^{**})$	$85 \pm 10^{**}$ $(47 \pm 10^{**})$	n.d.
4,4′-biphenol	$69 \pm 14^{**}$ $(64 \pm 8^{**})$	$101 \pm 8^{**}$ $(79 \pm 9^{**})$	n.d.
2-hydroxybenzoic acid	1 ± 3 (12 ± 5)	6 ± 2 (13 ± 7)	10 ± 7 (10 ± 6)
4-hydroxy-3-methoxybenz- aldehyde	4 ± 3 (11 ± 3)	$10 \pm 5^*$ (12 ± 5)	$22 \pm 10^*$ (12 ± 5)

Cells were plated and pretreated with increasing concentrations of the indicated various aromatic alcohols for 3 h (16 h) overnight. Then, glutamate (glut.) or hydrogen peroxide (H_2O_2) (data in parentheses) was added and 22 h later, 3- (4, 5-dimethyl-thiazol-2-y)-2,5-diphenol-teterazolium bromide (MTT) tests were performed. This test measures the reduction of MTT to a colored formazan. This assay was exactly employed as previously described (Behl et al., 1992). All results were expressed as percent MTT reduction in toxin/aromatic alcohols treated cultures compared to control cultures, which were treated with aromatic alcohols alone. The data were normalized to control values (no addition of toxin or aromatic alcohol) as 100%. Data are presented as means ± SEM of one representative quadruplicate determination. *n.d.* not determined; P-values
    * = 0.05, ** = 0.01

Table 2. Protection of primary rat cortical neurons against oxidative cell death by selected aromatic alcohols

Control	100	
250 µM H₂O₂ alone	23 ± 5	
250 µM H₂O₂ treatment after 3 h pre-incubation with	20 µM	200 µM
N-acetyl-5-methoxytryptamine	n.d.	14 ± 7
N-acetyl-5-hydroxytryptamine	n.d.	47 ± 7**
5-hydroxytryptamine	56 ± 5**	62 ± 10**
5-hydroxyindole	49 ± 4**	43 ± 7*
17-β estradiol	36 ± 8	n.d.
4,4'-biphenol	39 ± 4*	n.d.

Primary cortical neurons were prepared exactly as previously described (Behl et al., 1997) and were incubated with increasing concentrations of the various indicated aromatic alcohols. Then, hydrogen peroxide was added and 20-h later, MTT assays were performed. All results were normalized to control values (no addition of toxin) as 100%. The data are presented as means ± SEM of one representative quadruplicate determination. The P-values of $P < 0.05$ and $P < 0.01$ were considered as significant (*n.d.* not determined)

Table 3. Prevention of lipid peroxidation reactions by selected aromatic alcohols

Control	100		
	3 µM	30 µM	100 µM
N-acetyl-5-hydroxytryptamine	95 ± 4 (95 ± 9)	82 ± 9 (75 ± 10*)	31 ± 7** (41 ± 12**)
N-acetyl-5-methoxytryptamine	92 ± 5 (97 ± 9)	96 ± 5 (90 ± 14)	89 ± 4 (82 ± 11)
β-naphthol	73 ± 3** (78 ± 11)	4 ± 2** (14 ± 9**)	0 ± 0** (7 ± 5**)
2-methoxynaphthalene	95 ± 7 (95 ± 7)	87 ± 5 (85 ± 9)	80 ± 4 (81 ± 11)
17-β estradiol	46 ± 13* (45 ± 10**)	1 ± 1** (4 ± 2**)	6 ± 3** (8 ± 2**)

Pig brain membrane homogenates were prepared and lipid peroxidation reactions were detected. Chemiluminescence of the single photon-counting chemiluminescence assay (Reiber et al., 1994) is presented as relative light units (mean of 5 independent experiments) compared to the control after subtraction of the background luminescence (in %). The data on the detection of the TBARS are presented in parentheses. These data were calculated from 5 independent experiments each and were compared to the control values after subtraction of the baseline. The P-values of $P < 0.05$ and $P < 0.01$ were considered as significant

considerable structural differences, common to all these neuroprotective compounds is the presence of an intact phenolic group. Whenever this intact hydroxyl group at a mesomeric system is chemically modified, such as by methylation, the antioxidant activity in the lipid peroxidation reactions and, ultimately, the neuroprotective activity is completely lost.

We recently described neuroprotective activities against glutamate and hydrogen peroxide-induced oxidative neuronal cell death for various antioxidants (for review: Behl, 1997). These included also the phenolic molecule, estrogen (Behl et al., 1995, 1997). We also observed a potential neuroprotective activity in our toxicity paradigms for melatonin (Lezoualc'h et al., 1996). But melatonin had to be used at much higher concentrations in order to protect HT22 cells, compared to estrogens, which are neuroprotective at a low micromolar concentration. The pineal hormone melatonin has been shown to be an antioxidant with a poor capacity of preventing lipid peroxidations and can act as a cytoprotective antioxidant in vitro (for review: Marshall et al., 1996). Employing the aromatic alcohols normelatonin, serotonin and also 5-hydroxyindole, the precursor molecule of the latter molecules, with an intact phenolic hydroxyl group, now we were able to show a much higher protective potential for these compounds compared to melatonin. Consistently, while β-naphthol with an intact phenolic group has some protective potential, as shown in this study, its methylated counterpart, methoxynaphthalene, lacks these protective antioxidant properties.

With respect to the mechanism of this antioxidant activity, aromatic alcohols, such as estrogens, may donate hydrogen atoms from their intact phenolic hydroxyl groups to hydroxyl radicals or also to lipid peroxide radicals (for review: Halliwell and Gutteridge, 1989; Halliwell et al., 1992). We speculate that this mode of action may also apply to the active compounds tested in the presented study. Because we could show that the neuroprotective aromatic alcohols used can directly prevent lipid peroxidation reactions, very likely, it is this peroxidation inhibiting potential of the compounds that prevents oxidative neuronal cell death.

Antioxidants can be very potent neuroprotective molecules in vitro and in vivo (for review: Behl, 1997). The clinical importance and the clinical applicability of an antioxidant neuroprotection is clearly documented by very recent reports that the treatment of patients suffering from Alzheimer's disease with Vitamin E can slow the progression of the disease (Sano et al., 1997). Our data show for the first time the antioxidant potential of various aromatic alcohols in disease-related paradigms of oxidative neuronal cell death employing clonal and primary neurons. The presented data further strongly support and largely extend our previous findings that the structural prerequisite of a potent neuroprotective activity of steroids is an intact phenolic group (Behl et al., 1997). Therefore, our data may help in the design of novel antioxidative and neuroprotective compounds, which, ultimately, could prevent oxidative stress-associated neurodegenerative disorders.

Note added in proof

The main results of this study have been published in FEBS Letters (1997) 413: 467–472.

References

Behl C (1997) Amyloid β-protein toxicity and oxidative stress in Alzheimer's disease. Cell Tissue Res 290: 471–480

Behl C, Davis J, Cole GM, Schubert D (1992) Vitamin E protects nerve cells from amyloid β protein toxicity. Biochem Biophys Res Comm 186: 944–952

Behl C, Widmann M, Trapp T, Holsboer F (1995) 17-β Estradiol protects from oxidative stress-induced cell death in vitro. Biochem Biophys Res Comm 216: 473–482

Behl C, Skutella T, Lezoualc'h F, Post A, Widmann M, Newton CJ, Holsboer F (1997) Neuroprotection against oxidative stress by estrogens: structure-activity relationship. Mol Pharm 51: 535–541

Coyle JT, Puttfarcken P (1993) Oxidative stress, glutamate, and neurodegenerative disorders. Science 262: 689–695

Choi DW (1992) Excitotoxic cell death. J Neurobiol 23: 1261–1276

Davis JB, Maher P (1994) Protein kinase C activation inhibits glutamate-induced cytotoxicity in a neuronal cell line. Brain Res 652: 169–173

Fukunaga K, Takama K, Suzuki T (1995) High-performance liquid chromatographic determination of plasma malondialdehyde level without a solvent. Anal Biochem 230: 20–23

Halliwell B, Gutteridge JMC (1989) Free radicals in biology and medicine. Oxford University Press, Oxford

Halliwell B, Gutteridge JMC, Cross CE (1992) Free radicals, antioxidants, and human disease: where are we now? Lab Clin Med 119: 598–620

Lezoualc'h F, Skutella T, Widmann M, Behl C (1996) Melatonin prevents oxidative stress-induced cell death in hippocampal cells. NeuroReport 7: 2071–2077

Liu GT, Zhang TM, Wang BE, Wang YW (1992) Protective action of seven natural phenolic compounds against peroxidative damage to biomembranes. Biochem Pharmacol 43: 147–152

Marshall KA, Reiter RJ, Poeggeler B, Aruoma OI, Halliwell B (1996) Evaluation of the antioxidant activity of melatonin in vitro. Free Radic Biol Med 21: 307–315

Murphy TH, Miyamoto M, Sastre A, Schnaar RL, Coyle JT (1989) Glutamate toxicity in a neuronal cell line involves inhibition of cystine transport leading to oxidative stress. Neuron 2: 1547–1558

Nakano M, Sugioka K, Naito I, Takehoshi S, Niki E (1987) Novel and potent antioxidants on membrane phospholipid peroxidation: 2-hydroxy estrone and 2-hydroxy estradiol. Biochem Biophys Res Comm 142: 919–924

Reiber H, Martens U, Prall F, Uhr M (1994) Relevance of endogenous ascorbate and tocopherol for brain cell vitality indicated by photon emission. J Neurochem 62: 608–614

Sano M, Ernesto C, Thomas RG et al (1997) A controlled trial of selegiline, alphatocopherol, or both as treatment for Alzheimer's disease. N Engl J Med 336: 1216–1222

Sugioka K, Shimosegawa Y, Nakano M (1987) Estrogens as natural antioxidants of membrane phospholipid peroxidation. FEBS Lett 210: 37–39

Authors' address: Dr. C. Behl, Max-Planck-Institute of Psychiatry, Kraepelinstrasse 2-10, D-80804 Munich, Federal Republic of Germany

The therapeutic potential of tacrine

A. Kurz

Department of Psychiatry, Technical University, Munich,
Federal Republic of Germany

Summary. Tacrine, a non-competitive inhibitor of acetylcholine esterase, has been approved for the treatment of patients with mild to moderate Alzheimer's disease in 1995. The available evidence suggests that in a substantial proportion of patients tacrine has the potential to improve cognitive functions, to ameliorate behavioural problems, and to delay the time to significant clinical endpoints. Thus, tacrine meets realistic expectations from symptomatic treatment. The major safety concern about tacrine is the probability of liver enzyme elevations and the high frequency of adverse events, particularly gastrointestinal. Findings are presented from an open-label multicentre study showing that tacrine is a safe and manageable compound in private practice.

Introduction

Alzheimer's disease (AD) is a neurodegenerative disorder which affects primarily the older segment of the population. Clinical symptoms are caused by a significant loss of nerve cells and of synapses. The depletion in the cerebral cortex of the neurotransmitter acetylcholine is a secondary event. The clinical phenotype is characterized by gradual decline in cognitive functions, behaviour change, and loss of activities of daily living. The course of AD can be described in terms of annual rates of deterioration on cognitive instruments. On the Alzheimer's Disease Assessment Scale, cognitive section (ADAS-cog) (Mohs and Cohen, 1988) the mean annual change in untreated patients is approximately 7 points. On the Syndrom Kurztest (SKT), the mean annual untreated change is 3 points (Erzigkeit, 1989). Approximately 70 per cent of AD patients will be admitted to a nursing home, mostly in the advanced stage of the disease. Institutionalization is typically precipitated by problematic behaviours including incontinence, aggression or wandering. Given these features of the disease, realistic expectations from an effective treatment include improvement of cognitive functions, reduction of problematic behaviours, enhancement of activities of daily living, and delay of time to significant clinical endpoints. The present paper examines to what degree tacrine meets these expectations. This cholinesterase inhibitor has been approved for the treatment of Alzheimer's disease in the United States and in several European countries. The compound has a short half-life which necessitates four times daily dosing. The major safety concern about tacrine is the probability of reversible liver enzyme elevations.

Improvement of cognitive functions

The ability of tacrine to improve cognitive functions was examined in a 30-week randomized, double-blind, placebo-controlled parallel-group study (Gracon, 1996; Knapp et al., 1994). The study evaluated 663 patients with probable AD who were mildly to moderately impaired. Patients were divided into 4 groups receiving final doses of tacrine of 80, 120, and 160 mg per day, or placebo. A total of 263 patients were evaluable at 30 weeks. Before week 30, 384 patients withdrew from the study, 285 because of adverse events, 20 because of lack of compliance with the protocol, 19 because of lack of efficacy, and 60 for other reasons. In evaluable subjects, patients who received 160 mg per day improved by 2 points on the Alzheimer Disease Assessment Scale, cognitive section (ADAS-cog) (Mohs and Cohen, 1988) whereas placebo patients had a mean decline of 2 points. The cumulative distribution of change from baseline on the ADAS-cog showed that 40 per cent of patients who received the 160 mg per day tacrine dose improved by 4 or more points. This compared with 25 per cent of patients given placebo. A large proportion of the patients in this study reported adverse events (90 per cent).

Reduction of problematic behaviours

An open-label study was conducted on 28 AD patients to assess the effects of tacrine on behavioural changes (Kaufer et al., 1996). Patients completed a baseline evaluation and at least one assessment during treatment. Behavioural symptoms were assessed using the Neuropsychiatric Inventory (NPI) (Cummings et al., 1994). The mean NPI score at the maximum tolerated individual dose of tacrine was markedly decreased, indicating that behaviour had improved compared to baseline. Symptoms of anxiety, apathy, hallucinations, aberrant motor behaviours, and disinhibition were most responsive. These findings suggest that tacrine treatment may have beneficial effects on some of the most frequent behavioural symptoms in AD patients.

Enhancement of activities of daily living

In the 30-week study (Knapp et al., 1994) family members assessed patients on the Progressive Deterioration Scale (PDS). This instrument rates 26 instrumental activities of daily living on a visual analog scale (De Jong et al., 1989). Patients receiving 160 mg per day of tacrine showed a significant treatment difference from baseline of 4.6 points (Gracon, 1996).

Delay of time to significant clinical endpoints

After completion of the double-blind placebo-controlled 30-week study (Knapp et al., 1994) a total of 595 patients were followed up for a minimum of 2 years (Knopman et al., 1996). Patients who remained on tacrine and were treated with doses greater than 80 mg per day were less likely to have entered a nursing home than patients who had received doses less than 80 mg tacrine. The data suggest that long-term treatment with a dose of tacrine greater than 80 mg per day may delay institutionalization by more than 400 days. The findings must be interpreted with caution, however, because treatment assignment was not random nor was it blinded after 30 weeks. It cannot be excluded that patients who tolerated a high dose of tacrine were positively selected although their baseline data were comparable with the remaining patients.

Tacrine treatment in real life: an open-label study

The double-blind placebo-controlled study demonstrates that tacrine is an effective drug for the treatment of patients with mild to moderate AD. It leaves open the question, however, how tacrine treatment fits into real life. More specifically, the large dose-related drop-out rate casts doubt on whether tacrine treatment is safe, tolerable, and manageable under the conditions of private practice. We addressed this issue in an open-label study involving 314 patients (170 females, 144 males, mean age 71 years). Subjects were recruited in 45 centres. They met DSM-III-R criteria (American-Psychiatric-Association, 1987) for dementia of mild to moderate severity and NINCDS-ADRDA criteria for Probable Alzheimer's disease (McKhann et al., 1984). Patients were started on tacrine 40 mg per day and titrated upwards in increments of 40 mg per day up to a maximum dose of 160 mg per day. The dose was reduced to the previous level in case of intolerable gastrointestinal side effects. The total treatment period was 24 weeks. Alanine aminotransferase (ALT) was monitored bi-weekly during the first 3 months and monthly thereafter. Treatment was discontinued in patients showing ALT elevations over 5 times the upper limit of the norm (ULN). If patients had ALT elevations greater than 3 times ULN the dose was not increased, ALT was monitored weekly, and if values were still greater than 3 times ULN treatment was also discontinued. Approximately one half of the patients terminated treatment prematurely. The number of patients who completed the 24 week treatment period according to protocol was 135.

The conditional probability of experiencing an ALT elevation over 3 times ULN showed the same peak at treatment week 6 as in pooled US studies (Watkins et al., 1994). The frequency of ALT elevations, however, was significantly lower. Furthermore, the proportion of patients reporting adverse events was smaller than in the US studies. The most frequent adverse events were gastrointestinal, particularly nausea, vomiting, and diarrhea. Most adverse events were of mild or moderate severity. More than half of the patients dropped out of treatment before completion of the 24 week study period. However, only a minority of premature terminations were substance-related. The most frequent reasons for dropout were unwillingness to continue treatment, inability of the carer to ensure regular study visits, imminent nursing home admission, and holidays.

Of the 135 patients who completed the 24-week treatment period, almost 90 per cent reached a final dose of at least 120 mg per day and three out of four reached a final daily dose of 160 mg. In evaluable subjects cognitive functions showed a significant improvement over baseline values among patients receiving 120 mg and 160 mg tacrine per day. The improvement on the SKT during tacrine treatment was comparable to that observed on the ADAS-cog in the 30-week study (Gutzmann et al., 1997). Activities of daily living also showed a significant improvement over baseline values. According to the clinicians' global impression, 60 per cent of the patients were improved.

Discussion

According to the evidence documented in the literature tacrine is an effective treatment for patients with mild to moderate AD. In a substantial proportion of patients tacrine improves cognitive functions, clinician's global impression, and activities of daily living. Furthermore, tacrine ameliorates a number of relevant behavioural problems that occur in AD including anxiety, apathy, hallucinations, aberrant motor behaviours, and disinhibition. Long-term treatment with tacrine lowers the rate of nursing home admissions and significantly delays the time until that important clinical endpoint. Findings from the open-label study concerning the efficacy of tacrine were entirely consistent with published data although different outcome measures had been used. In addition, the open-label study has demonstrated that tacrine is a safe and manageable compound. Liver enzyme elevations were significantly less frequent than in the US studies. It should be noted that ALT monitoring was performed bi-weekly but no increased risk ensued from this procedure. Previous results were also confirmed regarding the temporal distribution of liver enzyme elevations. The probability for an individual patient to experience an ALT elevation greater than 3 times the upper limit of the norm was greatest in the sixth week after starting the treatment and was minimal after treatment week 12. Thus, the majority of liver enzyme elevations occur within a predictable and narrow time window. The proportion of patients on tacrine who reported adverse events was smaller than in the 30-week double-blind study. The relative frequencies of nausea, vomiting, and diarrhea were comparable. Unexpectedly, only a minority of premature terminations were substance-related. Most drop-outs were associated with difficulty of carers to carry on with regular study visits. This suggests that ALT elevations and cholinergic side effects of tacrine do not represent major limitations of tacrine treatment. Using a flexible dose escalation procedure which allowed physicians to return to the previous dose in the event of intolerable gastrointestinal side effects the majority of 24-week completers had a final dose of 160 mg per day. From this it follows that patients who do not drop out early in the course of treatment are very likely to reach the maximum effective dose of tacrine. In conclusion, the available evidence shows that tacrine is an effective, safe and manageable drug.

References

American Psychiatric Association (1987) Diagnostic and statistical manual of mental disorders, 3rd ed, rev. American Psychiatric Association, Washington

Cummings JL, Mega M, Gray K, Rosenberg-Thompson S, Carusi DA, Gornbein J (1994) The neuropsychiatric inventory: comprehensive assessment of psychopathology in dementia. Neurology 44: 2308–3214

De Jong R, Ostersund OW, Roy GW (1989) Measurement of quality-of-life changes in patients with Alzheimer's disease. Clin Ther 11: 545–554

Erzigkeit H (1989) SKT. Ein Kurztest zur Erfassung von Gedächtnis- und Aufmerksamkeitsstörungen. Beltz, Weinheim

Gracon SI (1996) Evaluation of tacrine hydrochloride (Cognex®) in two parallel-group studies. Acta Neurol Scand [Suppl] 165: 114–122

Gutzmann H, Hadler D, Erzigkeit H (1997) Long-term treatment of Alzheimer's disease with idebenone. In: Iqbal K, Winblad B, Nishimura T, Takeda M, Wisniewski HM (eds) Alzheimer's disease: biology, diagnosis and therapeutics. Wiley, New York, pp 688–705

Kaufer DI, Cummings JL, Christine D (1996) Effect of tacrine on behavioral symptoms in Alzheimer's disease: an open-label study. J Geriatr Psychiatry Neurol 9: 1–6

Knapp MJ, Knopman DS, Solomon PR, Pendlebury WW, Davis CS, Gracon SI (1994) A 30-week randomized controlled trial of high-dose tacrine in patients with Alzheimer's disease. JAMA 271(13): 985–991

Knopman D, Schneider L, Davis K, Talwalker S, Smith F, Hoover T, Gracon S (1996) Long-term tacrine (Cognex) treatment: effects on nursing home placement and mortality. Neurology 47: 166–177

McKhann G, Folstein M, Katzman R, Price D, Stadlan EM (1984) Clinical diagnosis of Alzheimer's disease: report of the NINCDS-ADRDA work group under the auspices of Department of health and Human Services Task Force on Alzheimer's Disease. Neurology 34: 939–944

Mohs RC, Cohen L (1988) Alzheimer's Disease Assessment Scale (ADAS). Psychopharmacol Bull 24(4): 627–628

Watkins PB, Zimmerman HJ, Knapp MG, Gracon SI, Lewis KW (1994) Hepatotoxic effecs of tacrine administration in patients with Alzheimer's disease. JAMA 271(13): 992–998

Author's address: Prof. Dr. A. Kurz, Department of Psychiatry, Technical University, Ismaninger Strasse 22, D-81675 München, Federal Republic of Germany

Sustained efficacy and safety of idebenone in the treatment of Alzheimer's disease: update on a 2-year double-blind multicentre study

H. Gutzmann[1] and **D. Hadler**[2]

[1] Krankenhaus Hellersdorf, ö.B. Wilhelm-Griesinger-Krankenhaus,
Abteilung für Gerontopsychiatrie, Berlin, and
[2] Takeda Europe, Research & Development Centre GmbH, Frankfurt/Main,
Federal Republic of Germany

Summary. The 2-year efficacy and safety of idebenone were studied in a prospective, randomized, double-blind multicentre study in 3 parallel groups of patients with dementia of the Alzheimer type (DAT) of mild to moderate degree. A total of 450 patients were randomized to either placebo for 12 months, followed by idebenone 90 mg tid for another 12 months (n = 153) or idebenone 90 mg tid for 24 months (n = 148) or 120 mg tid for 24 months (n = 149). The primary outcome measure was the total score of the Alzheimer's Disease Assessment Scale (ADAS-Total) at month 6. Secondary outcome measures were the ADAS cognitive (ADAS-Cog) and noncognitive score (ADAS-Noncog), the clinical global response (CGI-Improvement), the SKT neuropsychological test battery, and the Nurses' Observation Scale for Geriatric Patients (NOSGER-Total and IADL subscale). Safety parameters were adverse events, vital signs, ECG and clinical laboratory parameters. During the placebo controlled period (the first year of treatment), idebenone showed statistically significant dose-dependent improvement in the primary efficacy variable ADAS-Total and in all the secondary efficacy variables. There was no evidence for a loss of efficacy during the second year of treatment, as a further improvement of most efficacy variables was found in the second year in comparison to the results at the 12 months visit. Also, a clear dose effect relationship (placebo/90 mg < idebenone 90 mg < idebenone 120 mg) was maintained throughout the second year of treatment. This suggests that idebenone exerts its beneficial therapeutic effects on the course of the disease by slowing down its progression. Safety and tolerability of idebenone were good and similar to placebo during the first year of treatment and did not change during the second year.

Introduction

Idebenone (CV-2619) is a benzoquinone derivative that improves brain metabolism and protects the cell membranes against lipid peroxidation. It has already been investigated in various clinical studies for its effectiveness in dementia of the Alzheimer type (DAT) (Senin et al., 1992; Weyer et al., 1997; Gutzmann et al., 1997). We report on the 2-years results of one of these studies, whose 12 months results have already been reported and reviewed elsewhere (Weyer, 1996; Gutzmann, 1997).

Material and methods

Patient population

Study participants were inpatients and outpatients of both sexes, aged between 40 and 90 years with a diagnosis of primary degenerative dementia (DSM-III-R; American Psychiatric Association, 1987) and a diagnosis of probable Alzheimer's disease according to the criteria of the National Institute of Neurological and Communicative Disorders and Stroke-Alzheimer's Disease and Related Disorders Association (NINCDS-ADRDA; McKhann et al., 1984). Patients with a diagnosis of dementia of vascular or mixed (degenerative and vascular) origin were excluded as of a score of 5 or more on the Hachinski Ischemia Scale (Hachinski et al., 1975). The differential diagnosis was further supported by a CT- or MRI-scan without evidence of infarction or other focal lesions. Patients with a diagnosis of another type of dementia as evidenced by clinical or neurological examination or laboratory were also excluded. Mild to moderately severe degrees of dementia were defined by a score range of 10 to 24 points on the Mini Mental State Examination (MMSE; Folstein et al., 1975), a score of 9 points or above on the SKT neuropsychological test battery (Erzigkeit, 1989) and a total score of at least 20 points on the Alzheimer's Disease Assessment Scale [ADAS; Rosen et al., 1984; a validated German version (Weyer 1993) was used]. Each outpatient had a caregiver (close relative or professional caretaker) who ensured compliance with the protocol and served as informant for the patient's daily activities.

Written informed consent was obtained from the patient and from the caregiver who agreed to monitor the patient's compliance during the course of the study. The study was approved by the relevant ethics committee established at the "Ärztekammer Berlin" and conducted according to the provisions of the World Medical Association's Declaration of Helsinki (Version 1989).

Study design

The study was performed according to a double-blind, randomized parallel group design in 14 study centres throughout Germany. Patients were identified at an initial screening visit. The inclusion and exclusion criteria were reexamined after a 3 to 4-week placebo wash-out phase and thereupon, after having carried out baseline measurements, eligible patients were randomly assigned to one of three treatment groups: placebo for 12 months, followed by idebenone 90 mg tid for another 12 months or idebenone 90 mg tid for 24 months or 120 mg tid for 24 months. Assessments of efficacy and safety following baseline were scheduled after one and three months and subsequently in 3-month intervals during the entire treatment period.

Outcome measures

Instruments used by trained investigators for the evaluation of efficacy were the ADAS, the SKT, the Nurses' Observation Scale for Geriatric Patients (NOSGER; Spiegel et al.,

1991) and the Clinical Global Impressions Scale (CGI; National Institute of Mental Health [NIMH], 1976). The ADAS-Total score was predefined in the protocol as the primary variable in the evaluation of efficacy. The ADAS-Cog and -Noncog scores, the SKT total score, the NOSGER total and IADL subscale scores, and the CGI ratings were chosen as secondary efficacy variables. Changes from baseline to month 6 of double-blind treatment were defined per protocol as the main efficacy criteria for both the primary and the secondary outcome measures. The respective changes to month 12 were considered for an intermediate evaluation of long-term treatment effects. The patients who were randomized to placebo were given idebenone 90 mg t.i.d. during the second year of treatment. This offered the opportunity to see, whether

— the effect of idebenone is purely symptomatic (in which case the patients who had been treated with placebo in the first year should have caught up at months 18 with the patients receiving 90 mg t.i.d. from the beginning)
— or not (in which case a difference should be present even after 24 months of treatment)

This analysis is merely explorative. Its purpose is to provide preliminary evidence concerning a possible effect of idebenone on the progression of the disease. During this second year of treatment the study was still double blind and controlled. This design follows a rationale which has been proposed by Leber (1996) as an alternative to a withdrawal design. Safety evaluations included the assessment of adverse events with regard to frequency, severity, outcome, assumed relationship to study medication and clinical laboratory tests at each visit. Complete physical examinations were performed in 3-month intervals, 12-lead electrocardiograms at screening and at month 12.

Statistical analysis

Study sample size estimation required 100 patients in each treatment group in order to detect a minimal mean difference between treatments of 4 points (SD = 9) on ADAS-Total at the 5% level of significance (two-sided) with a power of 90%. The analyses of efficacy were performed on the data of all patients who were randomized to treatment, according to an intent-to-treat (ITT) principle, with (a) missing data replaced by the last available observation (last observation carried forward; LOCF) and (b) with the available observations only. The data of the ITT sample, last observation carried forward, were used for the primary confirmatory test of the efficacy hypothesis. The random code was opened for statistical analysis by an independent biometrician after completion of the 6-month treatment period. It was not released to investigators or patients, so treatment was continued under double-blind conditions.

The primary variable was analysed by two-way analysis of variance (ANOVA) with treatment and centre as main effect terms and differences from baseline to the endpoints at month 6 and at month 12 as dependent variables. Dose-response relationships for all secondary efficacy parameters were evaluated by means of regression analysis. Nonparametric techniques including Spearman's rank correlation coefficient and Cochran-Mantel-Haenszel Chi square methodology were used with categorical data and if the quasi-continuous data were not normally distributed.

In order to demonstrate the clinical relevance of statistically significant treatment effects (as revealed by group-statistical methods), a multidimensional analysis of therapy responder rates was performed, following recent recommendations of expert committees and regulatory bodies for the evaluation of efficacy of potential antidementia drugs (CPMP, 1992; Kanowski et al., 1990; Kern and Menges, 1992). Responders were identified according to their improvement in three target measures representing different levels of assessment. CGI-Improvement, ADAS-Cog and NOSGER-IADL were chosen to reflect (a) the overall clinical response, (b) an improvement in cognition and (c) an improvement in behaviour closely connected with activities of daily living. Criteria for relevant improvement on ADAS-Cog and NOSGER-IADL were derived from pre-treatment data of the study (screening and baseline) using estimates of test-retest reliability for the definition of critical cut-off scores for intraindividual changes (dcrit -values; Lienert, 1967) with a two-tailed 5% level of confidence. This resulted in critical differences of at least 7 for ADAS Cog and at least 2 for NOSGER IADL. Global ratings of change in the patient's condition signifying any degree of improvement according to the CGI were considered as relevant.

Results

Patient groups

A total of 450 patients (154 men, 296 women) entered the study, were randomized to double-blind treatment (153 on placebo/90 mg, 148 on 90 mg tid idebenone and 149 on 120 mg tid idebenone) and treated for up to 24 months. The characteristics of these patients at baseline, including test results, are summarised in Table 1, and the number of patients per visit is listed in Table 2. The treatment groups were comparable with respect to all their major characteristics at study entrance and the number of patients available at each visit.

Efficacy

First year of treatment

The confirmatory test (ADAS Total after 6 months treatment, LOCF sample) was significant at the 5% level ($F_{2,408}$ = 5.64, p = 0.0038). The treatment

Table 1. Patient characteristics and baseline test results per treatment group (ITT-population); mean values $\pm$ SD

	Plac./90 mg n = 153	90 mg n = 148	120 mg n = 149	Total N = 450
Patient characteristics				
Male: No (%)	55 (36)	42 (28)	57 (38)	154 (34)
Female: No (%)	98 (64)	106 (72)	92 (62)	296 (66)
Age (y)	68,9 $\pm$ 11,4	70,3 $\pm$ 11,6	70,4 $\pm$ 11,9	69,9 $\pm$ 11,6
MMSE (0–30)	16,8 $\pm$ 3,5	16,6 $\pm$ 3,2	17,1 $\pm$ 3,4	16,8 $\pm$ 3,4
CGI-severity (1–7)	5,2 $\pm$ 0.4	5,2 $\pm$ 0,5	5,1 $\pm$ 0,4	5,2 $\pm$ 0,4
Baseline test results (efficacy variables)				
ADAS-Total (0–120)	47,7 $\pm$ 15,3	48,3 $\pm$ 14,1	45,1 $\pm$ 13,6	47,0 $\pm$ 14,4
ADAS-Cog (0–70)	34,3 $\pm$ 9,3	35,3 $\pm$ 9,3	32,7 $\pm$ 8,0	34,1 $\pm$ 9,0
ADAS-Noncog (0–50)	13,5 $\pm$ 7,3	13,1 $\pm$ 6,5	12,3 $\pm$ 6,7	12,9 $\pm$ 6,9
SKT (0–27)	18,3 $\pm$ 5,1	19,2 $\pm$ 4,8	17,8 $\pm$ 4,6	18,4 $\pm$ 4,9
NOSGER (5–150)	78,8 $\pm$ 19,5	77,3 $\pm$ 20,0	74,4 $\pm$ 20,3	76,9 $\pm$ 20,0
NOSGER-IADL (1–25)	16,0 $\pm$ 4,8	16,0 $\pm$ 4,9	15,3 $\pm$ 4,9	15,8 $\pm$ 2,9

Table 2. Responder rates (%) for "relevant" differences at the 6, 12, 18 and 24 month visits (ITT-population)

| period | treatm. | n | Relevant improvement per level of assessment | | | Number of levels with relevant improvement | | | |
			ADAS Cog.	CGI improv.	IADL	0	1	2	3
6 m	Plac./90	141	30,7	60,3	28,1	36,9	25,5	26,2	11,3
	I 90	135	39,6	70,4	36,3	25,2	24,4	34,8	15,6
	I 120	139	53,2	87,8	41,0	10,1	29,5	38,1	22,3
	p-value*		0,0001	0,0000	0,0119	0,0000			
12 m	Plac./90	128	32,8	63,3	36,7	32,0	26,6	21,9	19,5
	I 90	125	45,6	73,4	41,1	20,8	21,6	37,6	20,0
	I 120	126	57,1	87,3	48,4	9,5	24,6	31,6	34,1
	p-value*		0,0000	0,0000	0,0298	0,0000			
18 m	Plac./90	104	52,9	86,5	51,9	13,5	22,1	34,6	29,8
	I 90	105	58,7	86,7	49,0	11,4	19,0	33,3	36,2
	I 120	102	63,7	95,1	62,7	3,9	18,6	36,3	41,2
	p-value*		0,0575	0,0236	0,0607	0,0061			
24 m	Plac./90	88	58,0	88,6	57,6	11,4	20,5	37,5	30,7
	I 90	85	65,9	94,1	48,8	3,5	15,3	45,9	35,3
	I 120	85	73,5	92,9	60,7	7,1	5,9	48,2	38,8
	p-value*		0,0164	0,1486	0,3463	0,0097			

Note: criteria of response were a change of at least -7 for ADAS-Cog, -2 for NOSGER-IADL, and "little" to "very much" for CGI imrpovement. *: descriptive p values for treatment differences from Mantel-Haenszel Chi-square test (1-sided)

response in the ITT sample is summarized in Fig. 1. Clear effects were demonstrated in favor of idebenone at the 6 and 12 months visits for all analysis populations (LOCF, ITT, PA) and for all dimensions of efficacy (1. Improvement in cognition {ADAS Cog and SKT, see Fig. 2,3}, 2. Overall clinical response {CGI, see Fig. 4}, 3. Improvement in behavior closely connected with activities of daily living {NOSGER-IADL see Fig. 5, NOSGER sum}) in a dose dependent manner. The differences between treatments tended to increase over time and reached their maximum at 12 months. The frequency of patients showing improvement across all of the three levels of assessment was well differentiated in favor of idebenone in a dose dependent manner (see Table 2). Only 9.5% of the patients in the idebenone 120 mg group showed no improvement in any variable after 12 months treatment, compared to 32% of the patients on placebo. On the other hand, 19.5% of the patients on placebo show a relevant improvement in all three variables, compared to 34.1% on idebenone 120 mg.

Second year of treatment

Patients who had been randomized to placebo received this treatment for 12 months, thereafter they were switched to idebenone 90 mg and treated for

ADAS Total, Diff, ITT

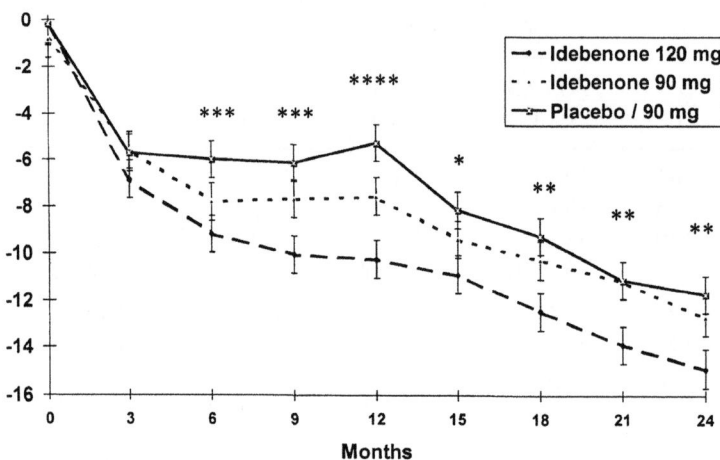

Fig. 1. Primary efficacy variable ADAS Total. Means ± SEM of the differences to baseline. ****: p < 0.0005, ***: p < 0.001, **: p < 0.01, *: p < 0.05. (test for dose-trend, onesided)

ADAS Cog, Diff, ITT

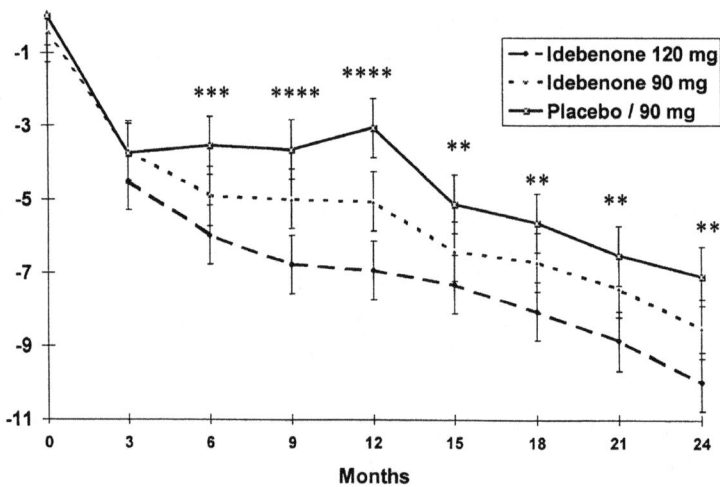

Fig. 2. Secondary efficacy variable ADAS Cog. Means ± SEM of the differences to baseline. Symbols explained in Fig. 1

further 12 months. There was no evidence for a loss of efficacy during the second year of treatment. The patients who had been switched from placebo to 90 mg idebenone after 12 months of treatment showed an improvement in most variable compared to their 12-month result. However, for some variables, including ADAS cog, a difference between the plac/90 group and the 90 mg group persisted throughout the second year of treatment. Furthermore, for many (but not all) efficacy variables, including ADAS Total (Fig. 1),

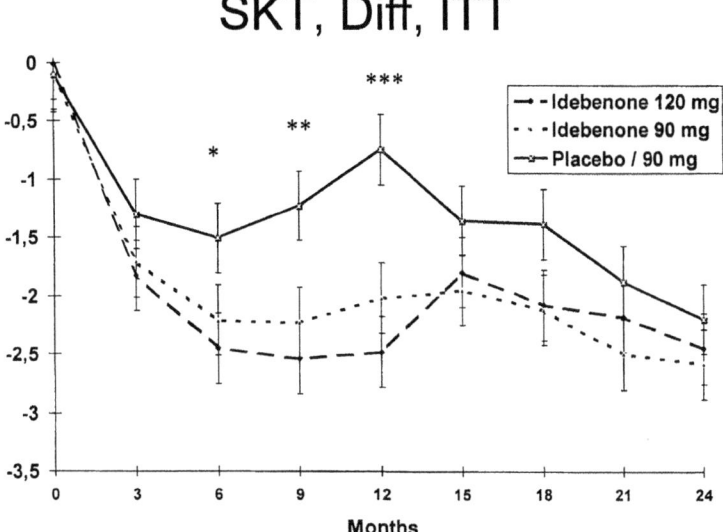

Fig. 3. Secondary efficacy variable SKT. Means ± SEM of the differences to baseline. Symbols explained in Fig. 1

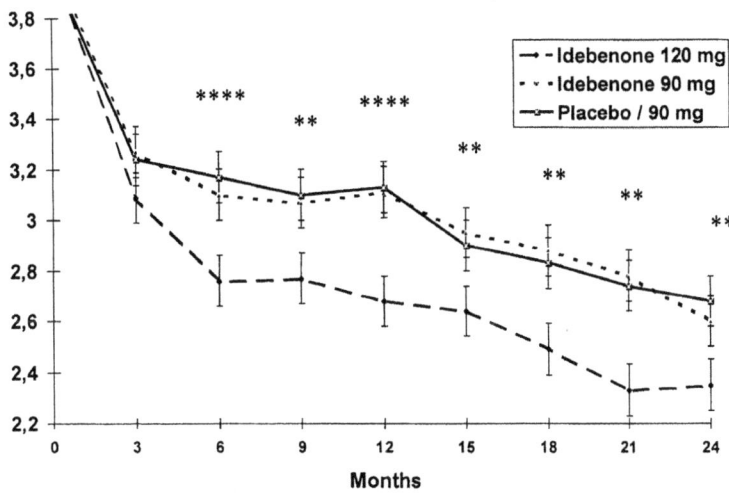

Fig. 4. Secondary efficacy variable CGI Global Improvement. Means ± SEM of the differences to baseline. Symbols explained in Fig. 1

ADAS Cog (Fig. 2), CGI Global Improvement (Fig. 4) and NOSGER IADL (Fig. 5), a clear dose effect relationship (placebo/90 mg < idebenone 90 mg < idebenone 120 mg) was observed throughout the second year of treatment. Again, the frequency of patients showing improvement across all of the three levels of assessment was well differentiated in favor of idebenone in a dose dependent manner (see Table 2). Only 13% of the patients in the idebenone

NOSGER IADL, Diff, ITT

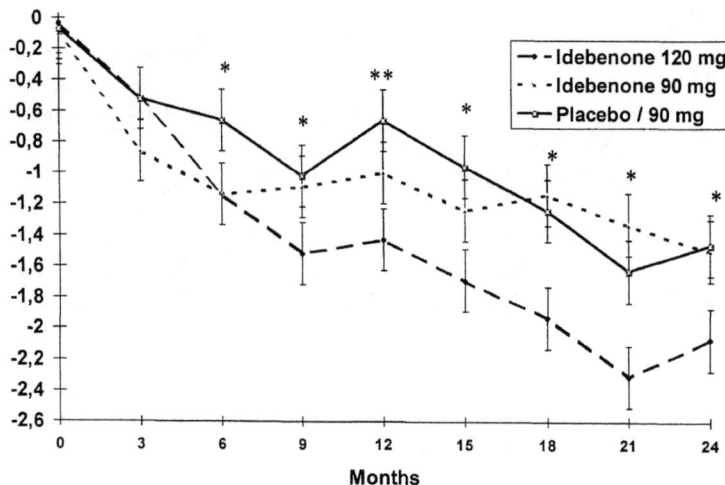

Fig. 5. Secondary efficacy variable NOSGER IADL. Means ± SEM of the differences to baseline. Symbols explained in Fig. 1

120 mg group showed improvement in no more than one variable after 24 months treatment, compared to 31.9% of the patients on placebo.

Safety

The most frequently reported adverse events were "dizziness", "influenza-like symptoms", "bronchitis" and "lumbar pain", each affecting more than 7% of the patients without clear differences between the treatment groups. No relevant differences of the adverse event profile were observed. Physical (including vital signs), neurological and standard laboratory examinations (including liver function tests) did not reveal any relevant differences between the treatment groups or systematic changes over time.

Discussion

Idebenone had a clear anti-dementia activity. Although the effects were clearly statistically significant when compared to placebo, this does not automatically settle the problem whether the effects are large enough to be clinically relevant. In this study the "relevant" differences were estimated by calculating intra-individual differences. This resulted in criteria which were quite demanding (e.g. 7 points improvement for ADAS-Cog), but may nevertheless indicate just the lower limit for an individual patient which would be noticeable (with certain probability) and therefore a meaningful threshold for clinical relevance. The superiority to placebo was evident in all measures. There was no evidence for a loss of efficacy during the second year of treatment, instead, a clear dose effect relationship (placebo/90 mg < idebenone 90 mg < idebenone 120 mg) was maintained. For most patients in all treatment groups, an improvement of most efficacy variables was found in comparison with the results at 12 months. When interpreting these results, the high drop-out rates during the second year must be kept in mind. Since mainly patients with an unsatisfactory response dropped out, most scores indicated continuing improvement, although one must assume that the overall population of randomized patients was deteriorating. Since the number of patients dropping out was very similar in all groups, comparisons between the groups still seem to be valid. For some of the variables (including ADAS Total, ADAS cog, CGI severity of disease and NOSGER total), a difference between the placebo/90 mg and the 90 mg group (and not just between the placebo/90 mg and the 120 mg group) persisted throughout the second year of treatment. This suggests, together with the late onset of action and the slowly increasing response during the first year of placebo-controlled treatment, that idebenone exerts its beneficial therapeutic effects on the course of the disease by slowing down its progression. It is remarkable in this context that another antioxidant, alpha-tocopherol, has recently been claimed to slow the progression of disease (Sano et al., 1997).

References

American Psychiatric Association (1987) Diagnostic and statistical manual of mental disorders, 3rd ed, rev. APA, Washington, DC

CPMP Working Party on Efficacy of Medicinal Products (1992) Antidementia medicinal products. Note for guidance (Draft 5). Commission of the European Communities, Brussels

Erzigkeit H (1989) SKT: Ein Kurztest zur Erfassung von Gedächtnis- und Aufmerksamkeitsstörungen (4th ed.) [SKT: A short test to assess impairment of memory and attention]. Beltz Test, Weinheim

Folstein MF, Folstein SE, McHugh PR (1975) "Mini-Mental State": a practical method for grading the cognitive state of patients for the clinician. J Psychiatr Res 12: 189–198

Gutzmann H, Hadler D, Erzigkeit H (1997) Long-term treatment of Alzheimer's disease with idebenone. In: Iqbal K, Winblad B, Nishimura T, Takeda M, Wisniewki HM (eds) Alzheimer's disease: biology, diagnosis and therapeutics. John Wiley & Sons, New York, pp 687–705

Hachinski VC, Illiff LD, Zihlka E, DuBoulay GH, McAllister VL, Marshall R, Ross-Russell RW, Symon L (1975) Cerebral blood flow in dementia. Arch Neurol 32: 632–637

Kanowski S, Ladurner G, Maurer K, Oswald WD, Stein U (1990) Empfehlungen zur Evaluierung der Wirksamkeit von Nootropika. Z Gerontopsychol-psychiatr 3: 67–79

Kern U, Menges K (1992) Proof of efficacy of nootropics for the indication "dementia" (Phase III) — Recommendations. Pharmacopsychiatry 25: 126–135

Leber P (1996) Observations and suggestions on antidementia drug development. Alzheimer Dis Assoc Disord 10 [Suppl 1]: 31–35

Lienert GA (1967) Testaufbau und Testanalyse, 2nd ed. [Test construction and test analysis]. Beltz, Weinheim

McKhann G, Drachman D, Folstein M, Katzman R, Price D, Stadlan EM (1984) Clinical diagnosis of Alzheimer's disease: report of the NINCDS-ADRDA work group under the auspices of Department Health & Human Services Task Force on Alzheimer's disease. Neurology 34: 939–944

National Institute of Mental Health (1976) Clinical Global Impressions. In: Guy W (ed) EDCEU assessment manual for psychopharmacology, rev ed. NIMH, Rockville, MD, pp 217–222

Rosen WG, Mohs RC, Davis KL (1984) A new rating scale for Alzheimer's disease. Am J Psychiatry 141: 1356–1364

Sano M, et al (1997) A controlled trial of selegiline, alpha-tocopherol, or both as treatment for Alzheimer's disease. N Engl J Med 336: 1216–1222

Senin U, Parnetti L, Barbagallo-Sangiorgi G, Bartorelli L, Bocola V, Capurso A, Cuzzupoli M, Denario M, Marigliano V, Tammaro A, Fioravanti M (1992) Idebenone in senile dementia of Alzheimer type: a multicentre study. Arch Gerontol Geriatr 15: 249–260

Spiegel R, Brunner C, Ermini-Fünfschilling D, Monsch A, Notter M, Puxty J, Tremmel L (1991) A new behavioral assessment scale for geriatric out- and in-patients: the NOSGER (Nurses' Observation Scale for Geriatric Patients). J Am Geriatr Soc 39: 339–347

Weyer G, Ihl R, Mohs RC, Schambach M, Denkel A, Kaiser-Kehl H (1993) Validierungsuntersuchungen zu einer deutschen Version der Alzheimer's Disease Assessment Scale ADAS [Investigations on the validity of a German version of the Alzheimer's Disease Assessment Scale ADAS]. Z Gerontopsychol-psychiatr 6: 67–81

Weyer G, Erzigkeit H, Hadler D, Kubicki S (1996) Efficacy and safety of idebenone in the long-term treatment of Alzheimer's disease: a double-blind, placebo-controlled multicentre study. Hum Psychopharmacol 11: 53–65

Weyer G, Babej-Dölle RM, Hadler D, Hofmann S, Herrmann W (1997) A controlled study of 2 doses of idebenone in the treatment of Alzheimer's disease. Neuropsychobiology 11: 340–350

World Medical Association (1989) Declaration of Helsinki: Recommendations guiding physicians in biomedical research involving human subjects (Amended by the 41st World Medical Assembly, Hong Kong, September 1989)

Authors' address: Dr. D. Hadler, Takeda Europe R & D Centre GmbH, Hamburger Allee 2-10, D-60486 Frankfurt, Federal Republic of Germany

Clinical experience with donepezil (Aricept™) in the UK

D. Wilkinson

Thornhill Research Unit, University of Southampton, United Kingdom

Summary. Experience of the use of Donepezil (Aricept™) in the UK since licencing is discussed. The results of a 30 week double blind parallel group study in the US of Donepezil 5 or 10 mg versus placebo show statistically significant improvements in cognitive and clinical global assessments. Beneficial effects were demonstrated in the absence of significant adverse effects on physical or laboratory values. The guidelines for use adopted in the UK are discussed with the emphasis on identifying non-cognitive behaviours, as significant improvements in these have been found and often have more impact on quality of life than cognitive improvements alone.

Donepezil Hydrochloride (Aricept™)

Donepezil has been licenced for the symptomatic treatment of mild to moderate Alzheimer's Disease in the UK since April 1997. Prior to that there had been no licenced treatment. Clinicians, whilst welcoming the arrival of the first rational treatment felt unsure as to what reaction this may have as experience of Acetyl-cholinesterase inhibitors was limited to a few specialist research units and the data on which the licence was based was from US studies.

The crucial evidence of efficacy came from a 30 week study designed to demonstrate the efficacy and safety of Aricept™ (Donepezil HCL) in patients with mild to moderate Alzheimer's disease (EISAI, 1996). The trial design was a 30 week, randomized, double-blind, multicenter, parallel group study of Donepezil HCL (5 or 10 mg) versus placebo, using 150 patients per group, 450 total patients. Test drug was administered for 24 weeks followed by a 6 week single-blind placebo washout. Primary measures of efficacy were the Alzheimer's Disease Assessment Scale-cognitive subscale (ADAS-cog) and the Clinicians Interview-based Impression of Change, incorporating caregiver input (CIBIC-Plus). Secondary measures of efficacy included the Minimental State Examination (MMSE) and the Clinical Dementia Rating sum-of-the-boxes (CDR-SB). Safety was assessed by physical examination, laboratory results, vital signs and adverse events.

After 24 weeks of treatment, the mean differences in the ADAS-cog scores for Aricept™ treated patients compared to patients treated with placebo were 2.49 ± 0.51 and 2.88 ± 0.51 units for the 5 mg/day and 10 mg/day treatments respectively. These differences were statistically significant (P < 0.001). Patients receiving Aricept™ also demonstrated statistically significant improvements in global function as measured by the CIBIC-plus. The mean drug-placebo difference for the 5 mg/day group was 0.36 ± 0.09 units and 0.44 ± 0.07 units for the 10 mg/day group. Secondary measures of efficacy were also statistically significant after 24 weeks of treatment. MMSE scores in placebo treated patients had deteriorated by 1.10 units, while Aricept™ treated patients scores improved by 0.34 and 0.44 units for 5 mg/day and 10 mg/day groups respectively. The CDR-SB also demonstrated significant change from placebo at the conclusion of treatment. After 24 weeks, placebo treated patients had declined by 0.59 units while Aricept™ treated patients improved by 0.07 units in both the 5 mg/day by 0.59 units while Aricept™ treated patients improved by 0.07 units in both the 5 mg/day and 10 mg/day groups. Aricept™ was well tolerated over the course of the study. The Aricept™ 10 mg/day group had a slightly higher incidence of nausea, diarrhoea and vomiting compared to placebo and the 5 mg/day treated patients. These adverse events were generally of mild severity, brief duration and typically resolved despite continued treatment.

The initial introduction to UK

Right from its launch, there was a wall of resistance to the prescription of Donepezil based not on the grounds of efficacy, but purely on cost. This was borne of an erroneous assumption that every one of the 650,000 dementia sufferers in the UK was likely to be prescribed a drug costing about £1,000 per annum.

Clearly this was a gross overestimate of the problem. The truth is that probably only 5–10% of all patients with dementia will be put on Donepezil until it becomes clearer from clinical practice what the benefits and side effects are likely to be in the general population. The subsequent drug costs will be correspondingly small, but where costs will occur is in the identification and management of the disease. It was clear to us in the UK that despite considerable public awareness of Alzheimer's Disease through the Alzheimer's Disease Society and media interest, general practitioners were still uncertain about making the diagnosis of AD and unhappy to institute treatment without specialist advice. It is also clear that many Health Authorities were reluctant to finance the use of Donepezil and this could be seen as a typically ageist response, as despite evidence from randomised controlled trials, purchasers were still debating the cost-effectiveness of the drug.

This created a further barrier to the introduction of this new treatment and we have developed guidelines to facilitate the diagnosis of dementia and use of anti-dementia drugs, which together with Health Department's directives to keep the prescription of the drug within the purview of secondary care services has helped allay irrational fears of runaway costs.

Guidelines have been published elsewhere (Wilcock, 1997) but essentially require a step-wise approach to patient identification.

Identification of dementia

Firstly primary care teams need to have a high index of suspicion in those presenting with symptoms which may indicate an underlying dementia. Initial clinical assessment should include a focussed history with the involvement of a reliable informant where possible, physical and mental state examination should be supported by brief standardised cognitive testing e.g. MMSE (Folstein, 1975). Diagnosis of dementia should be based on ICD-10 criteria (WHO, 1992). Factors that may cause or exacerbate the cognitive impairment should be identified and treated before reassessment. These include medication, depression and physical illnesses. Routine laboratory testing is recommended, with neuroimaging playing an increasingly important rôle. In the UK neuroimaging has not been routinely used to assess dementia, being used in atypical cases and where clinically indicated. However, with more sophisticated measurements and the need to diagnose very early cases if we are to reap maximum benefit from new treatments its use is likely to increase. These investigations insidiously, though quite justifiably and appropriately, increase the cost of introducing new treatments for this disease.

The diagnosis of Alzheimer's disease as a cause of dementia

Once any causative or exacerbating conditions are treated should any cognitive impairment have not fully resolved, the type of dementia should be identified. ICD-10 diagnostic guidelines are recommended for dementia in Alzheimer's disease and vascular dementia, and consensus criteria to diagnose dementia with Lewy Bodies (McKeith, 1996). The special problem having a treatment provides is the necessity for diagnostic accuracy in the early presentation of the disease. Hitherto with little to offer but the depressing prognosis early diagnosis was often avoided. More detailed neuro psychological testing perhaps combined with quantitative CT and SPECT scanning may be necessary, with regular review to measure change in doubtful cases.

General considerations in the utilization of therapeutic resources

Drug treatment of course should not be sole focus of our attention. There are many therapeutic options and support services available for patients and carers. A full range of services must be considered whether or not drug treatment is prescribed. The use of specific anti-Alzheimer medications should be subject to good clinical practice as with any other prescribed drug. The prescriber should have a thorough knowledge of the product, its indications side effects and expected outcomes. Informed consent, involvement of a carer and measures to ensure assessment of continuing needs and outcome should be arranged.

Patient selection for use of Donepezil

Donepezil has been licenced for use in patients with mild to moderate AD. Determining disease severity is essentially a clinical decision but may be assisted by using the Mini Mental State Examination (MMSE) (Folstein, 1975) where a score of greater than 10 out of 30 is usually associated with mild to moderate severity. Patients with severe dementia, as classified by research criteria, e.g. ICD-10 require continual supervision, are largely incoherent and are most likely to be in residential or nursing home care. There is no evidence yet as to efficacy in this group and testing any cognitive improvement would be very difficult.

The patient should be commenced on 5 mg daily and the patient and carer should be advised that, whilst the drug is well tolerated initially there may be some nausea, diarrhoea or vomiting which should pass off in 2–3 days. If it does not the carer should be instructed as to whom to contact for advice. Owing to the long half-life the patient should be reviewed at 4–6 weeks to assess response, and the dose should then be increased within the product prescribing guidelines unless significant side effects are present. Patients and carers should be advised that side effects may reappear for a few days after the dosage increase.

Assessment of efficacy

At the commencement of medication it is suggested that a baseline cognitive assessment e.g. MMSE or ADAS (Rosen, 1984) is undertaken and that three or four non-cognitive target symptoms are identified (e.g. apathy, restlessness, hallucinations). These should be used together to assess response. A formal assessment at 3 months should be made to determine clinical response. A consistent approach, preferably by the same clinician, is essential for improvements to be monitored most accurately. The decision to continue treatment should be based on feedback from patient and carer as well as the clinicians examination. If there is no evidence of improvement in cognitive function, target symptoms or quality of life then a trial of medication withdrawal is recommended. If further assessment 2–4 weeks later shows significant decline then medication should be restarted. Long term follow-up should be undertaken at least every 3 months. If the dementia progresses significantly, serious consideration should be given to a trial of discontinuing the medication especially if behavioural problems require the addition of neuroleptic, hypnotic or anti-depressant medication. The decision should take into account the patient's quality of life and the views of carers. It is our experience in the UK that whilst improvements in cognition are likely, the greatest improvements are seen in non-cognitive behaviours. Patients seem more alert, more likely to initiate conversation and more responsive. These behaviours are often far more important to carers than improvements in memory per se.

It should be noted that there is enormous individual variation in the progress of AD and a few points change on the MMSE should not be taken in isolation as evidence of response or deterioration. Some patients may gain benefit for a number of years despite a very gradual deterioration in cognitive function. This treatment is not a panacea and is one part of the overall management of AD but does present a significant advance and for some patients quite tangible benefits.

References

EISAI Corp (1996) Data on file. Teaneck N J., U.S.A.

Folstein MF, Folstein SE, McHugh PR (1975) Mini-Mental State: a practical method for grading the cognitive state of patients for the clinician. J Psychiatr Res 12: 189–198

McKeith, et al (1996) Consensus guidelines for the clinical and pathological diagnosis of dementia with Lewy Bodies (DLB): report of the consortium on DLB international workshop. Neurology 47: 1113–1124

Rosen WG, Mohs RC, Davis KL (1984) A new rating scale for Alzheimer's disease. Am J Psych 141/11: 1356–1364

Wilcock G, Banergee A, Burns A, Chubb A, Jones R, Lawlor B, Rossor M, Sharp D, Wilkinson DG (1997) Setting standards in Alzheimer's disease management in Primary and Secondary care. Geriatr Med 27 (part 3) [Suppl]

World Health Organisation (1992) The ICD-10 classification of mental and behavioural disorders: clinical descriptions and diagnostic guidelines. World Health Organization, Geneva

Author's address: Dr. D. G. Wilkinson, MBChB., MRCGP., FRCPsych., Thornhill Research Unit, Moorgreen Hospital, Botley Road, West End, Southampton, S030 3JB, United Kingdom

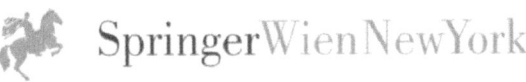

Springer Neurology

S. E. Daniel, F. F. Cruz-Sánchez, A. J. Lees (eds.)

Dementia in Parkinsonism

1997. 29 figures. VII, 204 pages.
Cloth DM 185,–, öS 1295,–. ISBN 3-211-82960-1
Special edition of "Journal of Neural Transmission, Supplement 51, 1997"
(Soft cover edition of Supplement 51 only available for subscribers to "Journal of Neural Transmission")

This supplement compiles the views of international experts dealing with dementia in parkinsonism. The subject is covered from a clinical, morphological and biochemical point of view and the diversity of terminology for dementia with Parkinson's Disease is emphasized. Subjects covered include normal brain function and the influence of age, investigation and treatment of dementia, pathological nomenclature and criteria for diagnosis, the relationship between dementia in Parkinson's Disease and Alzheimer's Disease, and biochemical and morphological substrates of dementia.

P. Riederer, D. B. Calne, R. Horowski,

Y. Mizuno, W. Poewe, M. B. H. Youdim (eds.)

Advances in Research on Neurodegeneration
Volume 5

1997. 45 figures. VIII, 215 pages.
Cloth DM 198,–, öS 1386,–. ISBN 3-211-82933-4
Special edition of "Journal of Neural Transmission, Supplement 50, 1997"
(Soft cover edition of Supplement 50 only available for subscribers to "Journal of Neural Transmission")

The "International Winter Conferences on Neurodegeneration" have become an established forum to discuss various aspects of basic and clinical topics related to the underlying mechanisms of neurodegenerative disorders. This volume focuses on brain imaging, endogenous and exogenous neurotoxins, programmed cell death, apoptosis and necrosis, and immunoinflammatory mechanisms, infective diseases causing neurological disorders. These topics have been reviewed by invited experts and the articles give an up-to-date reflection of the state of the art in these research fields.

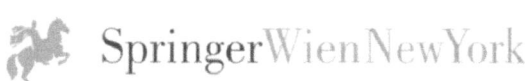

Springer Wien New York

Sachsenplatz 4-6, P.O.Box 89, A-1201 Wien, Fax +43-1-330 24 26, e-mail: order@springer.at. Internet: http.//www.springer.at
New York, NY 10010, 175 Fifth Avenue • D-14197 Berlin, Heidelberger Platz 3 • Tokyo 113, 3-13, Hongo 3-chome, Bunkyo-ku

Springer Neurology

Y. Mizuno, M. B. H. Youdim, D. B. Calne,

R. Horowski, W. Poewe, P. Riederer (eds.)

Advances in Research on Neurodegeneration

Volume 3 & 4

1997. 46 figures. VIII, 280 pages.

Cloth DM 215,–, öS 1505,–. ISBN 3-211-82935-0

Special edition of "Journal of Neural Transmission, Supplement 49, 1997"

(Soft cover edition of Supplement 49 only available for subscribers to "Journal of Neural Transmission")

The first part of the book focuses on disease models and mechanisms. The areas discussed include Alzheimer's disease, Parkinson's disease, glial and neuronal death, and demyelination/remyelination. The second part concentrates on the molecular biology of neurodegeneration. The topics include molecular genetics of neurological disorders, molecular biology of recognition sites, apoptosis, and neuroimmunology and multiple sclerosis. Leading experts have been invited to give state of the art presentations including their own recent data.

W. Kuhn, P. Kraus, H. Przuntek (eds.)

Deprenyl – Past and Future

1996. 16 figures. IX, 112 pages.

Cloth DM 130,–, öS 910,–. ISBN 3-211-82948-2

Special edition of "Journal of Neural Transmission, Supplement 48, 1996"

(Soft cover edition of Supplement 48 only available for subscribers to "Journal of Neural Transmission")

The clinical effect of L-Deprenyl was originally explained on the basis of irreversible and selective MAO-B inhibition and subsequent enhancement of dopaminergic neurotransmission. In recent years new experimental data have challenged this concept. In vitro and in vivo studies are suggesting that L-Deprenyl may have neuroprotective and/or neuroregenerative properties. Furthermore, controversial data of recently finished long-term clinical studies have brought forward a new discussion both on the clinical impact and the possible mode of action of L-Deprenyl in Parkinson's Disease and various other neurological and psychiatric disorders. This volume provides a forum for intensive discussions on the biochemical, pharmacological and clinical aspects of Parkinson's Disease.

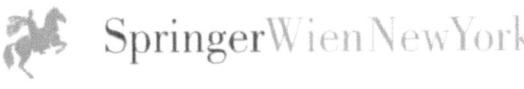 SpringerWien NewYork

Sachsenplatz 4-6, P.O.Box 89, A-1201 Wien, Fax +43-1-330 24 26, e-mail: order@springer.at, Internet· http://www.springer.at
New York, NY 10010, 175 Fifth Avenue • D-14197 Berlin, Heidelberger Platz 3 • Tokyo 113, 3-13, Hongo 3-chome, Bunkyo-ku